# Immunotherapy of Cancer

Yoshiyuki Yamaguchi
Editor

# Immunotherapy of Cancer

## An Innovative Treatment Comes of Age

Springer

*Editor*
Yoshiyuki Yamaguchi
Department of Clinical Oncology
Kawasaki Medical School
Kurashiki, Japan

ISBN 978-4-431-55030-3 ISBN 978-4-431-55031-0 (eBook)
DOI 10.1007/978-4-431-55031-0

Library of Congress Control Number: 2015960813

Springer Tokyo Heidelberg New York Dordrecht London


Printed on acid-free paper

Springer Japan KK is part of Springer Science+Business Media (www.springer.com)

# Preface

Preparation of this book started in October 2013, when the 51st Annual Meeting of the Japan Society of Clinical Oncology (JSCO) was held in Kyoto, Japan. When the editorship was offered to me, I thought, Why me? I was too inexperienced to complete such a great book, with so many Japanese experts in this field. However, I decided to take on the challenge of producing the book with much help from my dedicated older and younger colleagues. Here, I want to express my sincere thanks to all the authors who contributed.

This book contains the history, current status, and future perspective of cancer immunotherapy. The reader may understand easily, I hope, what you should know about the immune system when you treat a cancer patient. Immunotherapy has now come of age as the fourth modality of cancer treatment. Its role in cancer treatment, I believe, will grow day by day, and a future revolution in cancer treatment will occur as all the other treatments, including surgery, chemotherapy, and radiotherapy, may exist with and for the success of cancer immunotherapy.

About 30 years ago, when I was still a young surgeon, I was absorbed in research for tumor immunology. My Ph.D. thesis was titled "An Analysis of Suppressor Factor–Receptors on Peripheral Blood Lymphocyte Surfaces of Cancer Patients". My esteemed professors had thought in those days that there could be no success in cancer immunotherapy without modulation of immunosuppressive mechanisms. Now, they do seem to have been right! I dedicate this book to my two most important professors, the late Takao Hattori and the late Tetsuya Toge. I also dedicate this book to all my sincere researchers who helped me to develop in this field.

Kurashiki, Japan
July 2015

Yoshiyuki Yamaguchi

# Contents

# Part I
# Overview, History, Classification

# Chapter 1
# Overview of Current Cancer Immunotherapy

**Yoshiyuki Yamaguchi**

**Abstract** Immunotherapy has been investigated worldwide as the fourth cancer treatment modality, following the standard modalities of surgery, chemotherapy, and radiotherapy. Recently, the significant progress in our fundamental understanding of tumor immunology and the recent clinical advances in cancer immunotherapy trials have opened new avenues of cancer immunotherapy. At last, cancer immunotherapy has come of age, now. There is no longer any doubt that the immune system does work in tumor eradication. In this chapter, the progress made in cancer immunotherapy during the past half-century and the many types of cancer immunotherapy are summarized. A brief review of important nomenclature in tumor immunology is also provided, which may further facilitate the reader's understanding of the later chapters. Moreover, a future perspective for cancer immunotherapy development is discussed. Finally, I would say now that one lymphocyte, one dendritic cell, one antigen, and one drug can change the cancer treatment, immunotherapy, together.

**Keywords** Cancer immunotherapy • Mutation • Immunosurveillance • Immunocheckpoints • Personalized immunotherapy

## 1.1 Introduction

Immunotherapy has been investigated worldwide as the fourth cancer treatment modality, following the standard modalities of surgery, chemotherapy, and radiotherapy. Over the past five decades of research into cancer immunotherapy, several novel and promising discoveries have been investigated but then found to have disappointingly limited efficacy in clinical trials. Nevertheless, the significant progress in our fundamental understanding of tumor immunology and the recent clinical advances in cancer immunotherapy trials have opened new avenues of cancer immunotherapy, at last [1]. There is no longer any doubt that the immune system does work in tumor eradication.

Y. Yamaguchi, M.D., Ph.D. (✉)
Department of Clinical Oncology, Kawasaki Medical School, 577 Matsushima, Kurashiki, Okayama 701-0192, Japan
e-mail: shogo@med.kawasaki-m.ac.jp



Y. Yamaguchi (ed.), *Immunotherapy of Cancer*,
DOI 10.1007/978-4-431-55031-0_1

Cancer immunotherapy has only recently obtained a steady hold in the field of cancer treatment. Moreover, there is currently a fresh breeze of innovation in the field of immunotherapy as cancer treatment, and clinicians and researchers should thus be aware of the paradigm shift in our ways of thinking about how best to treat the many varieties of cancer. In this chapter, the progress made in cancer immunotherapy during the past half-century and the many types of cancer immunotherapy are summarized. A brief review of important nomenclature in tumor immunology is also provided, which may further facilitate the reader's understanding of the later chapters.

## 1.2 What Is the Immune System? Cells, Molecules, and Receptors Are Involved

The immune system plays a key role in human host-defense mechanisms, by which invaders such as viruses and bacteria are eradicated as not-self entities. Along with this eradication, antigenic information is saved in the memory of the host immune system, which can ensure the host's prompt immune response against the next attack of the same invaders. The host is also protected from cancer by this mechanism, which is known as the immunosurveillance mechanism [2].

The immune system consists of many types of functional cells, molecules, and receptors (Table 1.1), which together make the immune system quite complicated. The cells involved include granulocytes, natural killer (NK) cells, γδT cells, macrophages, T and B lymphocytes, and dendritic cells (DCs). Granulocytes and NK cells "look around" the body and attack invaders in an antigen-nonspecific manner. Macrophages are organ-specific phagocytes that also attack and collect the antigenic information of invaders as well as injured cells, old dying cells, and mutated cells, locoregionally. T lymphocytes work under the direction of DCs in an antigen-specific manner, and they can be classified into many functional cell types including helper T cells, cytotoxic T cells, inducer T cells, regulatory T cells, suppressor T cells, and more. It has been well established that T cells are highly involved in tumor eradication. B lymphocytes function as a producer cell of antigen-specific antibodies after antigenic stimulation through their differentiation into plasma cells. DCs are known as professional antigen-presenting cells (APCs). Immature DCs migrate, capture, and process antigens and then differentiate into mature DCs that present antigenic information to antigen-reactive T cells in regional lymph nodes, resulting in antigen-specific T-cell activation. DCs play a crucial role in the antigen-specific machinery of immune responses.

The immune molecules to be understood in cancer immunotherapy include antibodies, cytokines, and antigen peptides. Antibodies are molecules that are produced by B cells through their differentiation to plasma cells. Antibodies bind to antigens in an antigen-specific manner, and they then attack or neutralize the antigens. Antibodies also exist on the surface of B cells as a B-cell receptor (BCR).

**Table 1.1** Representative cells, molecules, receptors, and their functions in immune system

| | | |
|---|---|---|
| 1. Cells | Granulocytes, NK cells, γδT cells: | Systemic patrol |
| | Macrophages | Locoregional patrol |
| | T and B cells | Specific functions offered |
| | Dendritic cells | Director in immune reactions |
| 2. Molecules | Antibody | Bind to target and neutralize antigens |
| | Cytokine | Intercellular stimulatory or inhibitory signaling |
| | Peptide | Essential target recognized by effector T cells |
| 3. Receptors | TCR | Antigen-reactive receptor on T cells for recognition and signaling |
| | BCR | Antibody on B cells |
| | TLR | Danger signal transduction |
| | Cytokine receptor | Signaling specific for corresponding cytokine |

*NK* natural killer, *TCR* T-cell receptor, *BCR* B-cell receptor, *TLR* toll-like receptor

Cytokines are molecules that mediate intercellular communications such as stimulatory or inhibitory signals. Many cytokines have been identified to date, including interferons, interleukins, tumor necrosis factor, growth factors, colony-stimulating factors, and more. Some cytokines are directly cytotoxic to cancer cells, but a few cytokines are approved for use in cancer treatment. Antigen peptides are a part of the antigenic mother protein. They can stimulate antigen-reactive T-cell precursors in regional lymph nodes to become effector T cells, which then migrate to a target site and recognize the antigenic epitopes on target cells, including cancer cells. Many clinical trials using antigen peptides are now being conducted to determine the potential clinical benefits.

These immune molecules function in the immune system through their specific receptors. Antigen peptides are recognized by T-cell receptors (TCRs) specific to the antigen. A BCR is a receptor on B cells, a molecule of which is an antibody, as mentioned above. In addition, toll-like receptors (TLRs) are molecules that transduce danger signals of invaders into immune cells. Each cytokine has a corresponding receptor on the cell surface, through which functional signals are transduced into the cells.

## 1.3 Classification of Immune Systems and Cancer Immunotherapy

There are two different classifications with which one can understand the immune system in terms of the comparative counterpart nomenclatures of immunity: they are humoral immunity versus cellular immunity and innate immunity versus acquired immunity. Each of these types of immunity consists of the different cell types, molecules, and receptors mentioned above (Table 1.2).

**Table 1.2** Classification of immunity and cancer immunotherapy based on cells and molecules involved

| | | |
|---|---|---|
| 1. Humoral immunity versus cellular immunity | Humoral: | Antibody |
| | Cellular: | Functional T cells, macrophages, NK cells, NKT cells, γδT cells, DCs, granulocytes |
| 2. Innate immunity versus acquired immunity | Innate: | Granulocytes, NK cells, NKT cells, γδT cells, macrophages, DCs |
| | Acquired: | T cells, B cells |
| 3. Active immunotherapy versus adoptive immunotherapy | Active: | Vaccine, immunocheckpoint inhibitor |
| | Adoptive: | Antitumor antibody, antitumor cytokines, antitumor lymphocytes |

Humoral immunity is an immune response that depends on antigen-specific antibody production by B cells in concert with type 2 helper T cells (Table 1.2). Although there is evidence that the antibody response is involved in tumor responses, humoral response-based cancer immunotherapy has not been actively developed, except for research concerning monoclonal antibodies specific to tumor growth factors and growth factor receptors on the surfaces of tumor cells. Cellular immunity is an immune response involving many types of cells, including antigen-specific functional T cells (cytotoxic T cells and type 1 helper T cells) and antigen-nonspecific macrophages, NK cells, NKT cells, γδT cells, DCs, and granulocytes. Cellular immunity-based cancer treatment has been the main focus of investigation in the development of cancer immunotherapy.

The counterpart nomenclature, i.e., innate immunity versus acquired immunity, is also important. Innate immunity involves granulocytes, NK cells, NKT cells, γδT cells, macrophages, and DCs, whereas acquired immunity involves T- and B-cell responses (Table 1.2). Both of these types of immunity are quite important to the body's eradication of invaders including cancer cells, as well as in the overall understanding of cancer immunotherapy.

When we classify the current types of cancer immunotherapy, two nomenclatures of immunotherapy types are used: active immunotherapy and adoptive immunotherapy (Table 1.2). Active immunotherapy includes cancer vaccines, where therapeutic vaccines indirectly attack tumor cells with the emergence of immune activation specific to tumor antigens. Immune cells that are stimulated and activated by the cancer vaccines "actively" function in tumor eradication in a host. In terms of an "indirect" working property, the immunocheckpoint inhibitors described below can also be considered to belong to the active immunotherapy category. In contrast, adoptive immunotherapy is a treatment using tumor-reactive immune molecules (cytokines or antibodies) or cells, which themselves directly attack tumor cells for eradication. When treating a host undergoing cancer immunotherapy, more attention must be paid to the patient's immunocompetency in active immunotherapy compared to adoptive immunotherapy.

## 1.4 Eradication of Invaders Including Cancer by the Immune System

A scheme showing the eradication of invaders including cancer is shown in Fig. 1.1. When invaders enter a host, an initial response to the invaders is processed by the host's innate immunity, usually in an antigen-nonspecific manner. Antigenic information obtained in the initial response is further presented to the acquired immunity system by DCs, which are antigen-presenting cells. This presentation results in the activation and differentiation of T and B cells to function in an antigen-specific manner, which strengthens the eradication of invaders as a secondary response. After the initial and secondary immune responses, antigenic information is recorded in the memory of the host immune system to varying extents depending on the antigens. Thus, invaders including cancer can be completely eradicated with both initial and secondary immune responses in antigen-nonspecific and antigen-specific manners by the innate and acquired immunity, respectively. Cancer immunotherapy is a treatment that uses these precise machineries of the immune system.

Importantly, there is a regulatory immunity that controls both the initial and secondary immune responses (Fig. 1.1). The regulatory immunity consists of cellular and molecular systems, including regulatory T (Treg) cells, myeloid-derived suppressor cells (MDSCs), and immunocheckpoint molecules, for example, cytotoxic T-lymphocyte-associated protein (CTLA)-4 and programmed death (PD)-1. These cells and molecules are highly involved in the prevention of the emergence of effective antitumor immune responses (Fig. 1.1).

Thus, tumor eradication by the immune system is finally completed when the regulatory immune system of cellular and molecular interactions is overcome. The

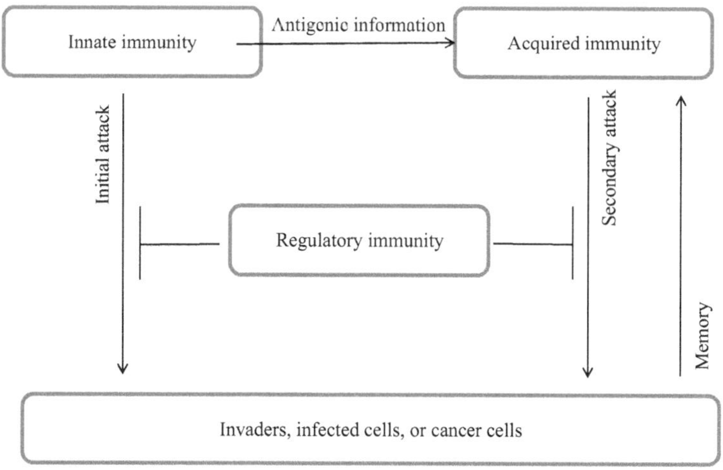


**Fig. 1.1** Scheme of effector and regulatory systems for eradication of invaders including cancer. Scheme of immune system against invaders including cancer is indicated. It consists of effector (innate and acquired immunity) and regulatory systems

concept of cancer "immunoediting" advocates that the "three Es" of elimination, equilibrium, and escape play dual roles in promoting host protection against cancer and facilitating tumor escape from immunosurveillance [3]. The immunoediting concept may help us to determine what is happening at the tumor site at the time of tumor recognition and eradication by the immune system.

## 1.5 Machinery of Antigen Presentation and Recognition

The machinery of antigen presentation and recognition is very important to the concept of cancer immunotherapy (Fig. 1.2). Exogenous and endogenous antigen proteins are processed randomly into peptides consisting of 8–12 amino acids at the proteasome of professional APCs, such as DCs. The processed antigen peptides meet with a human leukocyte antigen (HLA) molecule at the endoplasmic reticulum of the APCs to make an HLA-peptide complex that then moves to the cell surface of the APCs. The antigen peptides in context with an HLA molecule on APCs can stimulate antigen-reactive T-cell precursors to become effector T cells, in which HLA class I- and class II-peptide complexes can stimulate antigen-reactive

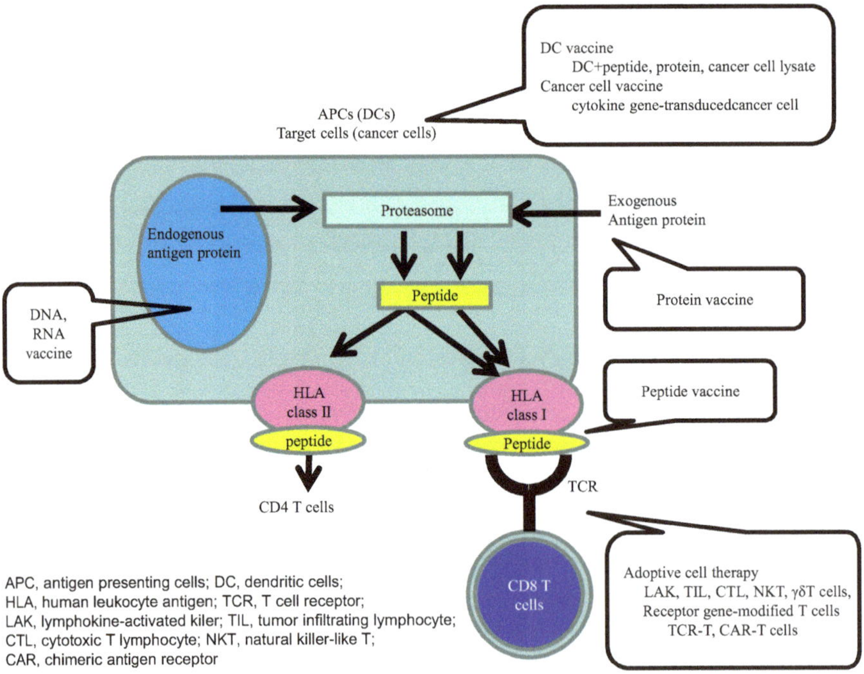


**Fig. 1.2** Machinery of antigen presentation and possible cancer immunotherapy. Machinery of antigen presentation and recognition is summarized. Possible cancer immunotherapies including vaccine therapy and adoptive cell therapy are also indicated

**Table 1.3** Molecules involved in antigen presentation and recognition

| Reaction | APC, target cell | Lymphocytes |
|---|---|---|
| Specific | HLA + peptide | TCR |
| Co-stimulatory | CD80 (B7-1), CD86 (B7-2) | CD28(stimulatory), CTLA-4 (inhibitory) |
| | CD40 | CD154 (CD40L) |
| Adhesion | HLA class II | CD4 |
| | HLA class I | CD8 |
| | CD54 (ICAM-1) | CD11a/CD18 (LFA-1) |
| | CD58 (LFA-3) | CD2 (LFA-2) |

*TCR* T-cell receptor, *CTLA-4* cytotoxic T-lymphocyte-associated protein-4, *LFA* lymphocyte function-associated antigen, *ICAM* intercellular adhesion molecule

CD8 and CD4 T cells, respectively (i.e., HLA restriction) [4]. Activated T cells then migrate to a target site and recognize the antigen epitopes on target cells, including cancer cells, to eradicate them.

Important molecules involved in the antigen presentation and recognition are summarized in Table 1.3. The machinery of antigen presentation and recognition consists of molecules needed for the antigen-specific reaction, co-stimulatory reaction, and adjunctive adhesion reaction, which together make a strong immunological synapse formation that can transduce efficient activation signals into antigen-reactive T cells [5].

Based on the above information, several treatment modalities for cancer immunotherapy have been proposed, including vaccines and adoptive cell therapy (ACT) (Fig. 1.2). The vaccine modalities include DC vaccines, cancer-cell vaccines, protein vaccines, peptide vaccines, and DNA/RNA vaccines. The ACT modality includes the transferal of cells of several effector cell types, including lymphokine-activated killer (LAK) cells, tumor-infiltrating lymphocytes (TILs), cytotoxic T lymphocytes (CTLs), NKT cells and γδT cells, and TCR gene and chimeric antigen receptor (CAR) gene-modified T cells, all of which are described in detail in the following chapters.

## 1.6 History of Cancer Immunotherapy Development

The history of the development of cancer immunotherapy is of interest. According to the literature, the first immunotherapy for cancer was conducted in 1891 by Dr. William Coley, who administered a bacterial preparation to patients [6]. I would say, however, that the development of cancer immunotherapy based on the current understanding of tumor immunology has been most active since the 1970s. Events that have contributed to the development of cancer immunotherapy are shown in Fig. 1.3, and the cancer immunotherapies currently approved in Japan are shown in Table 1.4.

| Years | Events | Therapies developed and examined |
|---|---|---|
| 1970s | | Plant extract, Bacterial preparation |
| 1980s | Cytokine cloning<br>Lymphocyte culture | Cytokine<br>ACT (LAK cells, TIL) |
| 1990s | MAGE discovery<br>DC culture<br>Antibody engineering<br>PD-1<br>CTLA-4<br>TLRs | Peptide vaccine<br>DC vaccine, ACT (DAK cells)<br>Anti-tumor antibody |
| 2000s | NKT, γδT cells<br>Regulatory T cells<br>MDSCs | ACT (NKT cells, γδT cells)<br><br><br>Immunoadjuvant<br>ACT (TCR-T cells, CAR-T cells) |
| 2010s | <br>Immunocheckpoint | Sipleucel-T<br>Ipilimumab (anti-CTLA-4 Ab)<br>Nivolumab (anti-PD-1 Ab) |

MAGE, melanoma antigen encoding gene; ACT, Adoptive cell therapy; DC, dendritic cell; DAK, DC-activated killer; PD-1, programmed death-1; CTLA-4, cytotoxic T lymphocyte-associated protein-4; TLR, toll-like receptor; NKT, natural killer-like T; MDSC, myeloid-derived suppressor T

**Fig. 1.3** History of cancer immunotherapy development. History of cancer immunotherapy development is shown. Milestone discoveries in tumor immunology are also indicated

First, crude biological response modifiers including plant extracts and bacterial preparations were investigated in clinical trials. Some agents demonstrated a clinical benefit, and they were consequently approved as drugs for cancer treatment in Japan. Most of them have been used in combination with cytotoxic chemotherapy or radiation therapy. However, none has become a standard cancer treatment except for bacillus Calmette-Guérin (BCG) for superficial bladder cancer, despite the accumulation of evidence of some agents' effectiveness (as described in Chaps. 2, 3, and 4).

In the 1980s, advances in molecular cloning and gene-engineering technology enabled the use of cytokines, including interferons and interleukins, in cancer treatment [7]. Some of these agents showed clinical benefit and were approved for use in clinical practice. A few of them have become a standard treatment for several cancer types including renal cell cancer (see Chap. 5). A crucial cytokine, interleukin (IL)-2, has permitted us to use ex vivo-activated autologous lymphocytes for cancer treatment as ACT. Representative treatments of ACT include LAK cell therapy [8], TIL therapy [9], and tumor-sensitized T cells [10] (see Chaps. 5, 6, 7, 8, and 9). ACT using TILs and tumor-sensitized T cells showed efficacy for treating malignant effusion and advanced cancer, resulting in their approval in Japan as the advanced medicine.

In addition to the clinical use of IL-2, studies of IL-2 enabled the establishment of tumor antigen-specific lymphocyte clones in vitro, which contributed to the first discovery of a melanoma antigen-encoding gene, MAGE, in 1991 [11]. This major

**Table 1.4** Cancer immunotherapy approved in Japan (at Nov. 2014)

| Immunotherapy | Diseases approved |
|---|---|
| 1st generation | |
| Polysaccharide-K | Stomach (PAC), colorectal (PAC), small cell LC (+C) |
| OK-432 | Stomach (PAC), NSLC (+C) |
| | Head and neck, thyroid, malignant effusion, ascites |
| Lentinan | Stomach (+C) |
| Ubenimex | Adult acute non-lymphatic leukemia (+C) |
| Sizophiran | Cervix (+R) |
| BCG | Bladder (superficial) |
| 2nd generation | |
| IFN-α-2β | RCC, MM, CML, Hairy cell, hepatitis B, hepatitis C |
| IFN-β | Brain tumor, melanoma, hepatitis B, hepatitis C |
| IFN-γ-1α | RCC |
| Teceleukin | RCC, angiosarcoma |
| 3rd generation | |
| Advanced medicine (A) | |
| ACT | Malignant effusion, advanced cancer |
| DC+peptide vaccine | Esophageal, stomach, colorectal, metastatic liver, pancreas, biliary, |
| | breast, lung |
| Advanced medicine (B) | |
| Tailer-made peptide vaccine | HLA-A24+ hormone-resistant prostatic cancer |
| NKT ACT | Lung, head and neck squamous cell cancer |
| γδT ACT | NSLC |
| 4th generation (immunocheckpoint inhibitor) | |
| Nivolumab | Melanoma |

Antitumor antibodies are excluded. Advanced medicine A is obligated to be reapplied for B until Mar. 2016

*PAC* postoperative adjuvant chemotherapy, *+C* with chemotherapy, *+R* with radiation, *RCC* renal cell cancer, *MM* multiple myeloma

discovery in concert with the establishment of DCs cultured in vitro [12] resulted in many new lines of research into cancer vaccine development (see Chaps. 10, 11, 12, 13, and 14). The technique of culturing DCs was also introduced in ACT for stimulating naïve T cells to generate antigen-reactive DC-activated killer (DAK) cells (see Chap. 5).

From the late 1990s to the 2000s, antibody-engineering technology enabled the use of antitumor monoclonal antibodies in cancer treatment, and nowadays, many antitumor antibodies are used in daily practice as a standard treatment for cancer. However, antitumor antibodies are not described in detail in this book.

In the 2000s, immunoadjuvants have been actively investigated, where TLRs play a key role [13] (see Chaps. 15, 16, and 17). In addition, novel effector cells including NKT cells [14] and γδT cells [15] were discovered and introduced into

ACT strategies as effector cells (see Chaps. 6, 7, and 8). ACT using NKT cells and γδT cells has been approved as the advanced medicine in Japan in tests of its efficacy for clinical use. The novel inhibitory cells, Treg cells, were also discovered in this period [16], and much attention has begun to be paid to their significance and to the establishment of conditioning strategies against Tregs in cancer immunotherapy.

In 2010, a DC vaccine was finally approved in the US for the treatment of castration-resistant prostate cancer [17] (see Chap. 14), although its low response rate once pricked the balloon of cancer vaccine development [18, 19]. On the other hand, ACT continued to progress with the development of antigen-specific TCR gene [20] and CAR gene transduction technology [21] that has made the irrelevant lymphocytes highly specific for the antigen (see Chap. 9). In addition, immunocheckpoint inhibitors have been providing exciting surprises each year since 2011 (see Chaps. 18, 19, and 20). Anti-CTLA-4 [22] and anti-PD-1/PD-ligand 1 (PD-L1) [23] antibodies and their combination [24] are very effective, showing objective tumor responses in melanoma. The anti-PD-1 antibody nivolumab was approved for melanoma treatment in September 2014 in Japan, the first such approval in the world. The novel inhibitory cells MDSCs were recently highlighted [25]; their reduction in the tumor microenvironment, as well as that of Treg cells (which may enhance antitumor immune responses for successful cancer immunotherapy), has been earnestly investigated in relation to the immunocheckpoint inhibitors (see Chaps. 21 and 22).

Cancer immunotherapy has thus progressed from the development of crude agents, followed by cytokines and antibodies, vaccines and effector lymphocytes, and now to immunocheckpoint inhibitors, all of which are classified as the first, second, third, and fourth generations of cancer immunotherapy, respectively (Table 1.4). Much of the progress that has been made is the result of the clarification of the fundamental molecular mechanisms of the immune system and the properties of immune-related tumor responses in clinical trials (see Chap. 23). It is very important when conducting cancer immunotherapy to validate and standardize the methods to monitor and examine immune responses and immune-related molecular expressions (see Chap. 25). The progress of cancer immunotherapy development is now contributing to the identification of biomarkers for personalized cancer immunotherapy as an even more effective form of cancer immunotherapy (see Chap. 24).

## 1.7 A Perspective on the Future of Cancer Immunotherapy

I would like emphasize several points regarding the current development of cancer immunotherapy, which differs significantly from cancer chemotherapy. First, cancer immunotherapy may result in limited tumor shrinkage but may also produce a prolongation of survival, which is the golden goal of cancer treatment. This has been shown clearly in a vaccine trial [26, 27]. The tumor shrinkage often takes a long time to observe, a phenomenon called the immune-related tumor response or delayed-type tumor shrinkage. A trial of immunocheckpoint inhibitors exemplifies this phenomenon [22]. Pseudo-progression, in which the tumor size increases compared to that seen at the beginning of the treatment period, has also been observed. In a sense, it is analogous to the idea that one ant cannot kill an elephant but an army of ants that develops (during a sufficient growth period of the tumor) could bring an elephant down. Physicians must bear in mind this property of the immune-related response in cancer immunotherapy, in daily clinical practice as well as in clinical trials. Immune-related response criteria (irRC) are essential to assessments of the true efficacy of cancer immunotherapy [28].

Second, I would point out that T cells really "know" cancer cells. Even a small number of T cells can cure or improve cancer patients. This has been shown in trials using antigen-reactive TCRs or CARs [20, 21]. In this treatment modality, however, we must pay more attention to the targeted antigens. Self-antigens, including cancer-testis antigens, differentiation antigens, and overexpression antigens, may not be appropriate for targeting, because the effector cells can make a response to them as on-target and/or off-target on normal cells [29]. From this point of view, mutated antigens must be targeted by T cells [30]. Whole-genome sequencing has demonstrated that tumor cells have at least one or more mutations as "neo-antigens" [31]. The identification of each mutation is one of the directions to be pursued toward the establishment of personalized immunotherapy; of course, doing so is not easy and it will take a long time to identify every cancer mutation for every individual. TILs themselves, on the other hand, may do identify each mutation in situ in the host, where passenger mutations may be a target for immune recognition [32]. Thus, cancer immunotherapy using TILs may become active again in light of its efficacy and safety in combination with a conditioning protocol to modify host immunocompetence [33].

Third, an immunosurveillance system does exist in a host, as shown in a trial using immunocheckpoint inhibitors [22]. Modifications of immunocheckpoint interactions between immune cells and tumor cells by inhibitory drugs could permit immune cells to attack the tumor cells. In cases in which there are no attenuation of immunocheckpoints on tumor cells, we could attempt to induce the upregulation of immunocheckpoints on the tumor cells using combinations of chemotherapy and radiotherapy. This means that it may be possible to create a trigger for a tumor-reactive immune response at the tumor site in situ, which may then spread to systemic immune responses for concomitant tumor eradication. Immunogenic cancer cell death at the tumor site may generate systemic antitumor responses, indicating the possibility of in situ cancer vaccination. In other words, this can be possible only when a tumor is present in the body. The time may come when we should not remove a tumor from the body for cure and prevention, based on our understanding of tumor immunology.

Finally, more attention should be focused on host immunocompetency in the development of personalized cancer immunotherapy [34]. Beyond the TNM staging system, I propose the establishment of an immune-related staging system (irStage) which would describe the locoregional values of effector cells, regulatory

**Table 1.5** Candidate factors for immune-related staging toward personalized cancer immunotherapy development

| | Biomarkers | |
|---|---|---|
| Site | Positive | Negative |
| Locoregional | CD8 T-cell infiltration | Treg, MDSCs |
| | | PD-L1 on tumor |
| Systemic | Lymphocyte count≧1,000 | Lymphocyte count<1,000 |
| | | G/L≧2 |
| | | CRP>0.5 mg/dl, IAP≧580 mg/dl |
| | | High tumor marker |
| | | Treg cells, MDSCs |

*Treg* regulatory T, *MDSC* myeloid-derived suppressor cell, *PD-L* programmed death-ligand, *G/L* granulocyte/lymphocyte ratio, *CRP* C-reactive protein, *IAP* immunosuppressive acidic protein

cells and their balances, the immunocheckpoint status on tumor cells, and systemic values including lymphocyte count, C-reactive protein, and tumor marker levels (Table 1.5). An appropriate modality of cancer immunotherapy may be chosen depending on this irStage level. For example, a vaccine strategy may be appropriate for patients with good immunocompetency and no immunosuppression. ACT may be preferable when patients have low effector precursors and low lymphocyte counts. Immunocheckpoint inhibitors may be active when effector cells are infiltrating at tumor sites and when the tumor cells express a counterpart ligand of the immunocheckpoint molecules. If a patient's immune system is in a depressed condition, a conditioning regimen may be necessary to modulate host immunosuppression. The use of such an irStaging system may enhance tumor responses with a concomitant survival benefit, resulting in the establishment of very effective personalized cancer immunotherapy.

## 1.8 Conclusions

As an important option for cancer treatment, cancer immunotherapy has come of age. It may be necessary to seek the best way to orchestrate cancer treatment with immunotherapy and other treatment modalities in order to identify the most effective cancer treatment for each patient. This will certainly contribute to cancer patients' survival and cure. We already have effective weapons and knowledge in the field of cancer immunotherapy. To paraphrase the recent Nobel Peace Prize speech by Miss Malala Yousafzai [35], I would say now that one lymphocyte, one dendritic cell, one antigen, and one drug can change the cancer treatment, immunotherapy, together.

# References


1. Couzin-Frankel J (2013) Breakthrough of the year 2013. Cancer immunotherapy. Science 342 (6165):1432–1433
2. Burnet FM (1970) The concept of immunological surveillance. Prog Exp Tumor Res 13:1–27
3. Dunn GP, Bruce AT, Ikeda H, Old LJ, Schreiber RD (2002) Cancer immunoediting: from immunosurveillance to tumor escape. Nat Immunol 3(11):991–998
4. Brodsky FM, Guagliardi LE (1991) The cell biology of antigen processing and presentation. Annu Rev Immunol 9:707–744
5. Goldstein JS, Chen T, Gubina E, Pastor RW, Kozlowski S (2000) ICAM-1 enhances MHC-peptide activation of CD8(+) T cells without an organized immunological synapse. Eur J Immunol 30(11):3266–3270
6. Coley WB (1891) Contribution to the knowledge of sarcoma. Ann Surg 14:199–220
7. Taniguchi T, Matsui H, Fujita T, Takaoka C, Kashima N, Yoshimoto R, Hamuro J (1983) Structure and expression of a cloned cDNA for human interleukin-2. Nature 302:305
8. Rosenberg SA, Lotze MT, Muul LM, Leitman S, Chang AE, Ettinghausen SE, Matory YL, Skibber JM, Shiloni E, Vetto JT, Seipp CA, Simpson C, Reichert CM (1985) Observations on the systemic administration of autologous lymphokine-activated killer cells and recombinant interleukin-2 to patients with metastatic cancer. N Eng J Med 313:1485–1492
9. Rosenberg SA, Spiess P, Lafreniere R (1986) A new approach to the adoptive immunotherapy of cancer with tumor-infiltrating lymphocytes. Science 233(4770):1318–1321
10. Aruga A, Yamauchi K, Takasaki K, Furukawa T, Hanyu F (1991) Induction of autologous tumor-specific cytotoxic T cells in patients with liver cancer. Characterizations and clinical utilization. Int J Cancer 49(1):19–24
11. van der Bruggen P, Traversari C, Chomez P, Lurquin C, De Plaen E, Van den Eynde B, Knuth A, Boon T (1991) A gene encoding an antigen recognized by cytolytic T lymphocytes on a human melanoma. Science 254(5038):1643–1647
12. Romani N, Gruner S, Brang D, Kämpgen E, Lenz A, Trockenbacher B, Konwalinka G, Fritsch PO, Steinman RM, Schuler G (1994) Proliferating dendritic cell progenitors in human blood. J Exp Med 180(1):83–93
13. Ishii KJ, Kawagoe T, Koyama S, Matsui K, Kumar H, Kawai T, Uematsu S, Takeuchi O, Takeshita F, Coban C, Akira S (2008) TANK-binding kinase-1 delineates innate and adaptive immune responses to DNA vaccines. Nature 451(7179):725–729
14. Kawano T, Cui J, Koezuka Y, Toura I, Kaneko Y, Motoki K, Ueno H, Nakagawa R, Sato H, Kondo E, Koseki H, Taniguchi M (1997) Natural killer-like nonspecific tumor cell lysis mediated by specific ligand-activated Valpha14 NKT cells. Science 278(5343):1626–1629
15. Tanaka Y, Morita CT, Tanaka Y, Nieves E, Brenner MB, Bloom BR (1995) Natural and synthetic non-peptide antigens recognized by human gamma delta T cells. Nature 375 (6527):155–158
16. Hori S, Nomura T, Sakaguchi S (2003) Control of regulatory T cell development by the transcription factor Foxp3. Science 299:1057
17. Kantoff PW, Higano CS, Shore ND, Berger ER, Small EJ, Penson DF, Redfern CH, Ferrari AC, Dreicer R, Sims RB, Xu Y, Frohlich MW, Schellhammer PF, IMPACT Study Investigators (2010) Sipuleucel-T immunotherapy for castration-resistant prostate cancer. N Engl J Med 363:411–422
18. Rosenberg SA, Yang JC, Restifo NP (2004) Cancer immunotherapy: moving beyond current vaccines. Nat Med 10(9):909–915
19. Eggermont AM (2009) Immunotherapy: vaccine trials in melanoma – time for reflection. Nat Rev Clin Oncol 6(5):256–258
20. Morgan RA, Dudley ME, Wunderlich JR, Hughes MS, Yang JC, Sherry RM, Royal RE, Topalian SL, Kammula US, Restifo NP, Zheng Z, Nahvi A, de Vries CR, Rogers-Freezer LJ, Mavroukakis SA, Rosenberg SA (2006) Cancer regression in patients after transfer of genetically engineered lymphocytes. Science 314:126–129

21. Porter DL, Levine BL, Kalos M, Bagg A, June CH (2011) Chimeric antigen receptor-modified T cells in chronic lymphoid leukemia. N Engl J Med 365:725
22. Hodi FS, O'Day SJ, McDermott DF, Weber RW, Sosman JA, Haanen JB, Gonzalez R, Robert C, Schadendorf D, Hassel JC, Akerley W, van den Eertwegh AJ, Lutzky J, Lorigan P, Vaubel JM, Linette GP, Hogg D, Ottensmeier CH, Lebbé C, Peschel C, Quirt I, Clark JI, Wolchok JD, Weber JS, Tian J, Yellin MJ, Nichol GM, Hoos A, Urba WJ (2010) Improved survival with ipilimumab in patients with metastatic melanoma. N Engl J Med 363 (8):711–723
23. Topalian SL, Hodi FS, Brahmer JR, Gettinger SN, Smith DC, McDermott DF, Powderly JD, Carvajal RD, Sosman JA, Atkins MB, Leming PD, Spigel DR, Antonia SJ, Horn L, Drake CG, Pardoll DM, Chen L, Sharfman WH, Anders RA, Taube JM, McMiller TL, Xu H, Korman AJ, Jure-Kunkel M, Agrawal S, McDonald D, Kollia GD, Gupta A, Wigginton JM, Sznol M (2012) Safety, activity, and immune correlates of anti-PD-1 antibody in cancer. N Engl J Med 366:2443
24. Wolchok JD, Kluger H, Callahan MK, Postow MA, Rizvi NA, Lesokhin AM, Segal NH, Ariyan CE, Gordon RA, Reed K, Burke MM, Caldwell A, Kronenberg SA, Agunwamba BU, Zhang X, Lowy I, Inzunza HD, Feely W, Horak CE, Hong Q, Korman AJ, Wigginton JM, Gupta A, Sznol M (2013) Nivolumab plus ipilimumab in advanced melanoma. N Engl J Med 369:122–133
25. Sinha P, Clements VK, Ostrand-Rosenberg S (2005) Reduction of myeloid-derived suppressor cells and induction of M1 macrophages facilitate the rejection of established metastatic disease. J Immunol 174(2):636–645
26. Hoos A, Eggermont AM, Janetzki S, Hodi FS, Ibrahim R, Anderson A, Humphrey R, Blumenstein B, Old L, Wolchok J (2010) Improved endpoints for cancer immunotherapy trials. J Natl Cancer Inst 102(18):1388–1397
27. Yamaguchi Y, Yamaue H, Okusaka T, Okuno K, Suzuki H, Fujioka T, Otsu A, Ohashi Y, Shimazawa R, Nishio K, Furuse J, Minami H, Tsunoda T, Hayashi Y, Nakamura Y, Committee of Guidance for Peptide Vaccines for the Treatment of Cancer, The Japanese Society for Biological Therapy (2014) Guidance for peptide vaccines for the treatment of cancer. Cancer Sci 105(7):924–931
28. Wolchok JD, Hoos A, O'Day S, Weber JS, Hamid O, Lebbé C, Maio M, Binder M, Bohnsack O, Nichol G, Humphrey R, Hodi FS (2009) Guidelines for the evaluation of immune therapy activity in solid tumors: immune-related response criteria. Clin Cancer Res 15 (23):7412–7420
29. Morgan RA, Chinnasamy N, Abate-Daga D, Gros A, Robbins PF, Zheng Z, Dudley ME, Feldman SA, Yang JC, Sherry RM, Phan GQ, Hughes MS, Kammula US, Miller AD, Hessman CJ, Stewart AA, Restifo NP, Quezado MM, Alimchandani M, Rosenberg AZ, Nath A, Wang T, Bielekova B, Wuest SC, Akula N, McMahon FJ, Wilde S, Mosetter B, Schendel DJ, Laurencot CM, Rosenberg SA (2013) Cancer regression and neurological toxicity following anti-MAGE-A3 TCR gene therapy. J Immunother 36(2):133–151
30. Tran E, Turcotte S, Gros A, Robbins PF, Lu YC, Dudley ME, Wunderlich JR, Somerville RP, Hogan K, Hinrichs CS, Parkhurst MR, Yang JC, Rosenberg SA (2014) Cancer immunotherapy based on mutation-specific CD4+ T cells in a patient with epithelial cancer. Science 344 (6184):641–645
31. Alexandrov LB, Nik-Zainal S, Wedge DC, Aparicio SA, Behjati S, Biankin AV, Bignell GR, Bolli N, Borg A, Børresen-Dale AL, Boyault S, Burkhardt B, Butler AP, Caldas C, Davies HR, Desmedt C, Eils R, Eyfjörd JE, Foekens JA, Greaves M, Hosoda F, Hutter B, Ilicic T, Imbeaud S, Imielinski M, Jäger N, Jones DT, Jones D, Knappskog S, Kool M, Lakhani SR, López-Otín C, Martin S, Munshi NC, Nakamura H, Northcott PA, Pajic M, Papaemmanuil E, Paradiso A, Pearson JV, Puente XS, Raine K, Ramakrishna M, Richardson AL, Richter J, Rosenstiel P, Schlesner M, Schumacher TN, Span PN, Teague JW, Totoki Y, Tutt AN, Valdés-Mas R, van Buuren MM, van't Veer L, Vincent-Salomon A, Waddell N, Yates LR, Australian Pancreatic Cancer Genome Initiative, ICGC Breast Cancer Consortium, ICGC MMML-Seq

Consortium, ICGC PedBrain, Zucman-Rossi J, Futreal PA, McDermott U, Lichter P, Meyerson M, Grimmond SM, Siebert R, Campo E, Shibata T, Pfister SM, Campbell PJ, Stratton MR (2013) Signatures of mutational processes in human cancer. Nature 500 (7463):415–21

32. Robbins PF, Lu YC, El-Gamil M, Li YF, Gross C, Gartner J, Lin JC, Teer JK, Cliften P, Tycksen E, Samuels Y, Rosenberg SA (2013) Mining exomic sequencing data to identify mutated antigens recognized by adoptively transferred tumor-reactive T cells. Nat Med 19 (6):747–752
33. Hinrichs CS, Rosenberg SA (2014) Exploiting the curative potential of adoptive T-cell therapy for cancer. Immunol Rev 257(1):56–71
34. Galon J, Mlecnik B, Bindea G, Angell HK, Berger A, Lagorce C, Lugli A, Zlobec I, Hartmann A, Bifulco C, Nagtegaal ID, Palmqvist R, Masucci GV, Botti G, Tatangelo F, Delrio P, Maio M, Laghi L, Grizzi F, Asslaber M, D'Arrigo C, Vidal-Vanaclocha F, Zavadova E, Chouchane L, Ohashi PS, Hafezi-Bakhtiari S, Wouters BG, Roehrl M, Nguyen L, Kawakami Y, Hazama S, Okuno K, Ogino S, Gibbs P, Waring P, Sato N, Torigoe T, Itoh K, Patel PS, Shukla SN, Wang Y, Kopetz S, Sinicrope FA, Scripcariu V, Ascierto PA, Marincola FM, Fox BA, Pagès F (2014) Towards the introduction of the 'Immunoscore' in the classification of malignant tumours. J Pathol 232(2):199–209
35. Malala Yousafzai. The full text: Malala Yousafzai delivers defiant riposte to Taliban militants with speech to the UN General Assembly. http://www.independent.co.uk/news/world/asia/the-full-text-malala-yousafzai-delivers-defiant-riposte-to-taliban-militants-with-speech-to-the-un-general-assembly-8706606.html

# Part II
# BRMs and Crude Agents

# Chapter 2
# Bacterial Preparations

**Junichi Sakamoto, Michitaka Honda, and Toru Aoyama**

**Abstract** From the era of Coley's toxin back in the beginning of the twentieth century, it was well known that certain acute bacterial infection might lead to the regression of malignant tumors in some cases. Many types of bacteria either in its crude form or with special preparation have been reported to possess immunotherapeutic activity against cancers. To date, experimental studies and clinical implications of those tumor immunotherapies have become more widely examined with more sophisticated methodology, utilizing activation of the two types of human immune system, i.e., innate and adaptive. In this chapter, various bacterial preparations that have been applied for tumor immunotherapy will be introduced, together with the new detailed mechanism of action of those two immune systems that have recently been elucidated. Of note, the efficacies of OK-432, a preparation derived from *streptococcus pyogenes*, are discussed by a tabulated data and individual patient data meta-analyses of randomized trials of adjuvant immunochemotherapy for lung and gastric cancers.

**Keywords** Bacterial preparation • Tumor immunity • Innate immune system • Adaptive immune system • Adjuvant immunochemotherapy clinical trials of OK-432

## 2.1 Everything Started from Coley's Toxin: Recent Findings Elucidating Mechanisms of Its Antitumor Activity

Spontaneous regressions of various types of cancer have been reported in the history of medical science. Regression is more commonly associated with groups of tumors like the embryonal tumors in children, breast cancer, chorioepithelioma,

J. Sakamoto, M.D., Ph.D., F.A.C.S. (✉)
Tokai Central Hospital, 4-6-2 Higashijimacho, Sohara, Kakamigahara, Gifu 504-8601, Japan
e-mail: sakamjun@tokaihp.jp

M. Honda, M.D., Ph.D.
Department of Gastroenterological Surgery, Cancer Institute Ariake Hospital, Tokyo, Japan

T. Aoyama, M.D.
Department of Gastrointestinal Surgery, Kanagawa Cancer Center, Kanagawa, Japan



Y. Yamaguchi (ed.), *Immunotherapy of Cancer*,
DOI 10.1007/978-4-431-55031-0_2

malignant melanoma, neuroblastoma, sarcomas, bladder cancer, skin cancer, and renal cancer [1, 2]. These phenomena are sometimes associated with infection, vaccine therapy, and incomplete surgical removal of the tumor [3, 4]. In line with those findings, presence of autologous cancer-specific antigens was enthusiastically pursued in melanoma and renal cancer patients in the 1970s and 1980s. Although scientifically intriguing, those studies could not have lead to any successful clinical implication [5, 6].

On the other hand, despite the assumption and fact that chronic infection may lead to cancer, it is presumed that acute infection, on the contrary, could have beneficial effects and often contributes to complete eradication of cancers even with a large tumor burden. In this regard, the use of microbial vaccines for immunotherapy is still being reexamined. This therapeutic concept is based on the early work of Coley, who reported infection-associated tumor regression over a century ago [7]. Inspired by the findings, he injected his first patients with vital Streptococcus pyogenes, a gram-positive organism causing erysipelas. By that attempt, although tumor shrinkage was observed, lethal systemic infections occurred. Thus, Coley modified his treatment regimen using a mixture of heat-inactivated Streptococcus pyogenes and Serratia marcescens. The inoculation of this bacterial vaccine, later known as "Coley's toxin" (CT), marked the origin of modern immunotherapy, and thus Coley is also referred to as "father of cancer immunotherapy" [8].

Recent comprehensive discoveries have deepened more precise understanding of the immune system. Coley himself believed that the effect of his bacterial mixture was based on the release of toxins affecting tumor but sparing normal cells [9]. In fact, CT activates the innate as well as the adaptive immune system by binding toll-like (TLR) and other pattern recognition receptors. With regard to the bacterial nature of CT, this mixture contains unmethylated cytosine phosphodiester guanine complex (CpG), lipoteichoic acid, and lipopolysaccharide (LPS), acting agonistic with several TLRs [10]. Engagement of TLRs induces an inflammatory cascade resulting in cytokine secretion and immune cell activation [11]. This proinflammatory milieu together with high fever breaks the tumor-induced immune tolerance and changes it to an antitumor immunity [12–14]. However, Coley's original hypothesis resting on an immune reaction against a "toxin" present in the microbial material that cross-reacts with and destroys the tumor cells fells more and more into oblivion and up to now has only partly been reexamined [7].

In the 1960s and 1970s, commercial CT preparations were tested on small patient cohorts. In these experiments, results were variable—presumably because of relatively short treatment courses. Also, most of the patients were immunocompromised due to prior or coadministered chemotherapy [15, 16]. Besides, plenty of immune mediators relevant for the inflammatory process were used as single agents in cancer immunotherapy [17–19]. But most of them failed to prove clinical efficiency.

Indeed, the benefit of CT treatment is supposed to be based on the chronological sequence of single immune mediators to induce an optimal antitumor immune response. These facts strengthen the usefulness of a comprehensive analysis regarding the therapeutic potential of the toxin, generated from the original protocol.

In 2005, a Canadian company (MBVax) started to produce CT and rekindle Coley's pioneer work. Since then, promising results for different tumor entities were obtained. These findings are an inducement for further investigations on the antitumor effect of CT.

Analysis of the potential of CT to affect tumor cell growth both in vivo and in vitro was implemented, taking advantage of its intrinsic immunestimulatory properties [20]. Examination of a direct impact on cell growth, proliferation, and viability was also performed. Of note, proapoptotic molecules in tumor target cells increased upon CT treatment [21]. In vivo, repetitive local CT applications effectively controlled tumor growth by stimulating immune responses.

The main objective of this chapter is to examine whether a purely microbial-based approach, or in combination with additional chemo- or targeted therapies, can cure non-immunogenic tumors. Picking up the historical idea of using Coley's toxin (CT), a complex mixture of gram-positive and gram-negative bacterial components as an active antineoplastic agent could be centered as a basis of immunotherapy or immunochemotherapy for cancers using bacterial preparations.

For potential clinical application of microbial-based vaccines, several requirements need to be complied. These include (I) reducing non-specific toxicity to normal cells, (II) preserving antitumor and tolerance-breaking immunostimulatory potential, and (III) applying a standardized treatment protocol. As for the latter, no such standardization was done in the past. Hence, Coley's work came under criticism, because at that time, 13 different preparations and various administration routes (i.v., i.m., and i.t.) existed, and some of these were more effective than others [9, 22]. This may explain why Coley's results could not be reproduced by others. In order to overcome this obstacle, CT should have been designed under constant, standardized conditions according to the original protocol.

Results of recent studies have demonstrated that this preparation acts as a potent antitumor and immune-activating agent. In a series of in vitro experiments, induction of cell death in tumor target cells was observed despite different susceptibility of cancer cells toward CT was demonstrated. In one of those studies, while AsPC-1 cells responded with substantial cell death, other cell lines were less affected. As central mechanisms of CT-induced growth alteration, an upregulation of p21waf gene expression and loss of G2/M phases, both indicative for cell cycle arrest, were reported [21]. In line with the established capacity of bacteria to induce apoptosis as well as necrosis in target cells, both kinds of cell death were observed. Proteins (i.e., LPS, Flagellin) delivered by *S. marcescens* may thus have preferentially induced necrosis, while factors provided by *S. pyogenes* (i.e., streptokinase, streptolysin, and lipoteichoic acid) led to apoptosis [7, 23, 24]. Accordingly, caspase 3/7 activation and DNA fragmentation were also detected in CT-treated tumor cells.

In addition to the capacity of directly compromising tumor viability, CT was also described as being a strong immune stimulator [9, 25–27]. The bacterial DNA (CpG ODN) present in this complex mixture may here be one of the best-known immune-activating candidates. CpG ODNs have been found to improve antigen-presenting cell functions and boost humoral as well as cellular Th1-directed immune responses. They have shown promising results as adjuvants for vaccines and in combination with radio- or immunotherapy [10, 12, 28]. Several CpG ODN-based agents were already included into clinical trials for exploring their safety and efficacy in hematological and solid cancers [28–30] [http://www.clinicaltrials.org/]. The underlying mechanism is due to activating TLRs, the most important innate immune receptors [12–14]. TLR signaling in immune cells is crucial for regulating innate and adaptive immune responses, such as DC maturation and antigen presentation as well as CD8+ T cell toxicity [31, 32]. 6#CT-stimulated leukocytes from healthy donors could be effectively activated and responded with upregulation of TLR 2, 5, and 9. Likewise, CD25 expression was significantly and sustainably induced in these short-time-mixed leukocyte cultures, suggesting a stimulation of γ/δ T cells [33]. Besides, secretion of Th1 and other proinflammatory cytokines (e.g., IFN-γ, IL12, and TNF-α) by immune cells belonging to both the innate and adaptive arm can also be anticipated. Hence, this mixture of TLR agonists likely stimulates a complex cascade, each of which plays a unique and vital role in orchestrating immune responses [34]. A boost of antitumor effects with a massive decrease in tumor cell numbers was also observed together with CT. That boosted antitumor effects could rather be dependent from tumor-specific than from the allotransplanted lymphocyte. T3M4 and BxPC-3 could be effectively killed by CT and leukocytes. However, comparable results were not obtained for AsPC-1 cells, which had been shown to be highly susceptible toward CT-mediated lysis alone. This can be attributed to a kind of tumor-escape mechanism. These cells probably secrete immunosuppressive factors (IL10, TGF-β), thereby preventing leukocyte stimulation and immune-mediated lysis.

In a subsequent syngeneic in vivo tumor model, CTs' potential to impact solid tumors was examined. Efficacy for a non-immunogenic tumor was examined although it is clearly established that low immunogenic tumors respond worse than their immunogenic counterpart [9]. As a result, in immunecompetent mice-bearing syngeneic tumor, strong oncopathic effects were demonstrated after repetitive challenge of CT. Of particular interest was the finding that maximal tumor growth control was obtained after six injections. Increasing the number of injections did not further boost therapeutic responses.

Hence, CT may thus be best combined with other (antineoplastic) drugs rather than used as a single agent. However, before further exploring such combinatorial approaches, possible intolerable toxic side effects (e.g., cardiac, gastrointestinal, and hematological toxicity, anorexia, neuropathy, arthralgia, and myalgia) have to be excluded or at least minimized. Additional to identifying the optimal nontoxic dose, a proper application route (i.e., systemic versus local), an appropriate and feasible time schedule (simultaneous versus consecutive therapy), and potential synergistic or antagonistic effects of selected combinations have to be evaluated. All in all, CT might still be worth being employed for cancer immunotherapy due to its direct antitumoral as well as indirect immunostimulatory capacity.

## 2.2 Various Bacterial Preparations for Cancer Therapy and Two Different System of Antitumor Activity

Role of bacterial infection involving immunotherapy of cancers has been investigated and reported. The most prominent agent is *Mycobacterium bovis* bacillus Calmette-Guérin (BCG). Molecular and cellular mechanisms of BCG involved in immunotherapy of cancers have been discovered in the past decades, and the details of the study will be precisely described in Chap. 4 of this book.

Although BCG has been widely used in experimental and clinical immunotherapy, in view of the problems associated with the use of a viable organism, more defined, nonliving mycobacterial products need to be examined. In this regard, various bacterial preparations have been examined for its efficacy as immunotherapeutic agents in experimental animals and in clinical studies (Table 2.1).

As listed on Table 2.1, infection of many types of bacteria, either in its crude form or with special preparation, has been reported to have immunotherapeutic activity against various cancers [35–69]. However, despite strenuous efforts of physicians and investigators, very few have actually been examined in clinical trials for humans [37, 38, 41, 44, 47, 50, 55, 56, 59, 62, 68, 69], and furthermore, most of those clinical studies so far could not have shown definitive effect of immunotherapy with bacterial preparation to date. In reality, therefore, the inherent inefficiency of the immune system has given rise to numerous and highly expensive cytotoxic cancer therapies over the past few decades with almost no real benefits translated to the patient such as a cure or decreasing the chances of patient dying from cancer [70].

The human immune system can be broadly divided into two parts, the innate and the adaptive. The evolutionarily older innate immune system reacts within minutes after the invading pathogens are encountered. The adaptive system, which employs evolutionarily younger and more customized tools, takes longer time from days to weeks to generate specialized antibodies and T cells to attack threats [71]. The innate system consists of natural anatomical barriers, such as skin and mucous membranes, and physiological barriers like elevation of temperature and acid in the stomach to digest harmful bacteria as well as the cells of first defense. Innate immunity is effective against a variety of infectious agents that have common features recognized by phagocytic cells but has no immunological memory against previous exposure and is antigen independent [72].

The innate system is composed mainly of natural killer (NK) cells, polymorphonucleocytes (PMN) and macrophages, and is most directly involved in tumor immunology. These cells also participate in the adaptive response and form an important and vital bridge between the two arms of the immune system [71]. It recognizes nonself molecules according to a specific pattern. Another feature of the innate immune system is the complement, a group of inactive proteins in the blood which are activated in the presence of pathogens and nonself cells and cause cell lysis [73]. Attenuated inactivated bacteria as nonspecific tumor immunotherapeutic agents have been investigated for centuries [74]. Among those, *Clostridium perfringens*, *Streptococcus pyogenes*, and *Mycobacterium bovis* (will be described

**Table 2.1** Bacterial preparations investigated for immunotherapy of cancers (excluding BCG)

| Bacteria | Target cancer | Model | References |
|---|---|---|---|
| *Corynebacterium parvum* | Mastocytoma | Mouse | [35] |
| | Melanoma | Mouse | [36] |
| | Lung cancer | Human | [37] |
| | AML | Human | [38] |
| *Nocardia rubra* | Fibrosarcoma | Rat | [39] |
| | Melanoma | Mouse | [40] |
| | Lung cancer | Human | [41] |
| *Serratia marcescens* | Fibrosarcoma | Mouse | [42] |
| | Sarcoma | Mouse | [43] |
| | Malignant astrocytoma | Human | [44] |
| *Lactobacillus casei* | Lung cancer | Mouse | [45] |
| | Fibrosarcoma | Mouse | [46] |
| | Cervical cancer | Human | [47] |
| *Staphylococcus aureus* | Breast cancer | Mouse | [48] |
| | Ehrlich ascites tumor | Mouse | [49] |
| | Malignant tumors | Human | [50] |
| *Listeria monocytogenes* | Breast cancer | Mouse | [51] |
| | Melanoma | Mouse | [52] |
| | Review | | [53] |
| *Mycobacterium smegmatis* | Bladder cancer | Mouse | [54] |
| | Melanoma | Human | [55] |
| | Lung cancer | Human | [56] |
| *Mycobacterium vaccae* | Non-small cell lung cancer | Human | [57] |
| | Melanoma | Human | [58] |
| | Renal cancer | Human | [59] |
| *Salmonella typhimurium* | Plasmacytoma | Mouse | [60] |
| | Review | | [61] |
| | Pancreatic cancer | Human | [62] |
| *Clostridium perfringens* | Sarcoma | Mouse | [63] |
| | Leukemia | Mouse | [64] |
| *Clostridium novyi* | Colon cancer | Mouse | [65] |
| | Colon cancer | Mouse | [66] |
| *Streptococcus pyogenes* | Leukemia | Mouse | [67] |
| | Sarcoma | Mouse | [68] |
| | Mammary cancer | Rat | [69] |
| | Lung cancer | Human | [70] |
| | Uterine cervical cancer | Human | [71] |

in Chap. 4) were considered to be the most active agents to induce tumor regressions for human tumors. Since we have already mentioned about the efficacy of Coley's vaccine in the previous paragraph, the other prominent nonspecific immunopotentiator OK-432, derived from *Streptococcus pyogenes*, will be introduced and discussed in the next paragraph [67–69].

The adaptive or acquired immunity is antigen specific, slower, and possesses immune memory against future attacks. The adaptive response follows the innate response and is dependent on specific recognition of antigen by antigen receptors present on the cell surface. The two types of adaptive immunity are cell-mediated immunity and humoral immunity. T lymphocytes are responsible for cell-mediated immunity and B lymphocytes for humoral immunity. B cells play a role in destroying tumor cells by complement-mediated lysis and facilitating antibody-dependent cell-mediated cytotoxicity [75]. The cytotoxic T cells (CTC) and the natural killer T (NKT) cells are two important T cells which are involved in lysis of tumor cells. The CTC kill and target cells with MHC–antigen complex on the cell wall, while the NKT cells actively search and kill tumor cells and play a crucial role in preventing metastasis of cancer. Affected cells which do not display MHC antigen complex are targeted by the NK cells [76, 77]. Linking the innate and adaptive immune systems are dendritic cells that hugely play an important role in restraining cancer. Dendritic cells migrate and are found patrolling below and within the epidermis and mucous membranes in the mouth, nose, ear, and colon. These cells produce antigens from ingested pathogens and cell debris, carry them to the lymph nodes, and display them on their surfaces to T cells. Thus, the T cells and B cells are stimulated to customize their immune attacks [73, 74] (Fig. 2.1). Briefly,

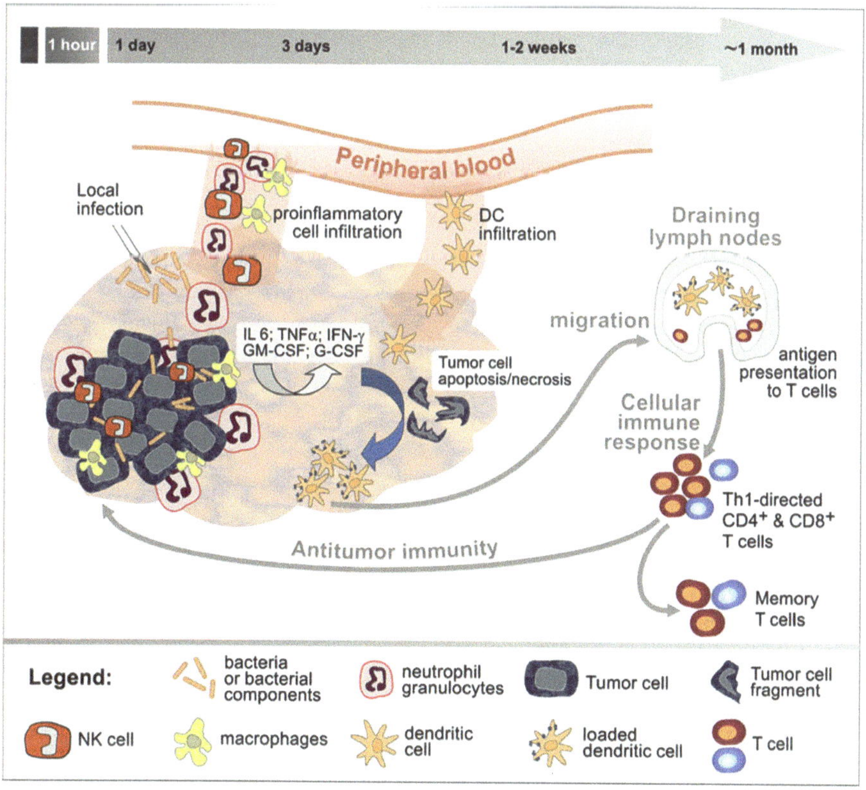


**Fig. 2.1** Schematic representation of bacterial immunotherapy's mode of action

intratumoral bacteria or bacterial components sensitized by the innate immune cells like NK cells, macrophages, and neutrophils, followed by secretion of proinflammatory cytokines and chemokines, attracting immature dendritic cells (DC) into the focus of infection. DCs take up bacterial material together with tumor fragments, mature while migrating to draining lymph nodes, where DCs present tumor antigens in addition to bacterial antigens to T cells. Those activated T cells infiltrate the tumor microenvironment and kill tumor cells, whereby the patient benefits from an active and powered immune response that fights the infection as well as the cancer. To be functionally active, DCs need certain danger signals to activate them, such as the pathogen-associated molecular patterns (PAMPs) that are present on bacteria and viruses but are absent on the cancer cells; that is clearly a situation of dual advantage [12]. Long-lasting antitumor immunity having the potential to control micro metastasis will be established when part of these T cells becomes memory cells.

## 2.3 OK-432, an Immunopotentiator Derived from *Streptococcus pyogenes*: Innate and Adaptive Function

OK-432, a preparation derived from *Streptococcus pyogenes* has been used for the treatment of curatively resected non-small cell cancers, and relatively favorable responses have been reported [68]. However, various clinical trials performed to assess the benefit of immunochemotherapy including OK-432 have not shown a significant benefit on survival of the cancer patients. Sakamoto et al. have collected results from randomized trial evaluating the superior effect of immunochemotherapy over chemotherapy alone. Meta-analysis to review all the relevant trials is considered to give rise to the best methods with a reasonable chance of detecting small, but humanly worthwhile, clinical benefits for lung cancer patients. In their meta-analysis, 1520 patients enrolled in 11 randomized clinical trials were examined comparing standard chemotherapy with the immunochemotherapy using the same chemotherapy regimen plus OK-432, the *Streptococcus pyogenes* preparation [78]. The 5-year survival rate was 51.2 % in the in the immunochemotherapy group versus 43.7 % in the chemotherapy-alone group. The odds ratio (OR) for 5-year overall survival was 0.70 (95 % CI = 0.56-0.87, $p = 0.001$) (Fig. 2.2).

In other meta-analysis, efficacy of OK-432 immunochemotherapy over chemotherapy-alone treatment was examined in 1522 patients enrolled in six clinical trials for curatively resected gastric cancer [79]. By this meta-analysis, the 3-year overall survival rate was 67.5 % in the immunochemotherapy group versus 62.6 % in the chemotherapy-alone group (OR; 0.81, 95 % CI; 0.65–0.99, $p = 0.044$) showing borderline effect of immunochemotherapy (Fig. 2.3).

Although the above mentioned two reports seem to have demonstrated the definite benefits of the addition of OK-432 for conventional chemotherapy, the possibility of bias due to several prognostic factors could not be excluded, since the

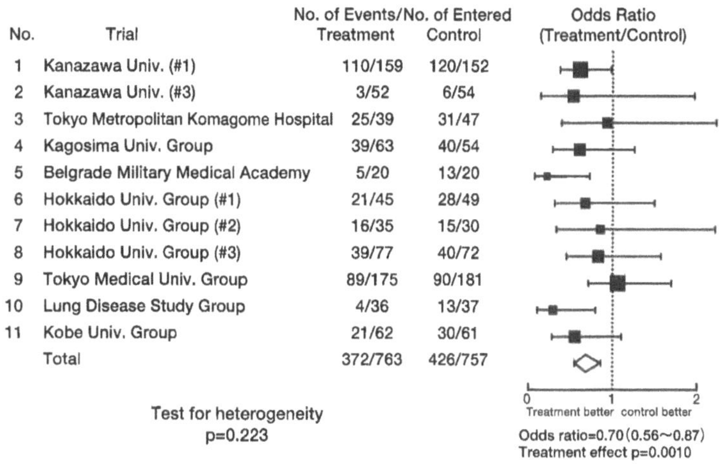


**Fig. 2.2** Survival odds ratios of non-small cell lung cancer patients in individual trials and overall. The overall test for treatment effect was significant ($p = 0.001$)

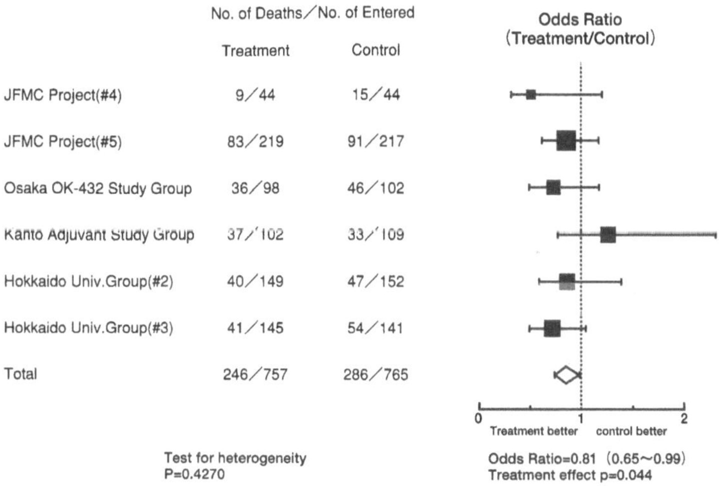


**Fig. 2.3** Survival odds ratios of curatively resected gastric cancer patients in individual trials and overall. The overall test for treatment effect showed borderline significant benefit of the addition of OK-432 ($p = 0.044$)

study was performed based on the tabulated data from a meta-analysis of the randomized trials.

In recent years, new aspects of OK-432 treatment have been investigated since the beginning of the twenty-first century, and multiple lines of evidence for the effects of OK-432 have been reported. With the increased attention on OK-432 therapy, a detailed reevaluation of the results of cancer therapy using OK-432 in previous clinical trials was determined to be important. In this regard, collection of the individual patients' data that were enrolled in eligible randomized trials and reexamination of the precise effects of immunotherapy using OK-432 in an adjuvant setting should be imperative. Since the current standard of treatment for patients with stage I or II gastric cancer after curative resection does not necessarily involve adjuvant chemotherapy, stage III or IV curatively resected gastric cancers have become the new target of the analysis. This reanalysis was important in order to clarify the immunological effects of OK-432, which has become widely utilized as a new immunotherapy and vaccine therapy for various cancers.

One thousand nine hundred and fifteen individual patients' data from 14 clinical trials were provided, and robust results showing a significant effect of OK-432 for locally advanced stage (III and IV) gastric cancers was confirmed and published [80].

Turning into the twenty-first century, more meticulous and diverse modes of action for OK-432 were investigated. Okamoto et al. precisely investigated the components of OK-432 and found that a lipoteichoic acid-related molecule is an active component of OK-432 stimulating TLR4/MD2 complex and Á-interferon production [81]. They have also reported that DC maturation and Th-1 cytokine stimulation by OK-432 are highly reliant on the expression of TLR4 and MD2 genes [82]. They have also shown the TLR4 expression-dependent anticancer immunity both in an OK-432-immunotherapy model using the TLR4- deficient mouse and in the OK-432 treatment of patients with head and neck cancer [83]. Taken together, these findings strongly suggest that the expression of TLR4, probably with MD2 on ascites cells could essentially be required for TNF induction in order to obtain positive clinical responses for locoregional immunotherapy with OK-432 to malignant ascites from gastric cancer.

Another aspect of antitumor effect of OK-432 has also been highlighted. Results from a trial in which the cancer vaccine NY-ESO-1 was mixed with OK-432 and Montanide® also suggested intervention in the immune tolerance system intercalated by PD-1 on CD4 lymphocytes [84]. Phase I clinical trials utilizing OK-432 plus HER2/neu and NY-ESO-1 have been started for the clinical implication against esophageal, lung, stomach, breast, and ovarian cancers [85].

## 2.4 Summary

Bacteria, either used as direct anticancer agent or as a vehicle for cytotoxic agents, mediate strong pro-inflammatory reactions that have beneficial effects for tumor therapy. In an acute phase, bacteria massively activate the immune system initiating an unspecific, often neutrophil-directed reaction that is followed by a Th1- or cytotoxic T cell-directed cellular response, eventually providing long-term protective immunity.

Bacteria and their components, mainly defined as TLR ligands or PAMPs, can be safely applied in humans with limited adverse side effects and are thus established in the clinic as immunestimulatory adjuvants. Combination therapies are also being investigated for potential future applications.

Those recent findings have been able to provide a ready basis for further expanding the concept of cancer immunotherapy for the clinical setting.

**Conflict of Interest** JS have been receiving honorarium from Takeda Pharmaceutical Inc. and from Merck Serono Co. Ltd.

**Acknowledgment** Collection of the materials and information for this review were supported, in part, by Epidemiological and Clinical Research Information Network (ECRIN).

## References

1. Everson TC (1967) Spontaneous regression of cancer. Prog Clin Cancer 3:79–95
2. Fauvet J, Campagne J, Chavy A, Piet G (1960) Cures, regressions and spontaneous remissions of cancer. Rev Prat 10:2349–2384
3. Hoption Cann SA, van Netten JP, van Netten C, Glover DW (2002) Spontaneous regression: a hidden treasure buried in time. Med Hypotheses 58:115–119
4. Rohdenburg GL (1918) Fluctuations in the growth energy of malignant tumors in man, with especial reference to spontaneous recession. J Cancer Res 3:193–225
5. Shiku H, Takahashi T, Resnick LA, Oettgen HF, Old LJ (1977) Cell surface antigens of human malignant melanoma. III. Recognition of autoantibodies with unusual characteristics. J Exp Med 145(3):784–789
6. Ueda R, Shiku H, Pfreundschuh M, Takahashi T, Li LT, Whitmore WF, Oettgen HF, Old LJ (1979) Cell surface antigens of human renal cancer defined by autologous typing. J Exp Med 150(3):564–579
7. Coley WB II (1891) Contribution to the knowledge of sarcoma. Ann Surg 14(3):199–220
8. Zacharski LR, Sukhatme VP (2005) Coley's toxin revisited: immunotherapy or plasminogen activator therapy of cancer? J Thromb Haemost 3(3):424–427
9. Wiemann B, Starnes CO (1994) Coley's toxins, tumor necrosis factor and cancer research: a historical perspective. Pharmacol Ther 64(3):529–564
10. Kumar H, Kawai T, Akira S (2009) Pathogen recognition in the innate immune response. Biochem J 420(1):1–16. doi:10.1042/BJ20090272
11. Rossol M, Heine H, Meusch U, Quandt D, Klein C, Sweet MJ, Hauschildt S (2011) LPS-induced cytokine production in human monocytes and macrophages. Crit Rev Immunol 31(5):379–446
12. Hobohm U, Stanford JL, Grange JM (2008) Pathogen-associated molecular pattern in cancer immunotherapy. Crit Rev Immunol 28(2):95–107
13. Skitzki JJ, Repasky EA, Evans SS (2009) Hyperthermia as an immunotherapy strategy for cancer. Curr Opin Investig Drugs 10(6):550–558
14. Oblak A, Jerala R (2011) Toll-like receptor 4 activation in cancer progression and therapy. Clin Dev Immunol 2011:609579. doi:10.1155/2011/609579, Epub 2011 Nov 3
15. Hobohm U (2001) Fever and cancer in perspective. Cancer Immunol Immunother 50(8): 391–396
16. Nauts HC, McLaren JR (1990) Coley toxins – the first century. Adv Exp Med Biol 267: 483–500
17. Belardelli F, Ferrantini M, Proietti E, Kirkwood JM (2002) Interferon-alpha in tumor immunity and immunotherapy. Cytokine Growth Factor Rev 13(2):119–134

18. Petrella T, Quirt I, Verma S, Haynes AE, Charette M, Bak K, Members of the Melanoma Disease Site Group of Cancer Care Ontario's Program in Evidence-Based Care (2007) Single-agent interleukin-2 in the treatment of metastatic melanoma. Curr Oncol 14(1):21–26
19. Perabo FG, Müller SC (2004) Current and new strategies in immunotherapy for superficial bladder cancer. Urology 64(3):409–421
20. Maletzki C, Klier U, Obst W, Kreikemeyer B, Linnebacher M (2012) Reevaluating the concept of treating experimental tumors with a mixed bacterial vaccine: Coley's toxin. Clin Dev Immunol 2012:230625. doi:10.1155/2012/230625, Epub 2012 Nov 11
21. Klier U, Maletzki C, Göttmann N, Kreikemeyer B, Linnebacher M (2011) Avitalized bacteria mediate tumor growth control via activation of innate immunity. Cell Immunol 269(2): 120–127. doi:10.1016/j.cellimm.2011.03.014, Epub 2011 Mar 17
22. Hobohm U (2005) Fever therapy revisited. Br J Cancer 92(3):421–425
23. Klenk M, Nakata M, Podbielski A, Skupin B, Schroten H, Kreikemeyer B (2007) Streptococcus pyogenes serotype-dependent and independent changes in infected HEp-2 epithelial cells. ISME J 1(8):678–692, Epub 2007 Oct 18
24. Tsung K, Norton JA (2006) Lessons from Coley's toxin. Surg Oncol 15(1):25–28, Epub 2006 Jun 30
25. Friedman H, Blanchard DK, Newton C, Klein T, Stewart W II, Keler T, Nowotny A (1987) Distinctive immunomodulatory effects of endotoxin and nontoxic lipopolysaccharide derivatives in lymphoid cell cultures. J Biol Response Modif 6(6):664–677
26. Park JM, Fisher DE (2010) Testimony from the bedside: from Coley's toxins to targeted immunotherapy. Cancer Cell 18(1):9–10. doi:10.1016/j.ccr.2010.06.010
27. Thomas JA, Badini M (2011) The role of innate immunity in spontaneous regression of cancer. Indian J Cancer 48(2):246–251. doi:10.4103/0019-509X.82887
28. Mason KA, Hunter NR (2012) CpG plus radiotherapy: a review of preclinical works leading to clinical trial. Front Oncol 2:101. doi:10.3389/fonc.2012.00101. eCollection 2012
29. Ursu R, Carpentier AF (2012) Immunotherapeutic approach with oligodeoxynucleotides containing CpG motifs (CpG-ODN) in malignant glioma. Adv Exp Med Biol 746:95–108, Review
30. Zent CS, Smith BJ, Ballas ZK, Wooldridge JE, Link BK, Call TG, Shanafelt TD, Bowen DA, Kay NE, Witzig TE, Weiner GJ (2012) Phase I clinical trial of CpG oligonucleotide 7909 (PF-03512676) in patients with previously treated chronic lymphocytic leukemia. Leuk Lymphoma 53(2):211–217. doi:10.3109/10428194.2011.608451, Epub 2011 Sep 19
31. Xu D, Liu H, Komai-Koma (2004) Direct and indirect role of Toll-like receptors in T cell mediated immunity. Cell Mol Immunol 1(4):239–246
32. Brown J, Wang H, Hajishengallis GN, Martin M (2011) TLR-signaling networks: an integration of adaptor molecules, kinases, and cross-talk. J Dent Res 90(4):417–427. doi:10.1177/0022034510381264, Epub 2010 Oct 12
33. Itoh T, Satoh H, Isono N, Rikiishi H, Kumagai K (1992) Mechanism of stimulation of T cells by Streptococcus pyogenes: isolation of a major mitogenic factor, cytoplasmic membrane-associated protein. Infect Immun 60(8):3128–3135
34. Decker WK, Safdar A (2009) Bioimmunoadjuvants for the treatment of neoplastic and infectious disease: Coley's legacy revisited. Cytokine Growth Factor Rev 20(4):271–281. doi:10.1016/j.cytogfr.2009.07.004, Epub 2009 Aug 4
35. Millman I, Scott AW, Halbherr T (1977) Antitumor activity of Propionibacterium acnes (Corynebacterium parvum) and isolated cytoplasmic fractions1. Cancer Res 37:4150–4155
36. Bowlin TL, Rosenberger AL, Sunkara PS (1985) The effect of combination treatment with alpha-difluoromethylornithine and Corynebacterium parvum on B16 melanoma growth and tumoricidal effector cell generation in vivo. Cancer Immunol Immunother 20(3):214–218
37. Woodruff M, Walbaum P (1983) A phase-II trial of Corynebacterium parvum as adjuvant to surgery in the treatment of operable lung cancer. Cancer Immunol Immunother 16(2):114–116
38. Ohno R, Nakamura H, Kodera Y, Ezaki K, Yokomaku S, Oguma S, Kubota Y, Shibata H, Ogawa N, Masaoka T (1986) Randomized controlled study of chemoimmunotherapy of

acute myelogenous leukemia (AML) in adults with Nocardia rubra cell-wall skeleton and irradiated allogeneic AML cells. Cancer 57(8):1483–1488
39. Ogura T, Namba N, Hirao F, Yamamura Y, Azuma I (1979) Association of macrophage activation with antitumor effect on rat syngeneic fibrosarcoma by Nocardia rubra cell wall skeleton. Cancer Res 39(11):4706–4712
40. Saijo N, Ozaki A, Beppu Y, Irimajiri N, Shibuya M, Shimizu E, Takizawa T, Taniguchi T, Hoshi A (1983) In vivo and in vitro effects of Nocardia rubra cell wall skeleton on natural killer activity in mice. Gann 74(1):137–142
41. Yamamura Y, Ogura T, Sakatani M, Hirao F, Kishimoto S, Fukuoka M, Takada M, Kawahara M, Furuse K, Kuwahara O (1983) Randomized controlled study of adjuvant immunotherapy with Nocardia rubra cell wall skeleton for inoperable lung cancer. Cancer Res 43(11): 5575–5579
42. Urban RW, Edwards BS, Segal W (1980) Tumor-immunotherapeutic efficacy of Serratia marcescens polyribosomes. Cancer Res 40(5):1501–1505
43. Ikekawa T, Ikeda Y, Fukuoka F (1975) Antitumor activity of polysaccharides from Serratia marcescens. Gann 66(3):317–318
44. Cress NB, Owens BM, Hill FH (1991) ImuVert therapy in the treatment of recurrent malignant astrocytomas: nursing implications. J Neurosci Nurs 23(1):29–33
45. Matsuzaki T, Yokokura T, Azuma I (1987) Antimetastatic effect of Lactobacillus casei YIT9018 (LC 9018) on a highly metastatic variant of B16 melanoma in C57BL/6J mice. Cancer Immunol Immunother 24(2):99–105
46. Yasutake N, Kato I, Ohwaki M, Yokokura T, Mutai M (1984) Host-mediated antitumor activity of Lactobacillus casei in mice. Gann 75(1):72–80
47. Okawa T1, Niibe H, Arai T, Sekiba K, Noda K, Takeuchi S, Hashimoto S, Ogawa N (1993) Effect of LC9018 combined with radiation therapy on carcinoma of the uterine cervix. A phase III, multicenter, randomized, controlled study. Cancer 72(6):1949–1954
48. Pulaski BA, Terman DS, Khan S, Muller E, Ostrand-Rosenberg S (2000) Cooperativity of Staphylococcal aureus enterotoxin B superantigen, major histocompatibility complex class II, and CD80 for immunotherapy of advanced spontaneous metastases in a clinically relevant postoperative mouse breast cancer model. Cancer Res 60(10):2710–2715
49. Mondal TK, Bhatta D, Biswas S, Pal P (2002) Repeated treatment with S. aureus superantigens expands the survival rate of Ehrlich ascites tumor bearing mice. Immunol Invest 31(1):13–28
50. Messerschmidt GL, Bowles CA, Henry DH, Deisseroth AB (1984) Clinical trials with Staphylococcus aureus and protein A in the treatment of malignant disease. J Biol Response Modif 3(3): 325–329
51. Kim SH, Castro F, Paterson Y, Gravekamp C (2009) High efficacy of a Listeria-based vaccine against metastatic breast cancer reveals a dual mode of action. Cancer Res 69(14):5860–5866. doi:10.1158/0008-5472.CAN-08-4855, Epub 2009 Jul 7
52. Wood LM, Guirnalda PD, Seavey MM, Paterson Y (2008) Cancer immunotherapy using Listeria monocytogenes and listerial virulence factors. Immunol Res 42(1–3):233–245. doi:10.1007/s12026-008-8087-0
53. Wood LM, Paterson Y (2014) Attenuated Listeria monocytogenes: a powerful and versatile vector for the future of tumor immunotherapy. Front Cell Infect Microbiol 4:51. doi:10.3389/fcimb.2014.00051
54. Young SL, Murphy M, Zhu XW, Harnden P, O'Donnell MA, James K, Patel PM, Selby PJ, Jackson AM (2004) Cytokine-modified Mycobacterium smegmatis as a novel anticancer immunotherapy. Int J Cancer 112(4):653–660
55. Vosika GJ, Schmidtke JR, Goldman A, Ribi E, Parker R, Gray GR (1979) Intralesional immunotherapy of malignant melanoma with mycobacterium smegmatis cell wall skeleton combined with trehalose dimycolate (P3). Cancer 44(2):495–503
56. Decroix G, Chastang C, Fichet D, Asselain B, Lebeau B, Morice V, Lepage T, Babo P, Fabre C, Rebischung JL (1984) Adjuvant immunotherapy with nonviable Mycobacterium

smegmatis in resected primary lung carcinoma. A randomized clinical trial of 219 patients. Cancer 53(4):906–912
57. O'Brien ME, Saini A, Smith IE, Webb A, Gregory K, Mendes R, Ryan C, Priest K, Bromelow KV, Palmer RD, Tuckwell N, Kennard DA, Souberbielle BE (2000) A randomized phase II study of SRL172 (Mycobacterium vaccae) combined with chemotherapy in patients with advanced inoperable non-small-cell lung cancer and mesothelioma. Br J Cancer 83(7): 853–857
58. Nicholson S, Guile K, John J, Clarke IA, Diffley J, Donnellan P, Michael A, Szlosarek P, Dalgleish AG (2003) A randomized phase II trial of SRL172 (Mycobacterium vaccae) +/− low-dose interleukin-2 in the treatment of metastatic malignant melanoma. Melanoma Res 13(4):389–393
59. Patel PM, Sim S, O'Donnell DO, Protheroe A, Beirne D, Stanley A, Tourani JM, Khayat D, Hancock B, Vasey P, Dalgleish A, Johnston C, Banks RE, Selby PJ (2008) An evaluation of a preparation of Mycobacterium vaccae (SRL172) as an immunotherapeutic agent in renal cancer. Eur J Cancer 44(2):216–223. doi:10.1016/j.ejca.2007.11.003
60. Eisenstein TK, Bushnell B, Meissler JJ Jr, Dalal N, Schafer R, Havas HF (1995) Immunotherapy of a plasmacytoma with attenuated salmonella. Med Oncol 12(2):103–108
61. Chorobik P, Marcinkiewicz J (2011) Therapeutic vaccines based on genetically modified Salmonella: a novel strategy in cancer immunotherapy. Pol Arch Med Wewn 121(12): 461–466, Review
62. Niethammer AG, Lubenau H, Mikus G, Knebel P, Hohmann N, Leowardi C, Beckhove P, Akhisaroglu M, Ge Y, Springer M, Grenacher L, Buchler MW, Koch M, Weitz J, Haefeli WE, Schmitz-Winnenthal FH (2012) Double-blind, placebo-controlled first in human study to investigate an oral vaccine aimed to elicit an immune reaction against the VEGF-Receptor 2 in patients with stage IV and locally advanced pancreatic cancer. BMC Cancer 12:361. doi:10.1186/1471-2407 -12-361
63. Sasaki T, Chihara G, Takasuka N, Suzuki S (1976) Effect of Clostridium toxoids, especially of Clostridium perfringens toxoid, on mouse transplanted tumors. Gann 67(2):275–277
64. Sethi KK, Brandis H (1973) Neuraminidase induced loss in the transplantability of murine leukaemia L 1210, induction of immunoprotection and the transfer of induced immunity to normal DBA-2 mice by serum and peritoneal cells. Br J Cancer 27(2):106–113
65. Dang LH, Bettegowda C, Huso DL, Kinzler KW, Vogelstein B (2001) Combination bacteriolytic therapy for the treatment of experimental tumors. Proc Natl Acad Sci U S A 98: 15155–15160
66. Agrawal N, Bettegowda C, Cheong I, Geschwind JF, Drake CG, Hipkiss EL, Tatsumi M, Dang LH, Diaz LA, Pomper M, Abusedera M, Wahl RL, Kinzler KW, Zhou S, Huso DL, Vogelstein B (2004) Bacteriolytic therapy can generate a potent immune response against experimental tumors. Proc Natl Acad Sci U S A 101:15172–15177
67. Aoki T, Kvedar JP, Hollis VW Jr, Bushar GS (1976) Streptococcus pyogenes preparation OK-432: immunoprophylactic and immunotherapeutic effects on the incidence of spontaneous leukemia in AKR mice. J Natl Cancer Inst 56(3):687–690
68. Higuchi Y (1986) Cytotoxic and antitumor activity of a soluble fraction of Streptococcus pyogenes against S180 sarcoma cells. Jpn J Med Sci Biol 39(4):169–175
69. Fukui H, Reynolds CW (1987) Antitumor activity of a Streptococcus pyogenes preparation (OK-432). I. Sequential effector mechanisms following a single OK-432 injection in F344 rats leading to the rejection of syngeneic MADB106 tumor cells. J Natl Cancer Inst 79(5): 1011–1017
70. Lee YC, Luh SP, Wu RM, Lee CJ (1994) Adjuvant immunotherapy with intrapleural Streptococcus pyogenes (OK-432) in lung cancer patients after resection. Cancer Immunol Immunother 39(4):269–274
71. Cervical Cancer Immunotherapy Study Group (1987) Immunotherapy using the streptococcal preparation OK-432 for the treatment of uterine cervical cancer. Cancer 60(10):2394–2402

72. MacAdam DH, Coley (eds) (2003) Spontaneous regression: cancer and the immune system, 1st edn. Xilibris, Philadelphia, pp 5–10
73. Hobohm U (2009) Healing heat: harnessing infection to fight cancer. Am Sci 97:34
74. Linnebacher, Maletzki C, Klier U, Klar E (2012) Bacterial immunotherapy of gastrointestinal tumors. Langenbeck's Arch Surg 397(4):557–568
75. Vivier E, Tomasello E, Baratin M, Walzer T, Ugolini S (2008) Functions of natural killer cells. Nat Immunol 9:503–510
76. Medzhitov R, Janeway CA Jr (1998) Innate immune recognition and control of adaptive immune responses. Semin Immunol 10:351–353
77. Hayakawa Y, Smyth MJ (2006) Innate immune recognition and suppression of tumors. Adv Cancer Res 95:293–322
78. Sakamoto J, Teramukai S, Watanabe Y, Hayata Y, Okayasu T, Nakazato H, Ohashi Y, Japanese Meta-Analysis Group in Cancer, Japanese Society of Strategies for Cancer Research and Therapy (2001) Meta-analysis of adjuvant immuno -chemotherapy using OK-432 in patients with resected non-small-cell lung cancer. J Immunother 24(3):250–256
79. Sakamoto J, Teramukai S, Nakazato H, Sato Y, Uchino J, Taguchi T, Ryoma Y, Ohashi Y (2002) Efficacy of adjuvant immunochemotherapy with OK-432 for patients with curatively resected gastric cancer: a meta-analysis of centrally randomized controlled clinical trials. J Immunother 25(5):405–412
80. Oba MS, Teramukai S, Ohashi Y, Ogawa K, Maehara Y, Sakamoto J (2015) The efficacy of adjuvant immunochemotherapy with OK-432 after curative resection of gastric cancer: an individual patient data meta-analysis of randomized controlled trials. Gastric Cancer [Epub ahead of print]
81. Okamoto M, Ohe G, Furuichi S, Nishikawa H, Oshikawa T, Tano T, Ahmed SU, Yoshida H, Moriya Y, Matsubara S, Ryoma Y, Saito M, Sato M (2002) Enhancement of anti-tumor immunity by lipoteichoic acid-related molecule isolated from OK-432, a streptococcal agent, in athymic nude mice bearing human salivary adenocarcinoma: role of natural killer cells. Anticancer Res 22:3229–3239
82. Okamoto M, Furuichi S, Nishioka Y, Oshikawa T, Tano T, Ahmed SU, Takeda K, Akira S, Ryoma Y, Moriya Y, Saito M, Sone S, Sato M (2004) Expression of toll-like receptor 4 on dendritic cells is significant for anticancer effect of dendritic cell-based immunotherapy in combination with an active component of OK-432, a streptococcal preparation. Cancer Res 64: 5461–5470
83. Okamoto M, Oshikawa T, Tano T, Ohe G, Furuichi S, Nishikawa H, Ahmed SU, Akashi S, Miyake K, Takeuchi O, Akira S, Moriya Y, Matsubara S, Ryoma Y, Saito M, Sato M (2003) Involvement of Toll-like receptor 4 signaling in interferon-gamma production and antitumor effect by streptococcal agent OK-432. J Natl Cancer Inst 95:316–326
84. Wada H, Isobe M, Kakimi K, Mizote Y, Eikawa S, Sato E et al (2014) Vaccination with NY-ESO-1 overlapping peptides mixed with Picibanil OK-432 and montanide ISA-51 in patients with cancers expressing the NY-ESO-1 antigen. J Immunother 37:84–92
85. www.cancer.gov/clinicaltrials

# Chapter 3
# Polysaccharides

**Yasuyuki Sugiyama**

**Abstract** Three kinds of polysaccharides, namely, polysaccharide kureha (PSK), lentinan (LNT), and schizophyllan (SPG), have been approved as anticancer drugs against several kinds of cancer in Japan. All of them are derived from mushrooms, and about 25 years has passed since their clinical approval. Since their mechanisms of action have become elucidated basically and clinically by many investigators, they are discussed here from an immunological point of view. Generally speaking, the immunological mechanisms of polysaccharides are as follows: (1) augmentation of the effect of either chemotherapy or radiotherapy, (2) direct actions on tumor cells, (3) modulation of both innate and acquired immune system, and (4) recovery from immune escape state in tumor-bearing hosts.

Even though polysaccharides might play an important role in immunomodulation under innate or acquired immune system of tumor-bearing host, the understanding of clinical oncologists in regard to polysaccharides is considerably poor. Alternatively the advances in molecular biology and tumor immunology have made a progress in immunotherapy against malignancy, especially in the field of immunological targeting therapy by use of monoclonal antibodies related to immune checkpoint pathway. It is no exaggeration to say that now is the chance for improving both specific and nonspecific immunotherapy against malignancies.

**Keywords** Biological response modifiers • Polysaccharides • Polysaccharide kureha • Lentinan • Schizophyllan

## 3.1 Introduction

In spite of considerable improvement in survival rates, prognosis of either advanced stage cancer or recurrent malignancies remains still poor. For the purpose of eradication, surgical resection, chemotherapy, and radiotherapy are main strategies against malignancy of relatively early stages, while they might be powerless against advanced systemic cancers. On the other hand, substantial number of oncologists, indeed, believes that so-called old immunotherapy might be one of unconventional

Y. Sugiyama, M.D., Ph.D. (✉)
Department of Surgery, Gifu Municipal Hospital, 7-1 Kashimacho, Gifu 500-8513, Japan
e-mail: ysugi@gmhosp.gifu.gifu.jp



Y. Yamaguchi (ed.), *Immunotherapy of Cancer*,
DOI 10.1007/978-4-431-55031-0_3

**Table 3.1** List of polysaccharides approved for cancer treatment in Japan

| Name | Raw material | Indications | Dosage | Administration | Others |
|---|---|---|---|---|---|
| PSK | Coliorus versicolor | Gastric ca. | 3.0 g/day | Oral | After curative resection |
| | | Colorectal ca. | 3 times | | In combination with chemotherapy |
| | | Small-cell lung ca. | | | In combination with chemotherapy |
| LNT | Lentinus edodes | Gastric ca. | 1 mg/body × 2/W or 2 mg/body/W | Intravenous | In combination with chemotherapy (tegafur:600 mg (400 mg/m$^2$)/day |
| SPG | Schizophyllum commune | Uterine cervical ca. | 20 mg/body × 2/W or 40 mg/body/W | Intramuscular | In combination with radiotherapy (Discontinuance of production at the end of March, 2011) |

anticancer therapies, and especially the nonspecific immunotherapy by use of polysaccharides, which belong to one category of biological response modifiers (BRMs), has been sometimes described as complementary and alternative medicine because of inappropriate early-phase trial development [1]. Recently, however, the mechanisms of action of polysaccharides have become elucidated basically and clinically by many investigators. Consequently immunotherapy by use of polysaccharides should be still thought one of the feasible strategies against malignancy.

Three kinds of polysaccharides, namely, polysaccharide kureha (PSK), lentinan (LNT), and schizophyllan (SPG), have been approved as anticancer drugs against several kinds of cancer in Japan (Table 3.1). All of them are derived from mushrooms, and about 25 years has passed since their clinical approval.

In this chapter, such polysaccharides are focused basically and clinically from an immunological point of view. Although it has been reported that antitumor activity of polysaccharides differs depending on the solubility in water, molecular weight, branching ratio, chemical structure, and chain combination, the details of structure-activity relationship should be discussed elsewhere [2].

## 3.2 Polysaccharide Kureha (PSK)

PSK is an extract from the fungus Colorius versicolor, and the molecular weight is approximately 100 kDa including 28–38 % of protein. Clinical use of PSK was approved in Japan on May, 1977, and reevaluation was done on December, 1989. Thereafter PSK has been used against either gastric cancer or colorectal cancer as postoperative adjuvant immunotherapy in combination with chemotherapy. It has also been used against small-cell lung cancer in combination with chemotherapy.

### 3.2.1 Basic Experiment and Translational Research

PSK showed various effects on immune cells and their cytokine production. When the lymphocytes derived from gastric cancer patients were cultured with PSK in vitro, the cytotoxicity against K562 and KATO-3 (human gastric cancer cell line) was augmented [3]. Culturing either peripheral blood mononuclear cells (PBMC) or tumor-infiltrating lymphocytes (TIL) with PSK in vitro induced autologous killing activity in human cancer patients [4]. In the induction of killer cells by interleukin-2 (IL-2), which is called lymphokine-activated killer cells (LAK), PSK enhanced the proliferation of LAK and their cytotoxic activity and inhibited the action of TGF-beta on LAK by blocking its receptors [5]. PSK was useful for maturation of dendritic cells derived from human PBMC [6], whereas it overcame defective maturation of dendritic cells exposed to tumor-derived factors in in vitro experiment of human gastric cancer model [7]. In murine experiment, it was demonstrated that PSK could augment IL-2 production from CD4+ T cell by modulating T cell receptor signaling [8]. Also PSK induced gene expression and production of immunomodulating cytokines in human peripheral blood lymphocytes (PBL) [9]. In addition, PSK was able to correct the Th1/Th2 imbalance shifted to Th1 dominant, followed by augmentation of antitumor immunity [10, 11]. Alternatively the fact that PSK directly enhanced immunoglobulin production in the human B cell line BALL-1 indicated that PSK might play some roles in humoral immunity [12].

In terms of antimetastatic effects of PSK, Kobayashi et al. overviewed precisely [13] the PSK-suppressed metastasis induced by hepatic ischemia and reperfusion injury in rat colon cancer model, in which the suppression of angiogenesis by PSK was thought to be one of the mechanisms of the inhibition of hepatic metastasis [14]. Indeed it was previously reported that inhibition of angiogenesis by direct binding of PSK with basic fibroblast growth factor (bFGF) could result in suppression of bFGF-induced proliferation of endothelial cells [15].

Since surgical stress should reduce the antitumor mechanisms to a certain extent, PSK could recover the immunosuppression [16]. When PSK was administered postoperatively to the patients with curatively resected stage III gastric cancer in combination with chemotherapeutic agent tegafur-gimeracil-oteracil potassium (TS-1), PSK partially prevented apoptosis of circulating T cells induced by TS-1 [17]. PSK might improve overall survival of the patients with stage III gastric cancer by decreasing the proportion of CD57+ suppressor T cells in their peripheral blood [18]. Administration of PSK in combination with chemotherapeutic agents (low-dose cisplatin and tegafur/uracil (UFT)) to the patients with advanced colorectal cancer for 2 months reduced the serum concentration of soluble receptors for interleukin-2 (sIL-2R) and the production of IL-10 by phytohemagglutinin (PHA)-stimulated PBMC [19].

As for direct action of PSK on tumor cells, PSK could induce apoptosis of tumor cells [16], but the mechanism seems different depending on the type of tumor [20]. In addition, PSK could augment the expression of HLA on human colon cancer cell line [21]. Furthermore PSK induced the alteration of gene expression in the experiment, in which the human colorectal cancer cell line was treated in vitro by PSK [22]. PSK inhibited the nuclear factor-kappa B activation by docetaxel when either human pancreatic cancer cell line or human gastric cancer cell line was treated with those two agents at the same time [23, 24].

### 3.2.2 Clinical Data

Nakazato et al. [25] assessed the efficacy of PSK in addition to standard chemotherapy (intravenous mitomycin C (MMC) plus oral fluorouracil) in 1980s. A total of 262 patients, who had undergone curative gastrectomy in Japan, were randomly assigned standard treatment alone or with PSK and were followed up for at least 5 years. PSK significantly improved the 5-year survival (73.0 % vs 60.0 %, $p = 0.044$) and 5-year disease-free rate (70.7 % vs 59.4 %, $p = 0.047$). In this randomized controlled trial (RCT), toxic effects were slight, and there were no significant differences between the treatment groups. In order to clarify the survival benefits of immunochemotherapy for patients with curative resections of gastric cancers, a meta-analysis to evaluate the effect of immunochemotherapy on survival in those patients was performed [26]. In this study 8,009 patients from eight RCTs after central randomization were included, and the results of chemotherapy and immunochemotherapy using PSK were compared. The result was that adjuvant immunochemotherapy with PSK improved the survival of patients after curative resection.

In regard to colorectal cancer, three RCTs were performed in Japan. Mitomi et al. reported the result of RCT on adjuvant immunochemotherapy with PSK in the patients who undergone macroscopic curative resection against stage III and stage IV colorectal cancer [27]. A total of 448 patients were randomly assigned either chemotherapy plus PSK or chemotherapy alone and were followed up for 5 years. PSK significantly improved the 5-year survival (78.5 % vs 69.7 %, $p = 0.0325$) and 5-year disease-free rate (72.3 % vs 63.2 %, $p = 0.0302$). Ito et al. reported the result of RCT on adjuvant immunochemotherapy with PSK in the patients who undergone curative resection against macroscopic Dukes' C colon cancer [28]. A total of 446 patients were randomly divided into two groups, the one was the group of alternating administration of 5-fluorouracil or PSK and the other was 5-fluorouracil alone, and were followed up for 7 years. PSK significantly improved the 7-year cancer death-free survival rate (83.4 % vs 78.5 %, $p = 0.019$). In addition, Ohwada et al. reported the result of RCT on adjuvant immunochemotherapy with PSK in the patients who undergone curative resection against stage II or III colorectal cancer [29]. A total of 205 patients were randomly assigned either UFT plus PSK or UFT alone and were followed up for 5 years. PSK significantly improved the 5-year disease-free survival rate (73.0 % vs 58.8 %, $p = 0.016$). For the purpose of evaluating the effect of immunochemotherapy by use of PSK on survival in the patients with curatively resected colorectal cancer, a meta-analysis was performed

[30]. In this study 1,094 patients from three RCTs after center randomization were included, and the survival of chemotherapy and that of immunochemotherapy using PSK was compared. The result was that adjuvant immunochemotherapy could improve both survival and disease-free survival of patients with curatively resected colorectal cancer.

As for lung cancer, Konno et al. reported the result of RCT on chemotherapy with vincristine, cyclophosphamide, and MMC in combination with PSK in patients with small-cell carcinoma [31]. A total of 93 patients were randomly assigned either chemotherapy plus PSK or chemotherapy alone. PSK significantly prolonged the median response duration (25 weeks vs 13 weeks, $p = 0.042$).

## 3.3 Lentinan (LNT)

LNT is isolated and purified from Lentinus edodes (the fruit body of shiitake mushroom) and a high molecular weight polysaccharide (400–800 Kda) containing a strictly purified beta-1,6: beta-1,3-glucan, the active component of which is beta-1,3-glucan. Clinical use of LNT was initially approved on November 1985 in Japan, and reappraisal was performed in 1994. LNT has been used against either unresectable or recurrent gastric cancer in combination with chemotherapeutic agent tegafur.

### *3.3.1 Basic Experiment and Translational Research*

While LNT by itself has no direct cytocidal effect on tumor cells, it induced apoptosis of human gastric cancer cell line in vitro [32].

Antitumor effect of LNT was reported in 1969 for the first time [33]. Thereafter many investigators demonstrated the inhibitory effects of LNT alone on tumor growth in animal experiments and in vitro studies. LNT inhibited the growth of sarcoma 180 implanted subcutaneously in mice without any sign of toxicity [34]. In murine syngeneic and autochthonous hosts, LNT showed both antitumor activity and suppressive effect on 3-methylcholanthrene-induced carcinogenesis [35]. LNT also inhibited significantly the growth of peritoneal carcinomatoses in a model of colon cancer in rat [36]. Likewise multiple pathways had been described for the effects observed in the immune system, including upregulation of T cell, increased production of various kinds of bioactive serum factors associated with immunity, and so on [37].

On the one hand, LNT activated the alternative pathway of complement system, in which C3b should be the essential component, and induced cytotoxic peritoneal exudate cells in vivo [38]. In in vitro and in vivo analysis of human leukocytes, LNT showed activation of complement 3b, followed by formation of lentinan-C3b complex, thereafter the complex bound to monocyte. This binding of LNT to human monocytes could initiate the influence of LNT on the immune system and might differ between individuals [39]. Also LNT showed the augmentation of antibody-dependent cell-mediated cytotoxicity (ADCC) [40].

The combination of LNT and IL-2 were more effective than either one alone for treatment of spontaneous pulmonary metastases in C57BL/6N mice model [41]. In addition synergistic antimetastatic effects of LNT and IL-2 with pre- and postoperative treatments were demonstrated in mice model [42]. Interestingly, combined administration of LNT and IL-2 was found to augment the endogenous LAK activity in tumor-bearing mice, whereas addition of LNT during culture in vitro did not augment LAK activity induced by IL-2 [43]. Experimentally LNT has proved prolongation of survival when it was administered in combination with TS-1, in which dendritic cells were thought to be one of key factors for eliciting antitumor effect by chemoimmunotherapy in vivo [44]. On the other hand Hamuro et al. reported the dual effects in the induction of resistance to immunochemotherapy by use of lentinan [45].

When human PBMC were cultured in vitro with LNT, natural killer cells were activated, whereas the generation of cytotoxic macrophages was noted by cultivation of macrophages separated from the spleens of gastric cancer patients [46]. Clinically single intravenous administration of LNT in dose of 2 mg to the patients with gastric cancer significantly augmented the LAK activity induced by in vitro activation of PBMC with IL-2 [47]. Moreover, when PBMC of either nine healthy volunteers or seven cancer patients were cultured with IL-2 and LNT, the expression of CD25 antigen, the alpha chain of the IL-2 receptor on the activated killer cells, was increased by LNT, followed by augmentation of killer activity against both autologous tumor and K562 cells [48]. Alternatively, LNT regulated the production of cytokine by PBMC derived from gastric cancer patients, such as tumor necrosis factor (TNF)-alpha, IL-1-alpha, and IL-1-beta [49].

In terms of macrophage, the oxidative macrophage could be dominant in cancer microenvironment, and these macrophages induced the production of cytokines, such as TNF-alpha, IL-6, and IL-10, which brought about the increase of malignant potential of tumor cells. Both oxidative type macrophages and tumor cells produced prostaglandin E2 and inflammatory cytokines and caused immunosuppressive state in host. LNT bound to macrophage and converted the redox status of macrophages, indexed by intracellular content of glutathione. Actually LNT induced reductive macrophages, which increased the production of IL-12 and nitrogen oxide (NO) resulting in skewing the Th1/Th2 imbalance to Th1 predominant state [50]. In digestive cancer patients, it is noted that LNT regulated the Th1/Th2 balance [51].

### *3.3.2 Clinical Data*

Phase I trial of LNT was conducted in Japan in 1979, and thereafter Phase II and Phase III trials were performed. In terms of Phase III trial against unresectable gastric cancer, it was first RCT in Japan, the primary end point of which was overall survival (OS). The result was reported that OS of immunochemotherapy group with chemotherapy (FT plus MMC) in combination with LNT was significantly better than the group with that of chemotherapy alone [52]. Thereafter individual patient data (IPD) meta-analysis of LNT for advanced gastric cancer was performed [53]. In this study, a total of 650 IPD from five trials were available, and it was shown that LNT prolonged significantly the overall survival ($p = 0.011$). The result was that the addition of LNT to standard chemotherapy offered a significant advantage over chemotherapy alone as to survival for patients with advanced gastric cancer.

It is noteworthy that LNT showed significant improvement of the general condition, symptoms and signs, and QOL when it was used in combination with chemotherapeutic agents in esophageal cancer patients [54]. On the one hand, TS-1 is recently the key drug in the chemotherapy against advanced gastric cancer, but there had been no RCT as to the combination of TS-1 with LNT. However, the pilot study of TS-1 combined with LNT in patient with unresectable or recurrent advanced gastric cancer was conducted by Nimura et al. [55]. In this study, a total of 19 patients from four institutes were eligible. In TS-1 plus LNT group, TS-1 was administered orally at the dose of 80 mg/m$^2$/day (bis in die) for 28 days, followed by 14-days rest, and LNT was administered intravenously at the dose of 2 mg/body in a week. This regimen was repeated four cycles and the median survival time was 400 days. The response ratio was 37.5 % and no toxicity of grade IV was observed. Based on this result, randomized phase III study of TS-1 alone versus TS-1 plus LNT in advanced or recurrent gastric cancer was planned in order to investigate the superiority of a combination of TS-1 and LNT compared to TS-1 in terms of survival benefit. This trial was kicked off on January, 2007 and a total of 309 patients were enrolled and completed in June, 2012 [56]. The result is, however, unpublished yet.

Since only intravenous administration of LNT was approved for its clinical use as a pharmaceutical product and LNT is commonly used as an adjuvant solely for treatment of advanced gastric cancer in Japan, superfine dispersed LNT was developed as food supplement for the purpose of easy availability and wider contribution to cancer immunotherapy. Several numbers of clinical trials were performed by using this supplement. The survival rates of patients with unresectable or recurrent hepatocellular carcinoma, who were administered superfine dispersed LNT-containing food supplements, were significantly improved [57]. In this trial, LNT-binding CD14 positive monocytes played an important role in clinical benefit. In addition, superfine dispersed LNT improved both the survival rate and the quality of life of pancreatic cancer patients [58]. Interestingly nutritional grade LNT improved the survival rates of the rats with acute myeloid leukemia when it was used in conjunction with chemotherapeutic agents [59]. Even though there were a lot of case reports and nonrandomized studies in Japan, they were thought to be sufficient to warrant further large-scale, quality trials [60]. On the other hand, oral administration of shiitake mushroom extract did not show any therapeutic effect in the case of prostatic cancer [61].

## 3.4 Schizophyllan

A polysaccharide schizophyllan (SPG) is derived from Schizophyllum commune and consisted of three beta-1, 3-linked glucoses and one beta-1, 6 glucose side chain linked at the every third main chain glucose. The molecular weight of SPG is 450 kDa. Clinical use of SPG was approved in Japan on June, 1986, and it had been used as an enhancer of radiotherapy against uterine cervical cancer. As a matter of fact, however, SPG is not available now because of discontinuation of its production at the end of March, 2011.

### *3.4.1 Basic Experiment and Translational Research*

Bioactivities of SPG had been studied in the fourth quarter of the twentieth century, and the promising immunological antitumor activities were elucidated. In experimental studies SPG showed host-mediated antitumor effect against different kinds of tumor [62]. Because SPG did not show any antitumor effect against sarcoma 180 in in vivo experiment when T cell was suppressed by cyclosporin A, T cell component should be necessary for induction of anti-tumor activity [63]. In addition SPG showed antitumor effect by stimulating cooperative role of T lymphocytes and macrophages in mice [64]. Furthermore SPG increased the cytokine production, such as IL-2 and interferon (IFN)-gamma by the mitogen-stimulated human PBMC [65]. Tsuchiya et al. also reported the cytokine-related immunomodulation by SPG [66]. Moreover SPG potentiated single or fractionated x-ray treatment against murine B-16 melanoma [67].

Recently Kobiyama K et al. reported a novel agent, a nanoparticulate cytosine-phosphodiester-guanine oligodeoxynucleotide (CpG ODN) (K3) wrapped by the nonagonistic Dectin-1 ligand SPG (K3-SPG) [68]. K3-SPG could increase the production of types I and II IFN by human PBMC, followed by induction of cytotoxic T cells in innate immunity. It is well known that SPG binds to Dectin-1 [69] and triggers a signaling cascade leading to the CARD9-dependent activation of NF-kappa B and MAP kinases [70]. Therefore K3-SPG is thought to be one of promising adjuvants for induction of both humoral and cellular immune responses.

### *3.4.2 Clinical Data*

Clinical trial of SPG with chemotherapy, in which MMC and tegafur or 5-FU were used, was conducted against a total of 367 recurrent or inoperable gastric cancer patients, and a significant prolongation of life span was noticed without serious side effects in spite of no influence on tumor size [71]. In head and neck cancer patients, the cumulative 5-year survival rate was 86.7 % in the SPG-treated group and 73.4 %

in the control group, and SPG quickly recovered the cellular immunity damaged by radiation, chemotherapy, and surgical procedure in SPG-treated group [72]. Concerning about uterine cervical cancer, SPG in combination with radiotherapy against stage II patients showed the significant prolongation of both the survival time and the time to recurrence in the randomized controlled trial, whereas in stage III patients such clinical effect was not noted [73]. In addition, a randomized controlled study of adjuvant immunotherapy by use of SPG for the patients with Stage II or III uterine cervical cancer was conducted, and time to recurrence and 5-year survival rate in 99 patients in the SPG group were significantly longer than in 96 patients in the control [74]. Even though Miyazaki et al. reported the usefulness of SPG in combination with surgery, radiotherapy, and chemotherapy against locally advanced uterine cervical carcinoma in a prospective, randomized clinical study, to which a total of 312 patients were enrolled [75], treatment protocols were too many to ensure the meaningfulness of the obtained results. However, this study demonstrated that SPG decreased the ratio of activated CD8+ cells/total CD8+ cells, while the disease progression of uterine cervical cancer was severe in proportion to that ratio, and radiotherapy should augment that ratio. Alternatively the ratio of activated CD4+ cells/total CD4+ cells was also the important factor for prolongation of survival time by SPG.

## 3.5 Conclusion

Three kinds of polysaccharides are discussed here from an immunological point of view. Generally speaking, the immunological mechanisms of polysaccharides are as follows: (1) augmentation of the effect of either chemotherapy or radiotherapy, (2) direct actions on tumor cells, (3) modulation of both innate and acquired immune system, and (4) recovery from immune escape state in tumor-bearing hosts (Fig. 3.1).

Even though there were many prospective randomized controlled trials in Japan, the understanding of clinical oncologists in regard to polysaccharides is considerably poor. Regrettably, none of the cancer treatment guidelines published in Japan has described the old immunotherapy at all. Notwithstanding relatively smaller part of investigators has continued to elucidate their antitumor mechanism in detail. Alternatively the advances in molecular biology and tumor immunology have made a progress in immunotherapy against malignancy, especially in the field of immunological targeting therapy by use of monoclonal antibodies related to immune checkpoint pathway. It is no exaggeration to say that now is the chance for making the progress in both specific and nonspecific immunotherapy against malignancies. Since polysaccharides might play an important role in immunomodulation under innate or acquired immune system of tumor-bearing host, it is urged that the identification of biomarkers in order to determine which type of patients and disease state could allow polysaccharides to perform their optimal effects.

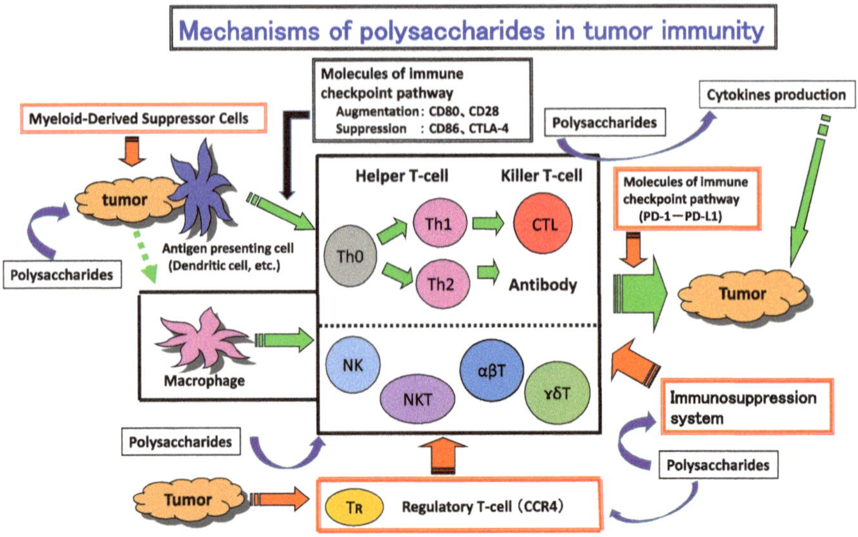


**Fig. 3.1** Mechanisms of polysaccharides in tumor immunity

# References


1. Vickers AJ, Kuo J, Cassileth BR (2006) Unconventional anticancer agents: a systematic review of clinical trials. J Clin Oncol 24:136–140
2. Zhang Y, Kong H, Fang Y et al (2013) Schizophyllan: a review on its structure, properties, bioactivities and recent developments. Bioact Carbohydrates Diet Fibre 1(1):53–71
3. Nio Y, Shiraishi T, Tsubono M et al (1991) In vitro immunimodulating effect of protein-bound polysaccharide, PSK on peripheral blood, regional nodes, and spleen lymphocytes in patients with gastric cancer. Cancer Immunol Immunother 32:335–341
4. Kariya Y, Okamoto N, Fujimoto N et al (1991) Lysis of fresh human cells by autologous peripheral blood lymphocytes activated PSK. Jpn J Cancer Res 82:1044–1050
5. Hirose K, Zachariae C, Oppenheim J et al (1990) Induction of gene expression and production of immunomodulating cytokines by PSK in human peripheral blood mononuclear cells. Lymphokine Res 94:475–483
6. Yamaguchi Y, Minami K, Ohshita A et al (2004) Enhancing effect of PS-K on IL-2-induced lymphocyte activation; possible involvement of antagonistic action against TGF-beta. Anticancer Res 24:639–647
7. Kanazawa M, Mori Y, Yoshihara K et al (2004) Effect of PSK on the maturation of dendritic cells derived from human peripheral blood monocytes. Immunol Lett 91:229–238
8. Okuzawa M, Shinohara H, Kobayashi T et al (2002) PSK, a protein-bound polysaccharide, overcomes defective maturation of dendritic cells exposed to tumor–derived factors in vitro. Int J Oncol 20:1189–1195
9. Asai H, Iijima H, Matsunaga K et al (2008) Protein-bound polysaccharide K augments IL-2 production from murine mesenteric lymph node CD4+ T cells by modulating T cell receptor signaling. Cancer Immunol Immunother 57:1647–1655
10. Sugiyama Y, Osada S, Yamaguchi K et al (2006) Evidence-based biotherapy by use of PSK. Biotherapy 20:396–402 (In Japanese with English abstract)

11. Yoshino S, Hazama S, Shimizu R et al (2005) Usefulness in predicting parameters for the selection of responders who received immunochemotherapy with PSK in patients with colorectal cancer. Jpn J Cancer Chemother 32:1568–1570 (In Japanese with English abstract)
12. Maruyama S, Akasaka T, Yamada K et al (2009) Protein-bound polysaccharide-K (PSK) directly enhanced IgM production in human B cell line BALL-1. Biomed Pharmacother 63:409–412
13. Kobayashi H, Matsunaga K, Oguchi Y (1995) Antimetastatic effects of PSK (Krestin), a protein-bound polysaccharide obtained from Basidiomycetes: an overview. Cancer Epidemiol Biomarkers Prev 4:275–281
14. Tamagawa K, Horiuchi T, Wada T et al (2012) Polysaccharide-K (PSK) may suppress surgical stress-induced metastasis in rat colon cancer. Langenbecks Arch Surg 397:475–480
15. Wada T, Wakamatsu Y, Bannai K et al (2002) Suppression mechanism of angiogenesis by PSK. Ann Cancer Res Ther 10:93–105
16. Sugiyama Y, Saji S, Kunieda K et al (1996) Effect of PSK on either immunocytes or tumor cells. Biotherapy 10:18–25 (In Japanese with English abstract)
17. Kono K, Kawaguchi Y, Mizukami Y et al (2008) Protein-bound polysaccharide K partially prevents apoptosis of circulating T cells induced by anti-cancer drugs S-1 in patients with gastric cancer. Oncology 74:143–149
18. Akagi J, Baba H (2010) PSK may suppress CD57+ T cells to improve survival of advanced gastric cancer patients. Int J Clin Oncol 15:145–152
19. Shibata M, Nezu T, Kanou H et al (2002) Immunomodulatory effects of low dose cis-diaminedichloroplatinum (cisplatin) combined with UFT and PSK in patients with advanced colorectal cancer. Cancer Invest 20:166–173
20. Maehara Y, Tsujitani S, Saeki H et al (2012) Biological mechanism and clinical effect of protein-bound polysaccharide K (Krestin®): review of development and future perspectives. Surg Today 42:8–28
21. Araya S, Nio Y, Hayashi H et al (1994) Various plant-derived polysaccharides augment the expression of HLA on Colo 205 human colonic cancer line. J Jpn Soc Cancer Ther 29:1965–1973 (In Japanese with English abstract)
22. Yoshikawa R, Yanagi H, Hashimoto T et al (2004) Gene expression in response to anti-tumor intervention by polysaccharide K (PSK) in colorectal carcinoma cells. Oncol Rep 12:1287–1293
23. Zhang H, Morisaki T, Nakahara C et al (2003) PSK-mediated NF-κB inhibition augments docetaxel-induced apoptosis in human pancreatic cancer cells NOR-P1. Oncogene 22:2088–2096
24. Kinoshita J, Fushida S, Harada S et al (2010) PSK enhances the efficacy of docetaxel in human gastric cancer cells through inhibition of nuclear factor-kappa B activation and surviving expression. Int J Oncol 36:593–600
25. Nakazato H, Koike A, Saji S et al (1994) Efficacy of immunochemotherapy as adjuvant treatment after curative resection of gastric cancer. Study group of immunochemo-therapy with PSK for gastric cancer. Lancet 343:1122–1126
26. Oba K, Teramukai S, Kobayashi M et al (2007) Efficacy of adjuvant immunochemotherapy with polysaccharides K for patients with curative resections of gastric cancer. Cancer Immunol Immunother 56:905–911
27. Mitomi T, Tsuchiya S, Iijima N et al (1993) Randomized controlled study on adjuvant immunochemotherapy with PSK in curatively resected colorectal cancer-5 years follow-up after surgery (a final report). J Jpn Soc Cancer Ther 28:71–83 (In Japanese with English abstract)
28. Ito K, Nakazato H, Takagi H et al (2004) Long-term effect of 5-fluorouracil enhanced by intermittent administration of polysaccharide K after curative resection of colon cancer. A randomized controlled trial for 7-year follow-up. Int J Colorectal Dis 19:157–164

29. Ohwada S, Ikeya T, Yokomori T et al (2004) Adjuvant immunochemotherapy with oral tegafur/uracil plus PSK in patients with stage II or IIIcolorectal cancer: a randomized controlled study. Br J Cancer 90:1003–1010
30. Sakamoto J, Morita S, Oba K et al (2006) Efficacy of adjuvant immunochemotherapy with polysaccharide K for patients with curatively resected colorectal cancer: a meta-analysis of centrally randomized controlled clinical trials. Cancer Immunol Immunother 55:404–411
31. Konno K, Motomiya M, Oizumi K et al (1998) Effects of protein-bound polysaccharide preparation (PSK) in small cell carcinoma of the lung. JJLC 28:19–28 (In Japanese with English abstract)
32. Sugiyama Y, Saji S, Yasuda K et al (2001) Tumor dormancy therapy against gastroenterological cancer by immunotherapy. Jpn J Gastroenterol Surg 34:397–402 (in Japanese with English abstract)
33. Chihara G, Maeda Y, Hamuro J et al (1969) Inhibition of mouse sarcoma 180 by polysaccharides from Lentinus edodes (Berk.) sing. Nature 222:687–688
34. Chihara G, Hamuro J, Maeda Y et al (1970) Fractionation and purification of the polysaccharides with marked antitumor activity, especially lentinan, from Lentinus edodes (Berk.) Sing (an edible mushroom). Cancer Res 30:2776
35. Suga T, Shiio T, Maeda Y et al (1984) Antitumor activity of lentinan in murine syngeneic and autochthonous hosts and its suppressive effect on 3-methylcholanthrene-induced carcinogenesis. Cancer Res 44:5132–5137
36. Jeannin JF, Lagadec P, Pelletier H et al (1988) Regression induced by lentinan, or peritoneal carcinomatoses in a model of colon cancer in rat. Int J Immunopharm 10:855–861
37. Chihara G, Hamuro J, Maeda Y et al (1987) Antitumor and metastasis-inhibitory activities of lentinan as an immunomodulator : an overview. Cancer Detect Prev Suppl 1:423–443
38. Hamuro J, Rollinghoff M, Wagner H (1980) Induction of cytotoxic peritoneal exudate cells by T-cell immune adjuvants of the beta(1 leads to 3) glucan-type lentinan and its analogues. Immunology 39:551–559
39. Oka M, Hazama S, Suzuki M et al (1996) In vitro and in vivo analysis of human leukocyte binding by the antitumor polysaccharide, lentinan. Int J Immunopharmacol 18:211–216
40. Herlyn D, Kaneko Y, Powe J et al (1985) Monoclonal antibody-dependent murine macrophage-mediated cytotoxicity against human tumors is stimulated by lentinan. Jpn J Cancer Res 76:37–42
41. Yamasaki K, Sone S, Yamashita T, Ogura T (1989) Synergistic induction of lymphokine (IL-2)-activated killer activity by IL-2 and the polysaccharide lentinan, and therapy of spontaneous pulmonary metastases. Cancer Immunol Immunother 29:87–92
42. Hamuro J, Takatsuki F, Suga T et al (1994) Synergistic antimetastatic effects of lentinan and interleukin 2 with pre-and post-operative treatments. Jpn J Cancer Res 85:1288–1297
43. Suzuki M, Higuchi S, Taki Y et al (1990) Induction of endogenous lymphokine-activated killer activity by combined administration of lentinan and interleukin 2. Int J Immunopharmacol 12:613–623
44. Mushiake H, Tsunoda T, Nukatsuka M et al (2005) Dendritic cells might be one of key factors for eliciting antitumor effect by chemoimmunotherapy in vivo. Cancer Immunol Immunother 54:120–128
45. Hamuro J, Kikuchi T, Takatsuki F, Suzuki M (1996) Cancer cell progression and chemoimmunotherapy—dual effects in the induction of resistance to therapy. Br J Cancer 73:465–471
46. Tani M, Tanimura H, Yamaue H et al (1992) In vitro generation of activated natural killer cells and cytotoxic macrophages with lentinan. Eur J Clin Pharmacol 42:623–627
47. Arinaga S, Karimine N, Takamuku K et al (1992) Enhanced induction of lymphokine-activated killer activity after lentinan administration in patients with gastric carcinoma. Int J Immunopharmacol 14:535–539
48. Tani M, Tanimura H, Yamaue H et al (1993) Augmentation of lymphokine-activated killer cell activity by lentinan. Anticancer Res 13:1773–1776

49. Arinaga S, Karimine N, Nanbara S et al (1992) Enhanced production of interleukin 1 and tumor necrosis factor by peripheral monocytes after lentinan administration in patients with gastric carcinoma. Int J Immunopharmacol 14:43–47
50. Murata Y, Shimamura T, Tagami T et al (2002) The skewing to Th1 induced by lentinan is directed through the distinctive cytokine production by macrophages with elevated intracellular glutathione content. Int Immunopharmacol 2:673–689
51. Yoshino S, Tabata T, Hazama S et al (2000) Immunoregulatory effects of the antitumor polysaccharide lentinan on Th1/Th2 balance in patients with digestive cancers. Anticancer Res 20:4707–4712
52. Taguchi T, Furue H, Kimura T et al (1985) Results of phase III study of lentinan. Gan To Kagaku Ryoho 12:366–378 (in Japanese with English abstract)
53. Oba K, Kobayashi M, Matsui T et al (2009) Individual patient based meta-analysis of lentinan for unresectable/recurrent gastric cancer. Anticancer Res 29:2739–2746
54. Wang JL, Bi Z, Zou JW, Gu XM (2012) Combination therapy with lentinan improves outcomes in patients with esophageal carcinoma. Mol Med Report 5:745–748
55. Nimura H, Mitsumori N, Tsukagoshi S et al (2003) Pilot study of TS-1 combined with lentinan in patients with unresectable or recurrent advanced gastric cancer. Gan To Kagaku Ryoho 30:1289–1296 (in Japanese with English abstract)
56. https://upload.umin.ac.jp/cgi-open-bin/ctr/ctr.cgi? function=brows&action=brows&recptno=R000000696&type=summary&language=E
57. Isoda N, Eguchi Y, Nukaya H et al (2009) Clinical efficacy of superfine dispersed lentinan (beta-1,3-glucan) in patients with hepatocellular carcinoma. Hepatogastroenterology 56:437–441
58. Shimizu K, Watanabe S, Watanabe S et al (2009) Efficacy of oral administered superfine dispersed lentinan for advanced pancreatic cancer. Hepatogastroenterology 56:240–244
59. McCormack E, Skavland J, Mujic M et al (2010) Lentinan; hematopoietic immunological, and efficacy studies in a syngeneic model of acute myeloid leukemia. Nutr Cancer 62:574–583
60. Sullivan R, Smith JE, Rowan NJ (2006) Medicinal mushrooms and cancer therapy: translating a traditional practice into Western medicine. Perspect Biol Med 49:159–170
61. deVere White RW, Hackman RM, Soares SE et al (2002) Effects of a mushroom mycelium extract on the treatment of prostate cancer. Urology 60:640–644
62. Komatsu N, Okubo S, Kikumoto S et al (1969) Host-mediated antitumor action of schizophyllan, a glucan produced by Schizophyllum commune. Gann 60:137–144
63. Kraus J, Franz G (1992) Immunomodulating effects of polysaccharides from medicinal plants. Adv Exp Med Biol 319:299–308
64. Suzuki M, Arika T, Amemiya K et al (1982) Cooperative role of T lymphocytes and macrophages in antitumor activity of mice pretreated with schizophyllan (SPG). Jpn J Exp Med 52:59–65
65. Sakagami Y, Mizoguchi Y, Shin T et al (1988) Effects of an anti-tumor polysaccharide, schizophyllan, on interferon γ and interleukin 2 production by peripheral blood mononuclear cells. Biochem Biophys Res Commun 155:650–655
66. Tsuchiya Y, Igarashi M, Inoue M et al (1989) Cytokin-related immunomodulating activities of an anti-tumor glucan, sizofiran (SPG). J Pharmacobiodyn 12:616–625
67. Takai Y, Goodman G, Chaplin D et al (1994) Combination therapy of single or fractionated x-rays and schizophyllan (SPG) for murine B-16 melanoma. Int J Oncol 4:385–389
68. Kobiyama K, Aoshi T, Narita H et al (2014) Nonagonistic Dectin-1 ligand transforms CpG into a multitask nanoparticulate TLR9 agonist. Proc Natl Acad Sci 11:3086–3091
69. Adachi Y et al (2004) Characterization of beta-glucan recognition site on C-type lectin, dectin-1. Infect Immun 72:4159–4171
70. Goodridge HS et al (2009) Beta-glucan recognition by the innate immune system. Immunol Rev 230:38–50

71. Furue H, Uchino H, Orita K et al (1985) Clinical evaluation of schizophyllan (SPG) in advanced gastric cancer (the second report) – a randomized controlled study. Gan To Kagaku Ryoho 12:1272–1277 (In Japanese with English abstract)
72. Kimura Y, Tojima H, Fukase S et al (1994) Clinical evaluation of sizofilan as assistant immunotherapy in treatment of head and neck cancer. Acta Otolaryngol Suppl 511:192–195
73. Okamura K, Suzuki M, Chihara T et al (1986) Clinical evaluation of schizophyllan combined with irradiation in patients with cervical cancer. A randomized controlled study. Cancer 58:865–872
74. Okamura K, Hamazaki Y, Yajima A et al (1989) Adjuvant immunotherapy: two randomized controlled studies of patients with cervical cancer. Biomed Pharmacother 43:177–181
75. Miyazaki K, Mizutani H, Katabuchi H et al (1995) Activated (HLA-DR+) T lymphocyte subsets in cervical carcinoma and effects of radiotherapy and immunotherapy with sizofiran on cell-mediated immunity and survival. Gynecol Oncol 56:412–420

# Chapter 4
# BCG

**Yoichi Mizutani**

**Abstract** Intravesical instillation therapy is currently being used in the management of non-muscle-invasive bladder cancer (NMIBC) and carcinoma in situ (CIS). Its main objectives constitute of treatment of existing or residual cancer, prevention of tumor recurrence, prevention of disease progression, and prolongation of survival. The initial clinical stage and grade of bladder cancer remains the main determinant factors in survival, irrespective of the treatments. Intravesical chemotherapy has shown a decrease in short-term tumor recurrence rates, but has had no positive impact on disease progression or prolongation of survival.

Bacillus Calmette-Guerin (BCG) immunotherapy remains the most effective treatment and prophylaxis modality for NMIBC and CIS and results in a positive outcome on tumor recurrence, disease progression, and prolongation of survival. Although intravesical treatment with BCG instillation is widely accepted as the therapy of choice, the development of BCG-resistant bladder cancer remains a major setback. Thus, there is an urgent need for a major effective therapy for bladder cancer patients who are unresponsive to BCG immunotherapy. This chapter summarizes briefly the recent highlights and advances in BCG immunotherapy against NMIBC and CIS.

**Keywords** BCG • Bladder cancer • Intravesical instillation

## Abbreviations

| | |
|---|---|
| ADR | Adriamycin |
| BCG | Bacillus Calmette-Guerin |
| CIS | Carcinoma in situ |
| CTL | Cytotoxic T lymphocyte |
| MIBC | Muscle-invasive bladder cancer |
| MMC | Mitomycin C |
| NK | Natural killer |

---

Y. Mizutani, M.D. (✉)
Department of Medical Engineering/Urology, Faculty of Health Science, Aino University, 4-5-4 Higashioda, Ibaraki, Osaka 567-0012, Japan
e-mail: y-mizutani@me-u.aino.ac.jp



Y. Yamaguchi (ed.), *Immunotherapy of Cancer*,
DOI 10.1007/978-4-431-55031-0_4

| | |
|---|---|
| NMIBC | Non-muscle-invasive bladder cancer |
| PC | Prostate cancer |
| RCC | Renal cell carcinoma |
| TUR | Transurethral resection |

## 4.1 Introduction

BCG was originally introduced as a vaccine for tuberculosis in 1921. Approximately a half century later, BCG started to be used as an immunotherapeutic agent especially for bladder cancer [1]. At present, intravesical BCG immunotherapy is the most effective treatment against non-muscle-invasive bladder cancer (NMIBC) and carcinoma in situ (CIS) [2, 3], especially for aggressive NMIBC. However, the current major problems are BCG-resistant bladder cancer and adverse events of BCG therapy. This review summarizes the history and development of BCG immunotherapy and its future direction.

## 4.2 Bacillus Calmette-Guerin (BCG)

Most of adults in the nineteenth century were infected with tuberculosis. Approximately one in seven deaths in the period was attributed to tuberculosis. A lot of scientists searched for effective vaccines for tuberculosis. Dr. Nocard isolated *Mycobacterium bovis* from the milk of an infected heifer. This strain was transferred to Dr. Calmette and Dr. Guerin. The primary strain was very virulent. However, the strain became avirulent by successive passages over a bile-potato medium for 13 years. The bacillus of the strain was named "bacillus Calmette-Guerin" [4].

## 4.3 History of BCG as an Anticancer Agent

BCG was first used as an antitumor drug for gastric cancer in 1935 [5]. After that, a lot of basic and clinical studies of BCG against various cancers such as leukemia and melanoma were performed [6, 7]. However, most of these clinical reports were uncontrolled studies, and controlled trials failed to demonstrate significant efficacy of BCG against various cancers.

## 4.4 Bladder Cancer

Bladder cancer accounts for approximately 4 % of all cancers worldwide. The incidence steadily continues to increase [8]. About 60 % of newly diagnosed bladder cancers consist of NMIBC. Half of stage Ta bladder cancer and 70 % of stage T1 bladder cancer recurred within 3 years after transurethral resection (TUR) [9]. The incidence of recurrence is also dependent on tumor grade. In addition, tumor multiplicity has been correlated with increased recurrence rates too [10]. - One-year recurrence rates of 31 %, 30 %, and 39 % were for bladder cancer less than 1 cm, 1–2 cm, and greater than 2 cm, respectively [11]. Other factors related to increased recurrence rates include the persistence of positive urinary cytology and the presence of dysplasia of the urothelium.

It has been reported that 4 % of Ta bladder cancer progressed to muscle-invasive bladder cancer (MIBC), while 30 % of T1 bladder cancer progressed [9]. Furthermore, tumor grade was also associated with increased progression rate.

The natural history of CIS is not as well defined as that of stage Ta and T1 bladder cancer. CIS has been demonstrated to be an aggressive form of superficial bladder cancer with rapid progression. A small focus of CIS may remain asymptomatic without for years, however, diffuse symptomatic CIS is likely to be related to tumor invasion [12, 13].

## 4.5 Basis of Treatment of Bladder Cancer with BCG

Success of BCG immunotherapy for cancers depends on fulfilling several criteria which are summarized in Table 4.1 [1, 3]. Patients with NMIBC seem to be suited to meet the criteria [1, 14]. Alternatively, when all these criteria are not met, intravesical BCG immunotherapy against bladder cancer is less effective, and bladder cancer develops resistance to BCG immunotherapy.

## 4.6 The Mechanisms Responsible for the Anticancer Effect of BCG

The major mechanism underlying the antitumor effect of BCG seems to be mediated by immunological responses. BCG shows little direct cytotoxic activity against cancer cells. However, BCG stimulates cytotoxic cells such as cytotoxic T lymphocytes (CTL), natural killer (NK) cells, and macrophages [15, 16].

**Table 4.1** Criteria for successful BCG immunotherapy against a variety of cancers

| | |
|---|---|
| 1. | Local administration of adequate number of viable BCG |
| 2. | Relatively small tumor burden |
| 3. | Close contact between BCG and cancer cells |
| 4. | Ability to develop an immune response to mycobacterial antigens |
| 5. | Good tolerance |

## 4.7 Selection of Patients for Intravesical BCG Immunotherapy

The potential benefit of a particular intervention has to be weighed against the risks of the therapy itself. Treatments that are nontoxic and inexpensive may be appropriately administered, even when the risks of tumor recurrence and progression are not low. However, intravesical BCG immunotherapy should not be given to patients who are at low risk of tumor recurrence and progression, adverse events of intravesical BCG instillation therapy are relatively heavy [17, 18]. On the other hand, patients with a high risk of tumor recurrence and progression such as CIS, stage T1, high grade, or positive urine cytology should be treated with intravesical BCG immunotherapy. Patients who cannot be classified as those who are at high risk or at low risk are considered to be an intermediate risk group. A common consensus on the optical therapy of these patients has not been reached. However, it has been agreed that some patients in this intermediate risk group require intravesical BCG instillation therapy.

## 4.8 Intravesical Immunotherapy with BCG for Bladder Cancer

BCG is currently the most effective intravesical agent known for the prevention of tumor recurrence and progression of NMIBC [2, 3]. A lot of studies have established that prophylaxis by intravesical BCG treatment, following transurethral resection (TUR) of bladder cancer, significantly reduces tumor recurrences and prolongs the tumor-free interval in comparison to TUR alone [17, 18]. A 32–65 % reduction in tumor recurrence was achieved in prospective and controlled studies that compared TUR in combination with intravesical BCG treatment to TUR alone. Ninety-one percent of patients with T1 bladder cancer treated with TUR and intravesical BCG instillation were free of tumor recurrence with a mean follow-up of approximately 5 years [19].

Several studies showed the effect of BCG on preventing tumor progression. The time to progression to muscle invasion or metastasis was significantly prolonged following intravesical BCG treatment [20]. Stage progression occurred in 35 % of controls and 28 % in patients treated with intravesical BCG instillation in this report. The mortality rate was reduced from 32 % to 14 % with the use of intravesical BCG, and radical cystectomy was required in 42 % of controls, while only in 26 % in patients treated with intravesical BCG. The other report compared the treatment between BCG and adriamycin (ADR) [21]. An increase in stage or extent of bladder cancer occurred in 15 % patients treated with intravesical BCG, as compared with 37 % patients treated with intravesical ADR. Another report demonstrated progression to stage T2 or higher to occur in 4 % of patients treated with intravesical BCG, compared with 17 % of control patients [22]. All of the above reports demonstrate significant reduction in tumor progression with the use of BCG, with the mean rate of progression being 14 % for patients receiving intravesical BCG and 28 % for control patients.

Intravesical BCG instillation is also effective for CIS. The average complete response rates were about 70 % [23, 24]. Furthermore, the overall complete response rates were increased to 87 %, when an additional 3-week course of intravesical BCG instillation at 3 months was performed. At present, intravesical BCG therapy is regarded as the first choice treatment for CIS, instead of cystectomy.

Randomized comparisons of intravesical BCG immunotherapy with intravesical chemotherapy have demonstrated that BCG is superior to chemotherapeutic agents. Significant decrease in tumor recurrence was observed with intravesical BCG, compared to intravesical thiotepa, ADR, or mitomycin C (MMC) [15, 20]. In addition, intravesical BCG immunotherapy improves the long-term therapeutic outcomes, compared with intravesical chemotherapy.

## 4.9 Strategies to Overcome Resistance of NMIBC to Intravesical BCG Immunotherapy

A lot of studies tried to increase the efficacy of intravesical BCG immunotherapy and to reduce the toxicity of BCG therapy as follows:

1. High doses of BCG

   High doses of BCG might be more effective for NMIBC than standard doses of BCG. However, BCG at high concentrations inhibited NK activity [25]. In addition, the other study showed that high doses of BCG unfavorably influenced its anticancer effect on bladder cancer [26].
2. Low doses of BCG

   A phase III randomized controlled trial compared a low dose (Pasteur strain of BCG: 75 mg) versus a standard dose (150 mg). This trial showed that response rates were better in patients submitted to a low dose of BCG administration than a standard dose [27]. In addition, most of common adverse events obtained with a standard dose of BCG were significantly reduced with a low dose of BCG. However, no significant difference in progression rate was seen between a low dose and a standard dose of BCG. In contrast to the above finding, another manuscript showed that no significant difference was observed between low and standard doses BCG immunotherapy in recurrence and progression rates [28]. However, the safety of intravesical BCG immunotherapy was improved.

3. Additional BCG immunotherapy
   When patients with NMIBC failed the 6-week BCG induction course, an additional 6-week course showed additional response [27]. The other paper demonstrated that 69 % of the prophylaxis group and 50 % of the therapy group in patients underwent an additional course achieved complete response [29].
4. Maintenance intravesical immunotherapy with BCG
   Maintenance intravesical BCG immunotherapy improved long-term results. Complete response at 6-months post-therapy was increased from 73 to 87 % with three additional instillations given at three monthly intervals in patients with CIS treated with intravesical BCG immunotherapy [23]. Maintenance BCG given in a series of 3 weekly therapy at 3 months, 6 months, and every 6 months for 3 years significantly decreased tumor recurrence in patients with NMIBC, compared to a single 6-week course [30]. In addition, this maintenance immunotherapy demonstrated significant improved survival, when compared to induction therapy alone. Eighty-six percent survival at 4 years in patients with induction BCG therapy was improved to 92 % in patients with maintenance BCG therapy in a randomized study [31].
5. Combination with high doses of vitamins
   In NMIBC patients treated with a suboptimal maintenance BCG therapy, there was a significant reduction in tumor recurrence in patients randomized to high doses of vitamins A, B6, C, and E, compared with recommended daily allowance vitamins [32]. Vitamins were most effective in patients with low-grade/stage NMIBC. High-dose vitamins may improve immune systems such as enhancing NK activity.
6. Combined therapy with anticancer chemotherapeutic agents
   To improve the efficacy of BCG immunotherapy, a lot of studies on BCG in combination with antitumor chemotherapeutic drugs or other immunotherapeutic agents have been largely unsuccessful [31]. Combined sequential use of MMC and BCG for CIS showed as effective as BCG alone [33]. However, combined therapy with MMC and BCG produced a few adverse events, compared with BCG monotherapy.

## 4.10 BCG for Other Cancers

1. Renal cell carcinoma (RCC)
   Several studies support BCG immunotherapy for RCC. Twenty patients with metastatic RCC who received intradermal BCG was compared with 36 historical controls in a nonrandomized study [34, 35]. All control patients died within 4 years. However, 35 % of RCC patients treated with BCG were alive up to 5 years after the therapy. In addition, complete response and long-term survival were observed in 10 % of patients treated with BCG; in contrast, no complete

response was seen in control patients. A randomized study demonstrated that 48 and 60.5 % survival were noted in control patients and patients with BCG immunotherapy [36, 37]. Since molecular-targeted therapeutic agents are relatively effective against RCC at present, the role of BCG in RCC therapy might be adjuvant.

2. Prostate cancer (PC)

   Direct injection of BCG into PC induced a granulomatous response related to tumor necrosis [38, 39]. However, adverse events such as fatal septic shock were heavy. Percutaneous BCG immunotherapy prolonged survival in patients with PC [40]. A randomized controlled study confirmed the above results in patients with advanced PC treated with hormonal therapy [41]. Since sample size in these reports are small, larger trials are needed.

## 4.11 Future Directions of BCG Immunotherapy

Several tumor-associated genes such as MAGE-1, MAGE-3, and BAGE on melanoma cells have been characterized and demonstrated to be recognized by autologous CTL. These antigens are also expressed on bladder cancer [40, 41]. Therefore, immunotherapy to generate CTL for these antigens might be useful for BCG therapy against on melanoma cells.

The present management of NMIBC consists of two complementary but separate treatment goals: treatment of existing bladder cancer and prevention of recurrence and progression of bladder cancer. Intravesical BCG instillation therapy has been used for more than 40 years. However, optimal doses, schedules, strains, and mechanisms of action are still now being evaluated. In addition, innovative therapeutic approaches are necessary to improve prognosis.

## 4.12 Conclusions

Currently, there are important unresolved questions on BCG immunotherapy against NMIBC: [1]. Does BCG immunotherapy for NMIBC affect overall survival? [2]. What is the optimal concentration of BCG, time of exposure, and duration of BCG therapy? [3]. What is the appropriate therapy for BCG-resistant bladder cancer? These issues should be explored in the near future. Furthermore, it is hopeful to identify high-risk patients, to select the best protocol for each patient, and to use alternative strategies for patients with BCG-resistant bladder cancer. Thus, additional research and clinical trials are necessary to identify more effective and less toxic BCG immunotherapy. These innovative approaches will lead to further improvement in the management of NMIBC.

## References


1. Morales A, Eidinger D, Bruce AW (1976) Intracavitary Bacillus Calmette-Guerin in the treatment of superficial bladder tumors. J Urol 116:180–183
2. Gandhi NM, Molales A, Lamm DL (2013) Bacillus Calmette-Guerin immunotherapy for genitourinary cancer. BJU Int 112:288–297
3. Mizutani Y, Yoshida O, Bonavida B (1997) Bacillus Calmette-Guerin (BCG) in the treatment of superficial bladder cancer: development of resistance to BCG and strategies for overcoming resistance to BCG. Int J Oncol 11:79–86
4. Calmette A, Bocquet A, Negre L (1921) Contribution a l'etude du bacilli tuberculuex bilie. Ann Inst Pasteur 9:561–570
5. Holmgren I (1936) Employment of BCG, especially in intravenous injection. Acta Med Scand 90:350–361
6. Old LJ, Clarke DA, Benacerraf B (1959) Effect of bacillus Calmette-Guerin infection on transplanted tumours in the mouse. Nature 184:291
7. Morton DL (1974) BCG immunotherapy of malignant melanoma: summary of a seven-year experience. Ann Surg 180:635–641
8. Cohen SM, Johansson SL (1992) Epidemiology and etiology of bladder cancer. Urol Clin North Am 12:421–428
9. Heney NM, Ahmed S, Flanagan MJ, Frable W, Corder MP, Hafermann MD et al (1983) Superficial bladder cancer. Progression and recurrence. J Urol 130:1083–1086
10. Prout GR Jr, Barton BA, Griffin PP, Fridell GH, National Bladder Cancer Group (1992) Treated history of non-invasive grade one transitional cell carcinoma. J Urol 148:1413–1419
11. National Bladder Cancer Collaborative Group A (1977) Surveillance, initial assessment, and subsequent progress of patients with superficial bladder cancer in a prospective longitudinal study. Cancer Res 37:2907–2910
12. Riddle PR, Chrishol GD, Trott PA (1976) Flat carcinoma *in situ* of the bladder. Br J Urol 47:829–834
13. Utz DC, Farrow GM (1980) Management of carcinoma *in situ* of the bladder. Urol Clin North Am 7:533–541
14. Zbar B, Rapp HJ (1974) Immunotherapy of guinea pig cancer with BCG. Cancer 34:1532–1540
15. Haaf BO, Catalona WJ, Ratliff TL (1986) Detection of interleukin-2 in the urine of patients with superficial bladder tumors after treatment with intravesical BCG. J Urol 136:970–975
16. Mizutani Y, Nio Y, Fukumoto M, Yoshida O (1992) Effects of bacillus Calmette-Guerin on cytotoxic activities of peripheral blood lymphocytes against human T24 lined and freshly isolated autologous urinary bladder transitional carcinoma cells in patients with urinary bladder cancer. Cancer 69:537–545
17. Lamm DL, Griffith JG (1992) Intravesical therapy: does it affect the natural history of superficial bladder cancer? Semin Urol 10:39–44
18. Nseyo UO, Lamm DL (1996) Therapy of superficial bladder cancer. Semin Oncol 23:598–604
19. Cookson MS, Sarosdy MF (1992) Management of stage T1 superficial bladder cancer with intravesical bacillus Calmette-Guerin therapy. J Urol 148:797–800
20. Herr HW, Laudone VP, Badalament RA (1988) Bacillus Calmette-Guerin therapy alters the progression of superficial bladder cancer. J Clin Oncol 6:1450–1455
21. Lamm DL, Crissman J, Blumenstein B, Crawford ED, Montie J, Scardino P et al (1989) Adriamycin versus BCG in superficial bladder cancer: a Southwest Oncology Group study. Prog Clin Biol Res 310:263–270
22. Pagano F, Bassi P, Milani C (1991) A low dose bacillus Calmette-Guerin regimen in superficial bladder cancer therapy: is it effective? J Urol 146:32–36
23. Lamm DL (1992) Long-term results of intravesical therapy for superficial bladder cancer. Urol Clin North Am 19:573–580

24. Morales A (1996) Intravesical therapy of bladder cancer: an immunotherapy success story. Int J Urol 3:329–333
25. Mizutani Y, Yoshida O (1994) *In vitro* dose-dependent enhancement of natural killer cell activity by bacillus Calmette-Guerin and the antagonistic inhibition of the susceptibility of K562 cells to lysis by peripheral blood lymphocytes in patients with urinary bladder tumor. Int J Urol 1:49–56
26. Lamm DL, Reichert DF, Harris SC, Lucio RM (1982) Immunotherapy of murine transitional cell carcinoma. J Urol 1982:1104–1108
27. Pagamo F, Bassi P, Piazza N, Abatangelo G, Drago Ferrante GL et al (1995) Improving efficacy of BCG immunotherapy by dose reduction. Eur Urol 27:19–22
28. Martinez-Pineiro JA, Solsona E, Flores N, Isorna S, Cooperative Group CUETO (1995) Improving the safety of BCG immunotherapy by dose reduction. Eur Urol 27:19–22
29. Catalona WJ, Hudson ML, Gillen DP, Andriole GL, Ratliff TL (1987) Risks and benefits of repeated courses of intravesical bacillus Calmette-Guerin therapy for superficial bladder cancer. J Urol 137:220–223
30. Lamm DL (1995) BCG in perspective: advances in the treatment of superficial bladder cancer. Eur Urol 27:2–8
31. Witjes JA, Fransen MPH, van der Meijden (1993) Use of maintenance intravesical bacillus Calmette-Guerin (BCG), with or without intradermal BCG, in patients with recurrent superficial bladder cancer. Urol Int 51:67–72
32. Lamm DL, Riggs DR, Shriver JS, VanGilder PF, Rach JI, DeHaven JI (1994) Megadose vitamins in bladder cancer. J Urol 151:21–26
33. Rintala E, Jauhiainen K, Rajala P, Ruutu M, Kaasinen E, Alfthan O et al (1995) Alternating mitomycin C and bacillus Calmette-Guerin instillation therapy for carcinoma in situ of the bladder. J Urol 154:2050–2053
34. Morales A, Wilson JL, Pater JL, Loeb M (1982) Cytoreductive surgery and systemic bacillus Calmette-Guerin therapy in metastatic renal cancer. J Urol 127:230–235
35. Dagnone AJ, Young I, Morales A (1999) Metastatic renal cell carcinoma regression after nephrectomy and BCG immunotherapy. Can J Urol 6:749–750
36. Mavrichev AS, Grigorovich NA, Sukonko OG (1990) The late results of the combined treatment of kidney cancer patients. Urol Nephrol 5:13–16
37. Wirch MP (1993) Immunotherapy for metastatic renal cell carcinoma. Urol Clin North Am 20:283–295
38. Merrin C, Han T, Klein E, Wajsman Z, Murphy GP (1975) Immunotherapy of prostatic carcinoma with bacillus Calmette-Guerin. Cancer Chemother Rep 59:157–163
39. Rubinson MR, Rigby CC, Pugh RC, Dumonde DC (1978) Prostate carcinoma; intratumor BCG immunotherapy. Natl Cancer Inst Monogr 49:351–353
40. Patard JJ, Brasseur F, Gil-Diez S, Radvanyi F, Marchand M, Francois P et al (1995) Expression of MAGE genes in transitional-cell carcinoma of the urinary bladder. Int J Cancer 64:60–64
41. Boel P, Wilkdmann C, Sensi ML, Brasseur R, Renauld JC, Coulie P et al (1995) BAGE: a new gene encoding an antigen recognized on human melanomas by cytotoxic T lymphocytes. Immunity 2:167–175

# Part III
# Adoptive Cell Therapy

# Chapter 5
# αβ-T Cells

**Atsushi Aruga**

**Abstract** Adoptive cell therapy using autologous αβ-T cells is one of the most effective treatments for various cancers and has minimal side effects. αβ-T cells have the ability to recognize the cancer antigens that present with human leukocyte antigen (HLA) molecules on the cancer cells and kill them by secreting several granules, such as perforin, granzyme, or granulysin. Several clinical effects have been defined in clinical trials, but standardized treatment approaches have not been established. Because of the difficulty of dealing with several regulations and the high costs, there have been very few large clinical trials. Even so, recent technical advances in such fields as genetic engineering may make it possible to cure various cancers using new candidates for αβ-T-cell therapy. It is expected that safe and effective αβ-T-cell therapy will be developed as a standard cancer therapy in the near future.

**Keywords** Adoptive transfer • Immunotherapy • TIL • CTL • ATVAC

## 5.1 Introduction

There has been a revival of interest in the field of cancer immunotherapy in recent years, and adoptive cell therapy is one of the most important approaches [1, 2]. In particular, it is expected that adoptive cell therapy will be developed for several malignant diseases which have very few treatment options [3, 4]. In humans, both "innate immunity" and an "acquired immunity" can be present. Components of innate immunity include natural killer cells (NK cells; Chap. 8), natural killer T cells (NKT cells; Chap. 7), and γδ-T cells (Chap. 9), and all these cells show nonspecific immunity which is present at birth. The acquired immunity is derived from αβ-T cells that have αβ-T-cell receptors (TCRs), which can recognize antigen-derived peptides within human leukocyte antigen (HLA) molecules (Fig. 5.1). Numerous cancer antigens have been discovered in the last decade and have

A. Aruga (✉)
Institute of Advanced Biomedical Engineering and Science, Tokyo Women's Medical University, 8-1 Kawada-cho, Shinjuku-ku, Tokyo 162-8666, Japan
e-mail: aruga.atsushi@twmu.ac.jp


Y. Yamaguchi (ed.), *Immunotherapy of Cancer*,
DOI 10.1007/978-4-431-55031-0_5

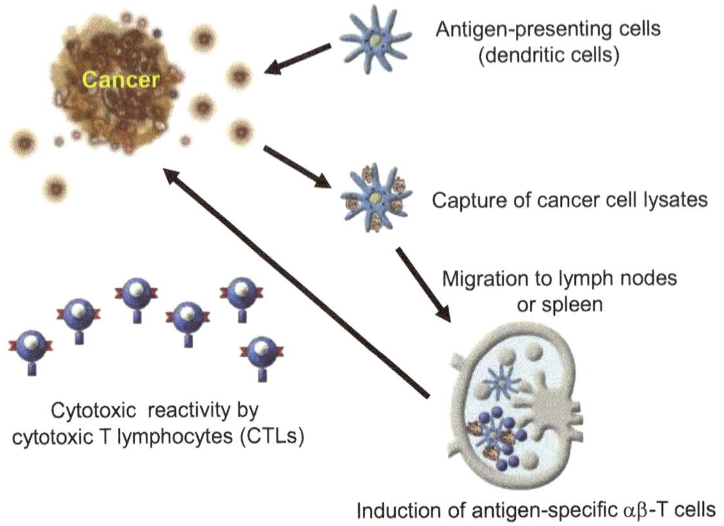


**Fig. 5.1** Acquired immunity for cancer by αβ-T cells in human

enabled progress in cancer antigen-specific cell therapies. In this chapter, adoptive cell therapy using αβ-T cells is discussed.

## 5.2 Recognition of Cancer Antigens by αβ-TCR

αβ-TCRs consist of an α chain and a β chain and recognize antigen-derived peptides displayed in the HLA molecules of antigen-presenting cells (APC) such as dendritic cells, resulting in the induction of antigen-specific T cells (Fig. 5.2). When the TCRs combine with the HLAs presenting on cancer cells, several granules, including perforin, granzyme, and granulysin, are released from CD8-positive T cells and kill the cancer cells (Fig. 5.3). This cytotoxicity is mainly shown by CD8-positive T cells that are called cytotoxic T lymphocytes (CTLs). CD4-positive T cells may assist the CTLs by releasing Th1 cytokines such as interleukin-2 (IL-2) and interferon-γ (IFN-γ). Cancer antigens are categorized into cancer-testis antigens, cancer-related gene-derived antigens, tissue-specific antigens, oncofetal antigens, overexpressed antigens, and virus-related antigens (Table 5.1). Cancer antigen-derived epitope peptides exist within HLA molecules and become a target of CTLs. To date, many cancer antigens have been identified, and some of them are expected to be useful tools for cancer immunotherapy [5].

Induction of cancer antigen-specific CTLs would be expected to be one of the most important issues in the field of adoptive cell therapy and is now becoming a clinical reality.

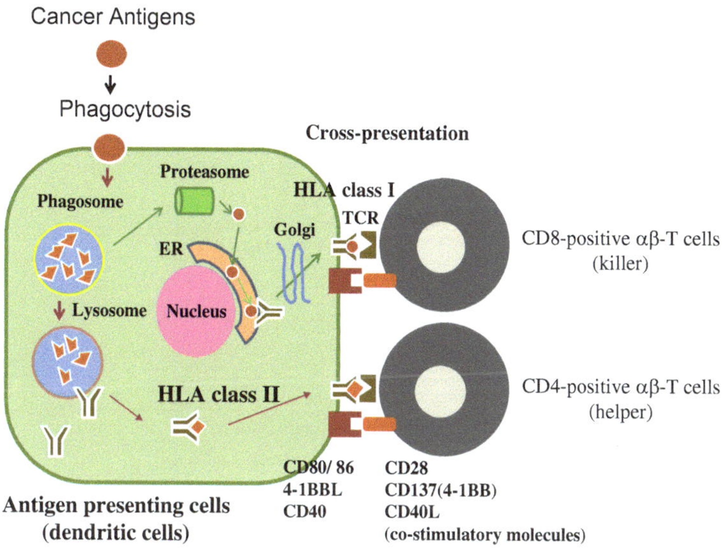


**Fig. 5.2** Induction of cancer antigen-specific CD8-positive αβ-T cells and CD4-positive αβ-T cells with antigen-presenting cells

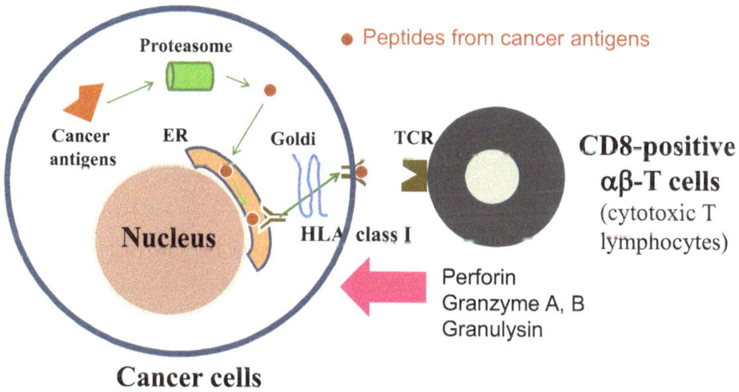


**Fig. 5.3** Recognition of cancer antigens expressed on cancer cells and release of cytotoxic granules by CD8-positive αβ-T cells

## 5.3 Adoptive Cell Therapy of αβ-T Cells

To date, six types of protocol to induce αβ-T-cell activation have been reported (Table 5.2). All the methods require ex vivo activation or stimulation to expand the cell number. In vivo or ex vivo sensitization of αβ-T cells with cancer cells has generally been required for the induction of cancer antigen-specific immunity. Recently, cancer vaccines composed of dendritic cells (see Chap. 15), peptides

**Table 5.1** Categorization of cancer antigens

| Categorization | Antigens |
| --- | --- |
| Cancer-testis antigen | MAGE A1, MAGE A3, NY-ESO-1, LY6K |
| Cancer-related gene-derived antigen | Ras, p53, bcr-abl, HER2, WT1 |
| Tissue-specific antigen | MART1, MelanA, gp100, PSA, PSMA, TRP-2 |
| Oncofetal antigen | AFP, CEA |
| Overexpressed antigen | MUC1, EpCAM, mesothelin, survivin |
| Virus-related antigen | HPV E6, HPV E7, LMP2 |

**Table 5.2** Designation and activation protocol of effector cells

| Designation | Activation protocol | References |
| --- | --- | --- |
| TIL | Harvest from cancer tissues followed by IL-2 expansion | [6–9] |
| CTL | Ex vivo stimulation with cancer cells plus IL-2 | [10–12] |
| PDAK/DCAT | Ex vivo stimulation with antigen-presenting DCs | [13] |
| CAT/CD3-LAK/T-LAK | Ex vivo stimulation with anti-CD3 mAb plus IL-2 (optional addition: IFN-γ, retronectin, fibronectin) | [14–19] |
| VPLN | Harvest vaccine-primed LNs followed by anti-CD3/IL-2 expansion | [20, 21] |
| ATVAC | Combination with dendritic cell vaccine plus T-cell transfer | [22–29] |

(see Chaps. 11, 12, and 13), or proteins (see Chap. 14) have been expected to induce strong antigen-specific immunity in vivo.

### *5.3.1 TILs (Tumor-Infiltrating Lymphocytes)*

Tumor-infiltrating lymphocytes (TILs) are mechanically collected from autologous cancer tissues followed by ex vivo expansion with interleukin-2 (IL-2). Adoptive transfer of TILs has demonstrated some clinical effects in melanoma, lung cancer, and other diseases [6–9]. However, despite these clear clinical effects, the techniques are difficult and limited to a few specific carcinomas, which have hindered the diffusion of TIL therapy. Thus, while TIL has long been investigated, there is currently no approved product by the FDA or EMA.

### *5.3.2 CTLs (Cytotoxic T Lymphocytes)*

Induction of cancer antigen-specific T cells can be induced ex vivo by using a mixed culture of αβ-T cells and cancer cells in some cases [10–12]. The expression of HLA molecules and co-stimulatory molecules is needed to induce antigen-specific T cells in ex vivo culture. However, some cancer cells lack the expression of HLA molecules, and most of them do not express the co-stimulatory molecules such as CD80 or CD86. This is why the mixed cultures of cancer cells and T cells can only rarely induce antigen-specific CTLs in practice.

### 5.3.3 PDAK (Peptide-Pulsed Dendritic Cell-Activated Killer)/ DCAT (Dendritic Cell-Activated T Cells)

It is efficient and effective to use antigen-presenting cells (APCs) for the induction of antigen-specific CTLs, because the APCs can express both HLA molecules and co-stimulatory molecules such as CD80, CD86, and CD40 [13]. The use of APCs such as dendritic cells would be ideal, but the protocol for the ex vivo culture of dendritic cells is cumbersome and expensive. For this reason, there have been no large trials using this technique.

### 5.3.4 CAT/CD3-LAK/T-LAK

αβ-T cells could be activated and expanded by the immobilized anti-CD3 monoclonal antibody (mAb) plus recombinant interleukin-2 (rIL-2) ex vivo. These anti-CD3 mAb activated T cells (CAT) have been used in some clinical trials and showed some clinical effects. Clinical effects in the recurrence-free survival of patients with hepatocellular carcinoma (HCC) are well known [18], and other reports have described cases of clinical effects on tumor regression. This protocol is more convenient for the activation and expansion of T cells for adoptive transfer. These cells are also termed CD3-LAK (lymphocyte-activated killer), T-LAK, or activated T cells and have been used in several clinical trials. Recently, the refinement of culture conditions with IFN-γ [14], retronectin [15], and fibronectin [16] has been attempted. Activation with not only anti-CD3 mAb but anti-CD28/CD137 mAbs might be a good idea [17]. While CAT has a distinct advantage in terms of its clinical simplicity because it does not require antigen stimulation, its antigen-specific cytotoxicity is limited. It is therefore not expected that this modality will achieve an excellent response, but an increase in the number of T cells after adoptive transfer would be helpful for patients with immunosuppression caused by leukopenia or for type 2 dominant hosts [19] in order to improve the host immune condition.

### 5.3.5 VPLNs (Vaccine-Primed Lymph nodes)

In vivo sensitization of T cells with cancer antigens is one method for inducing antigen-specific T cells and followed by activation ex vivo with anti-CD3 mAb plus rIL-2. The patients are first treated with irradiated autologous cancer cells, and then the vaccine-primed lymph nodes are removed for activation with anti-CD3 mAb followed by expansion in rIL-2. Activated T cells are administered intravenously and result in some clinical effects. These activated T cells show cancer-specific IFN-γ release to autologous cancer cells in an HLA class I-restricted manner [20, 21].

### *5.3.6 ATVAC (Adoptive Transfer of T Cells Plus Dendritic Cell Vaccine)*

Recently, new types of cancer vaccines have been under increasing study. One of the most anticipated candidates is the dendritic cell vaccine (see Chap. 15). In vivo vaccination of antigen-pulsed dendritic cells could induce antigen-specific CTLs in vivo, and some clinical effects have been reported in clinical trials. However, it has often been suggested that the leukopenia in patients with advanced cancer would counteract the effect of cancer vaccines. An increase in the number of T cells in vivo is needed to ensure the efficacy of cancer vaccines. On the other hand, dendritic cell vaccines could induce antigen-specific CTLs in vivo, and this would be a good way to induce ex vivo activation in a large number of antigen-specific T cells. The combination of dendritic cell vaccine and activated T-cell transfer should be the best way to treat cancer with immunotherapy [22]. We have reported the clinical utilization of an adoptive transfer of T cells plus dendritic cell vaccine (ATVAC) in patients with intrahepatic cholangiocarcinoma (ICC) [23] and hepatocellular carcinoma (HCC) [24]. Postoperative ATVAC could improve both recurrence-free survival (RFS) and overall survival (OS). In order to assess the effect of ATVAC immunotherapy, further randomized control trials are needed. There have been several similar trials using a combination of cancer vaccine plus adoptive T-cell transfer [25–29], and all of these trials showed an improved outcome.

## 5.4 Future Perspectives of Adoptive αβ-T-Cell Transfer

Several refinements will be needed for the clinical trials to succeed, such as the use of irRC [30] (see Chap. 25), suitable statistical methods [31], or suitable immunomonitoring (see Chap. 24). Therefore, we will next consider various means of achieving optimum therapeutic results using adoptive αβ-T-cell therapy.

### 5.4.1 Improvement of Immunosuppression

To date, the enhancement of immunity has been tended to search for a desirable response. However, it is becoming known that the improvement of immunosuppression is more important (Fig. 5.4). The use of immunocheckpoint blockades actually could result in remarkable progress in the field of cancer immunotherapy and might influence adoptive cell therapy in the near future (see Chaps. 19, 20, and 21). The combination of immunocheckpoint blockades and adoptive cell therapy would be expected to demonstrate a beneficial effect. In addition, the reduction of regulatory T cells (Treg cells) (see Chap. 22) or myeloid-derived suppressor cells (MDSCs) (see Chap. 23) might be effective to enhance the clinical responses of cancer immunotherapy. Trafficking of activated T cells to the cancer site is also an important issue to be solved [32].

### 5.4.2 Artificial Manipulation of TCRs

CTL would be the most efficient method in cancer immunotherapy, but the induction is often difficult. The artificial manipulation of TCRs has recently been studied intensively with the goal of making a large number of cancer antigen-specific CTLs. Genetically engineered T cells bearing chimeric antigen receptors (CARs) [33] or recombinant TCR technology [34] are expected to be candidates for future immunotherapy (see Chap. 10).

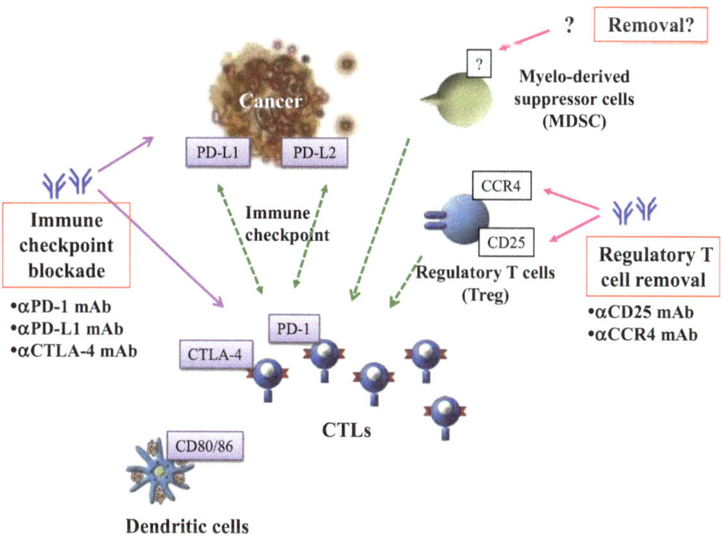


**Fig. 5.4** New approaches to relieve immunosuppression in cancer patients

### 5.4.3 Combination with Bispecific Antibody

CAT has been shown to have poor antigen specificity, and therefore, a new approach to acquire the antigen specificity by using the bispecific antibody has been investigated [35–37]. The bispecific antibody has two antigen-specific sites, one is a receptor for CD3 molecules on T cells and the other accepts cancer-specific antigens. The combination of treatment with a bispecific antibody could enable T cells to respond to the cancer antigen in specific manner. Although the construction of the bispecific antibody might be technically difficult, advances in techniques could lead to an improved ability to treat cancers.

### 5.4.4 Regeneration of T Cells or Dendritic Cells from iPS

In the distant future, T cells or dendritic cells might be regenerated from induced pluripotent stem cells (iPS) or embryonic stem cells (ES). At this time, the regeneration of antigen-specific T cells from iPS derived from mature CD8-positive T cells and dendritic cells has already been succeeded [38, 39]. CTLs with standardized quality will be safely and easily mass produced for widespread use by such generations.

## 5.5 Conclusions

The approval of adoptive cell therapy has been minimal because of the difficulty in maintaining the quality of the treatment. Several criteria should be considered when using adoptive cell therapy that are not considered when using pharmaceutical drugs. In Japan, a new governmental regulatory system for stem cell-based therapies has just established [40]. The new law regulates not only regenerative medicine but also adoptive cell therapy for cancer patients. Physicians who handle human cells for medicine are required to report to the Ministry of Health, Labour and Welfare (MHLW) after the approval of a particular committee. On the other hand, the new law will shorten the approval process in some cases. To date, many clinical studies have been performed by using αβ-T cells. It is hoped that a safe and effective αβ-T-cell therapy will be developed as a standard therapy for cancer as soon as possible.

# References


1. Vacchelli E, Eggermont A, Fridman WH, Galon J, Tartour E, Zitvogel L et al (2013) Adoptive cell transfer for anticancer immunotherapy. Oncoimmunology. doi:10.4161/onci.24238
2. Aranda F, Vacchelli E, Obrist F, Eggermont A, Galon J, Fridman WH et al (2014) Adoptive cell transfer for anticancer immunotherapy. Oncoimmunology. doi:10.4161/onci.28344
3. Chung DS, Shin HJ, Hong YK (2014) A new hope immunotherapy for malignant gliomas: adoptive T cell transfer therapy. J Immunol Res. doi:10.1155/2014/326545
4. Xie F, Zhang X, Li H, Zheng T, Xu F, Shen R et al (2012) Adoptive immunotherapy in postoperative hepatocellular carcinoma: a systemic review. PLoS One. doi:10.1371/journal.pone.0042879
5. Cheever MA et al (2009) The prioritization of cancer antigens: a National Cancer Institute pilot project for the acceleration of translational research. Clin Cancer Res 15(17):5323–5337
6. Wu R, Forget MA, Chacon J, Bernatchez C, Haymaker C, Chen JQ et al (2012) Adoptive T-cell therapy using autologous tumor-infiltrating lymphocytes for metastatic melanoma: current status and future outlook. Cancer J 18(2):160–175. doi:10.1097/PPO.0b013e31824d4465
7. Kvistborg P, Shu CJ, Heemskerk B, Fankhauser M, Thre CA, Tobes M et al (2012) TIL therapy broadens the tumor-reactive CD8+ T cell compartment in melanoma patients. Oncoimmunology 1(4):409–418. doi:10.4161/onci.18851
8. Goff SL, Smith FO, Klapper JA, Sherry R, Wunderlich JR, Steinberg SM et al (2013) Tumor infiltrating lymphocyte therapy for metastatic melanoma: analysis of tumors resected for TIL. J Immunother 33(8):840–847. doi:10.1097/CJI.0b013e3181f05b91
9. Khammari A, Knol AC, Nguyen JM, Bossard C, Denis MG, Pandolfino MC et al (2014) Adoptive TIL transfer in the adjuvant setting of melanoma: long-term patient survival. J Immunol Res. doi:10.1155/2014/186212
10. Aruga A, Yamauchi K, Takasaki K, Furukawa T, Hanyu F (1991) Induction of autologous tumor-specific cytotoxic T cells in patients with liver cancer. Characterizations and clinical utilization. Int J Cancer 49:19–24
11. Toh U, Yamana H, Sueyoshi S, Tanaka T, Niiya F, Katagiri K et al (2000) Locoregional cellular immunotherapy for patients with advanced esophageal cancer. Clin Cancer Res 6:4663–4673
12. Lutzky V, Crooks P, Morrison L, Stevens N, Davis JE, Corban M et al (2014) Cytotoxic T cell adoptive immunotherapy as a treatment for nasopharyngeal carcinoma. Clin Vac Immunol 21 (2):256–259
13. Yamaguchi Y, Ohta K, Kawabuchi Y, Ohshita A, Okita R, Okawaki M et al (2005) Feasibility study of adoptive immunotherapy for metastatic lung tumors using peptide-pulsed dendritic cell-activated killer (PDAK) cells. Anticancer Res 25:2407–2416
14. Zhang Y, Wang J, Wang Y, Lu XC, Fan H, Liu Y et al (2013) Autologous CIK cell immunotherapy in patients with renal cell carcinoma after radical nephrectomy. Clin Dev Immunol. doi:10.1155/2013/195691
15. Ma H, Zhang Y, Wang Q, Li Y, He J, Wang H et al (2010) Therapeutic safety and effects of adjuvant autologous RetroNectin activated killer cell immunotherapy for patients with primary hepatocellular carcinoma after radiofrequency ablation. Cancer Biol Ther 9(11):903–907
16. Ishikawa T, Kokura S, Enoki T, Sakamoto N, Okayama T, Ideno M et al (2014) Phase I clinical trial of fibronectin CH296-stimulated T cell therapy in patients with advanced cancer. PLoS One. doi:10.1371/journal.pone.0083786
17. Teschner D, Wenzel G, Distler E, Schnurer E, Theobald M, Neurauter AA et al (2011) In vitro stimulation and expansion of human tumour-reactive CD8+ cytotoxic T lymphocytes by anti-CD3/CD28/CD137 magnetic beads. Scand J Immunol 74:155–164. doi:10.1111/j.1365-3083.2011.02564.x

18. Takayama T, Sekine T, Makuuchi M, Yamasaki S, Kosuge T, Yamamoto J et al (2000) Adoptive immunotherapy to lower postsurgical recurrence rates of hepatocellular carcinoma: a randomised trial. Lancet 356:802–807
19. Noguchi A, Kaneko T, Naitoh K, Saito M, Iwai K, Maekawa R et al (2014) Impaired and imbalanced cellular immunological status assessed in advanced cancer patients and restoration of the T cell immune status by adoptive T-cell immunotherapy. Int Immunopharmacol 18:90–97. doi:10.1016/j.intimp.2013.11.009
20. Chang AE, Aruga A, Cameron MJ, Sondak VK, Normolle DP, Fox BA et al (1997) Adoptive immunotherapy with vaccine-primed lymph node cells secondarily activated with anti-CD3 and interleukin-2. J Clin Oncol 15(2):796–807
21. Chang AE, Li Q, Jiang G, Sayre DM, Braun TM, Redman BG (2003) Phase II trial of autologous tumor vaccination, anti-CD3^activated vaccine-primed lymphocytes, and interleukin-2 in stage IV renal cell cancer. J Clin Oncol 21(5):884–890. doi:10.1200/JCO.2003.08.023
22. Tanigawa K, Takeshita N, Eickhoff GA, Shimizu K, Chang AE (2001) Antitumor reactivity of lymph node cells primed in vivo with dendritic cell-based vaccines. J Immunother 24 (6):493–501
23. Shimizu K, Kotera Y, Aruga A, Takeshita N, Takasaki K, Yamamoto M (2012) Clinical utilization of postoperative dendritic cell vaccine plus activated T-cell transfer in patients with intrahepatic cholangiocarcinoma. J Hepato-Biliary-Pancreat Sci 19:171–178. doi:10.1007/s00534-011-0437-y
24. Shimizu K, Kotera Y, Aruga A, Takeshita N, Katagiri S, Ariizumi S et al (2014) Postoperative dendritic cell vaccine plus activated T-cell transfer improves the survival of patients with invasive hepatocellular carcinoma. Hum Vac Immunother. doi:10.4161/hv.27678
25. Poschke I, Lovgren T, Adamson L, Nystrom M, Andersson E, Hansson J et al (2014) A phase I clinical trial combining dendritic cell vaccination with adoptive T cell transfer in patients with stage IV melanoma. Cancer Immunol Immunother 63:1061–1071. doi:10.1007/s00262-014-1575-2
26. Niu J, Ren Y, Zhang T, Yang X, Zju W, Zhu H et al (2014) Retrospective comparative study of the effects of dendritic cell vaccine and cytokine-induced killer cell immunotherapy with that of chemotherapy alone and in combination for colorectal cancer. Biomed Res Int. doi:10.1155/2014/214727
27. Kandalaft LE, Powell EJ Jr, Chiang CL, Tnyi J, Kim S, Bosch M et al (2013) Autologous lysate-pulsed dendritic cell vaccination followed by adoptive transfer of vaccine^primed ex vivo co-stimulated T cells in recurrent ovarian cancer. Oncoimmunology 2:1. doi:10.4161/onci.22664
28. Rapoport AP, Aqui NA, Stadtmauer EA, VOgi DT, Xu YY, Kalos M et al (2014) Combination immunotherapy after ASCT for multiple myeloma using MAGE-A3/Poly-ICLC immunizations followed by adoptive transfer of vaccine-primed and costimulated autologous T cells. Clin Cancer Res. doi:10.1158/1078-0432.CCR-13-2817
29. Shindo Y, Hazama S, Maeda Y, Matsui H, Iida M, Suzuki N et al (2014) Adoptive immunotherapy with MUC1-mRNA transfected dendritic cells and cytotoxic lymphocytes plus gemcitabine for unresectable pancreatic cancer. J Transl Med. doi:10.1186/1479-5876-12-175
30. Wolchok JD et al (2009) Guidelines for the evaluation of immune therapy activity in solid tumors: immune-related response criteria. Clin Cancer Res 15(23):7412–7420
31. Chen TT (2013) Statistical issues and challenges in immuno-oncology. J Immunother Cancer 1:18
32. Abastado JP (2012) The next challenge in cancer immunotherapy: controlling T-cell traffic to the tumor. Cancer Res 72(9):2159–2161. doi:10.1158/0008-5472.CAN-11-3538
33. Grupp SA, Kalos M, Barrett D et al (2013) Chimeric antigen receptor-modified T cells for acute lymphoid leukemia. N Engl J Med 368(16):1509–1518. doi:10.1056/NEJMoa1215134

34. Morgan RA, Chinnasamy N, Abate-Daga D, Gros A, Robbins PF, Zheng Z et al (2013) Cancer regression and neurological toxicity following anti-MAGE-A3 TCR gene therapy. J Immunother 36(2):133–151. doi:10.1097/CJI.0b013e3182829903
35. Buhmann R, Michael S, Juergen H, Horst L, Peschel C, Kolb HJ (2013) Immunotherapy with FBTA05(Bi20), a trifunctional bispecific anti-CD3 xanti-CD20 antibody and donor lymphocyte infusion (DLI) in relapsed or refractory B-cell lymphoma after allogeneic stem cell transplantation: study protocol of an investigator-driven, open-label, non-randomized, uncontrolled, dose-escalating Phase I/II-trial. J Transl Med. doi:10.1186/1479-5876-11-160
36. Thakur A, Schalk D, Sarkar SH, AL-Khadimi Z, Sarkar FH, Lum LG (2012) A Th1 cytokine-enriched microenvironment enhances tumor killing by activated T cells armed with bispecific antibodies and inhibits the development of myeloid-derived suppressor cells. Cancer Immunol Immunother 61:497–509. doi:10.1007/s00262-011-1116-1
37. Araki K, Noguchi Y, Hirouchi T, Yoshikawa E, Kataoka S, Silverni L et al (2000) Cancer regression induced by modified CTL therapy is regulated by HLA class II and class I antigens in Japanese patients with advanced cancer. Int J Oncol 17(6):1107–1118
38. Vizcardo R, Masuda K, Yamada D, Ikawa T, Shimizu K, Fujii S et al (2013) Regeneration of human tumor antigen-specific T cells from iPSCs derived from mature CD8+ T cells. Cell Stem Cell 12(1):31–36. doi:10.1016/j.stem.2012.12.006
39. Nishimura T, Kaneko S, Kawana-Tachikawa A, Tajima Y, Goto H, Zhu D et al (2013) Generation of rejuvenated antigen-specific T cells by reprogramming to pluripotency and redifferentiation. Cell Stem Cell 12(1):114–126. doi:10.1016/j.stem.2012.11.002
40. Hara A, Sato D, Sahara Y (2014) New governmental regulatory system for stem cell-based therapies in Japan. Ther Innov Regul Sci. doi:10.1177/2168479014526877

# Chapter 6
# NKT Cell-Based Immunotherapy

**Shinichiro Motohashi**

**Abstract** CD1d-restricted invariant natural killer T (NKT) cells are a specialized innate lymphocyte subset that recognizes a glycolipid antigen via the invariant T-cell receptor. Ligand-activated NKT cells display direct antitumor activities against various tumors. In addition, NKT cells are spontaneously poised to display the rapid effector function, which enables them to produce a wide variety of cytokines expeditiously following activation and to modulate the function of other immune cells, including those responsible for antitumor immunity. Numerical and/or functional changes in the numbers of NKT cells have been observed in patients with various malignant diseases, which correlate with a patient clinical outcome. Therefore, the restoration of the NKT cell system in tumor-bearing patients would be a rational treatment for malignant disease. This chapter summarizes the results of our recent passive or active immunotherapy aimed at augmenting the NKT cell function in vivo in patients with non-small cell lung cancer and discusses the role of NKT cell-induced immune responses.

**Keywords** NKT cell • α-Galactosylceramide • Antigen-presenting cell • Clinical trial • Non-small cell lung cancer

## 6.1 Introduction

Cancer immunotherapy has been investigated to mobilize the immune system to control tumor growth and provide a survival benefit. Early clinical trials of active immunotherapeutic, such as those employing dendritic cells (DCs) or adoptive cell therapy, including tumor-infiltrating lymphocytes or genetically engineered T cells, provided a proof of concept that therapeutic immunity can be elicited and lead to some clinical benefit [1–5]. In 2010, the US Food and Drug Administration (FDA) approved Provenge (sipuleucel-T) as the first active cellular immunotherapy derived from autologous antigen-presenting cells for the treatment of advanced prostate cancer [6, 7]. Another dramatic development in the field of cancer

---

S. Motohashi (✉)
Department of Medical Immunology, Graduate School of Medicine, Chiba University, 1-8-1 Inohana, Chuo-ku, Chiba 260-8670, Japan
e-mail: motohashi@faculty.chiba-u.jp



Y. Yamaguchi (ed.), *Immunotherapy of Cancer*,
DOI 10.1007/978-4-431-55031-0_6

immunotherapy was the results of recent clinical trials using immune checkpoint inhibitors such as anti-cytotoxic T-lymphocyte-associated antigen 4 (CTLA-4) or anti-programmed cell death protein-1 (PD-1) antibodies, which showed an obvious survival benefit [8, 9]. The anti-CTLA-4 antibody or anti-PD-1 antibody blocks the inhibitory signals of T cells and modulates the endogenous T-cell response [10]. The most important point is that these molecules are expressed on T cells, not on tumor cells, and the mechanism underlying the clinical benefits is the existence of an endogenous immune system that substantively acts as an anticancer drug.

Invariant (or type I) natural killer T (NKT) cells are a unique innate lymphocyte subpopulation, characterized by a unique T-cell receptor (TCR)-α chain (Vα14-Jα18 in mice and Vα24-Jα18 in humans) paired with a restricted number of TCR-β chains, mostly with a Vβ11 in humans. Unlike conventional T cells, which recognize peptide antigens, NKT cells recognize a glycolipid antigen presented by the major histocompatibility complex (MHC) class I-like CD1d molecules expressed

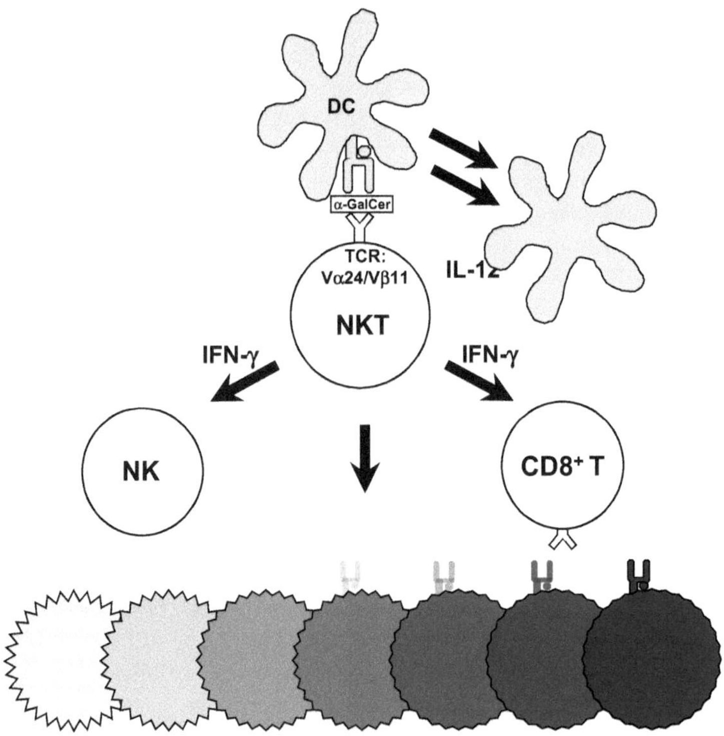


**Fig. 6.1** NKT cell-mediated antitumor immune responses induced by α-GalCer activation. α-GalCer-presenting APCs such as immature DCs activate NKT cells. Activated NKT cells exhibit various kinds of direct and indirect effects, including maturation of DCs, activation and recruitment of NK cells, and cytotoxic $CD8^+$ T cells to eradicate malignant tumors

on antigen-presenting cells (APC). The first glycolipid antigen identified for NKT cells was α-galactosylceramide (α-GalCer, KRN7000) [11]. α-GalCer was originally extracted from the marine sponge *Agelas mauritianus*, and the potent antitumor effects were demonstrated in several mouse models after treatment with this compound [12]. After activation with α-GalCer, NKT cells show the potential to produce or express cytotoxic molecules, such as perforin, granzymes, Fas ligand and TNF-related apoptosis-inducing ligand (TRAIL), and directly disrupt malignant tumor cells [13–15]. At the same time, activated NKT cells promptly produce an enormous amount of cytokines such as IFN-γ, which exerts indirect antitumor activities mainly through the subsequent activation of downstream immune effector cells, including NK cells, $CD8^+$ CTLs, B cells, and DCs (Fig. 6.1) [16–19]. Therefore, NKT cells play a key role in the immune regulation that links the innate and adaptive immune responses [20, 21]. Several ligands for invariant NKT cells have now been identified from microbial pathogens or synthetic screening studies; however, α-GalCer is currently only antigen used for clinical trials of NKT cell-targeted cancer immunotherapy [22–25].

This chapter summarizes the results of NKT cell-targeted clinical studies of not only adoptive cell therapy such as adoptive transfer of ex vivo-activated NKT cells but also active immunotherapy including injection of ligand-loaded antigen-presenting cells for non-small cell lung cancer (NSCLC). The progress of the latest ongoing clinical trial is also described in detail.

## 6.2 NKT Cell-Based Immunotherapy for NSCLC

Lung cancer is the most common and lethal cancer worldwide [26]. The number of newly diagnosed lung cancer cases each year is increasing, and NSCLC accounts for 80 % of the total cases. NSCLC is classified according to the histological findings, including mainly adenocarcinoma, squamous cell carcinoma, and large cell carcinoma, and it is treated based on this classification. Cytotoxic chemotherapy remains the standard treatment for inoperable advanced or recurrent NSCLC and is associated with an absolute increase in the median survival of 1.5 months [27]. The median survival time (MST) after first-line chemotherapy is around 8–12 months, which is not considered satisfactory by patients.

Intravenously injected α-GalCer-pulsed DCs effectively activated endogenous murine NKT cells in the lung parenchyma and inhibited tumor metastasis in a murine lung metastatic model [28, 29]. These murine experimental findings suggested that similar antitumor effects of NKT cells activated with α-GalCer-pulsed DCs might be expected in patients with lung cancer. Moreover, a complete inhibition of B16 melanoma metastasis in the liver was obtained even by delayed treatment with α-GalCer-pulsed DCs. Based on these in vivo effects of α-GalCer-pulsed DCs, we considered performing a clinical trial using α-GalCer-pulsed autologous DCs in patients with lung cancer.

### 6.2.1 The Preparation of APCs for NKT Cell Stimulation

We explored the autologous APC preparation method that would best present the glycolipid antigen to NKT cells, thereby inducing efficient activation of NKT cell-specific immune responses. We established an alternative APC preparation procedure that maintained the ability to activate NKT cells in vivo [30]. Briefly, peripheral blood mononuclear cells (PBMCs) were collected and cultured with granulocyte-macrophage colony-stimulating factor (GM-CSF) and interleukin-2 (IL-2) for 1 or 2 weeks, and then all cultured cells were loaded with α-GalCer and used as antigen-presenting cells. These α-GalCer-pulsed whole PBMCs cultured with GM-CSF and IL-2 are referred to as "α-GalCer-pulsed APCs" throughout the rest of this article.

These α-GalCer-pulsed APCs could induce superior expansion and activation capacity of NKT cells compared to the monocyte-derived DCs developed with IL-4 and GM-CSF. The TNF-α produced by $CD3^+$ T cells in the culture induced DC maturation during the culture period, and these matured DCs exerted potent stimulatory activity on NKT cells that enabled them to preferentially produce IFN-γ. Moreover, the cell preparation is simple, since discarding non-adherent cells or purification of $CD14^+$ monocytes is not required, which leads to minimum cell loss during the cell preparation. Therefore, the use of α-GalCer-pulsed APCs may be an ideal method for producing active NKT cell-targeted immunotherapy.

### 6.2.2 Induction of Active Immunotherapy with α-GalCer-Pulsed APCs

We have started a phase I study of α-GalCer-pulsed APCs in patients with unresectable NSCLC at Chiba University Hospital, Japan [31]. In this early clinical study, patients with no other therapeutic options after the standard treatments were enrolled (Table 6.1). Four intravenous infusions of α-GalCer-pulsed APCs were carried out with three doses, including 50 million cells (level 1), 250 million cells (level 2), and 1 billion cells (level 3)/$m^2$/injection. We first administered α-GalCer-non-pulsed APCs to test the effects of APCs themselves. No severe adverse events were observed in any of the patients, and some grade 1 or 2 adverse events were recorded. The number of circulating NKT cells number and the expression level of IFN-γ mRNA in the circulating NKT cells were enhanced after the injections of α-GalCer-pulsed APCs in one patient in the level 3 dosing group. This patient showed long-term stable disease with lung and plural metastases for more than 2 years without additional chemotherapy and survived for 59 months. The number of circulating NKT cells was modestly increased in the remaining two cases at the level 3 dose. Nine cases were clinically evaluable. Five cases had stable disease, and four cases had disease progression at the end of the study period.

**Table 6.1** The summary of NKT cell-based immunotherapy for NSCLC

| Clinical stage | Number of patients | Treatment (number of injection) | Immunological responses (number of patients) | Antitumor effects (number of patients) | References |
|---|---|---|---|---|---|
| Non-resectable c-stage IIIB, IV, recurrence | 11 | APC only (1) | NKT cell expansion in PBMC (3) | SD (3) | [28] |
| | | α-GalCer APC (4) | Elevated IFN-γ spot-forming cell number (1) | | |
| Non-resectable c-stage IIIB, IV, recurrence | 17 | α-GalCer APC (4) | NKT cell expansion in PBMC (6) | SD (5) | [29] |
| | | | Elevated IFN-γ spot-forming cell number (10) | | |
| Recurrence | 6 | α-GalCer activated NKT cell (2) | NKT cell expansion in PBMC (2) | SD (2) | [38] |
| | | | Elevated IFN-γ spot-forming cell number (3) | | |
| Resectable stage IIB, IIIA | 4 | α-GalCer APC (1) | NKT cell expansion in PBMC (2) | SD (4) | [31] |
| | | | Elevated IFN-γ spot-forming cell number (1) | | |
| | | | NKT cell accumulation and elevated IFN-γ spot-forming cell number in the tumor (4) | | |
| Non-resectable c-stage IIIB, IV, recurrence | 35 | α-GalCer APC (4) | Ongoing trial, under evaluation | Under evaluation | – |

A phase I–II study of α-GalCer-pulsed APCs was performed in patients with NSCLC in 2004–2007 [32]. The cell dose was 1 billion cells/m$^2$/injection, based on the results of the previous study. In this study, advanced or recurrent NSCLC patients refractory to standard treatment, with no other therapeutic options, were enrolled, and 17 patients completed the four injection of α-GalCer-pulsed APCs (Table 6.1). A severe adverse event occurred in one patient, who needed hospitalization to undergo anticoagulant therapy due to the exacerbation of deep vein thrombosis, which was estimated to have no clear relationship with the cell therapy by the Chiba University Quality Assurance Committee on Cell Therapy. In other patients, only minor adverse events occurred.

The peripheral blood NKT cell number was increased in six patients, and the number of α-GalCer-specific IFN-γ-producing cells in PBMCs detected by an enzyme-linked immunospot (ELISPOT) assay was elevated in ten patients. The IFN-γ producers were NKT cells and NK cells, which are subsequently stimulated by in vivo-activated NKT cells [33]. The median overall survival time of the elevated IFN-γ production group (good responder group) was significantly better than that of the IFN-γ non-elevated group (nonresponder group) (29.3 months

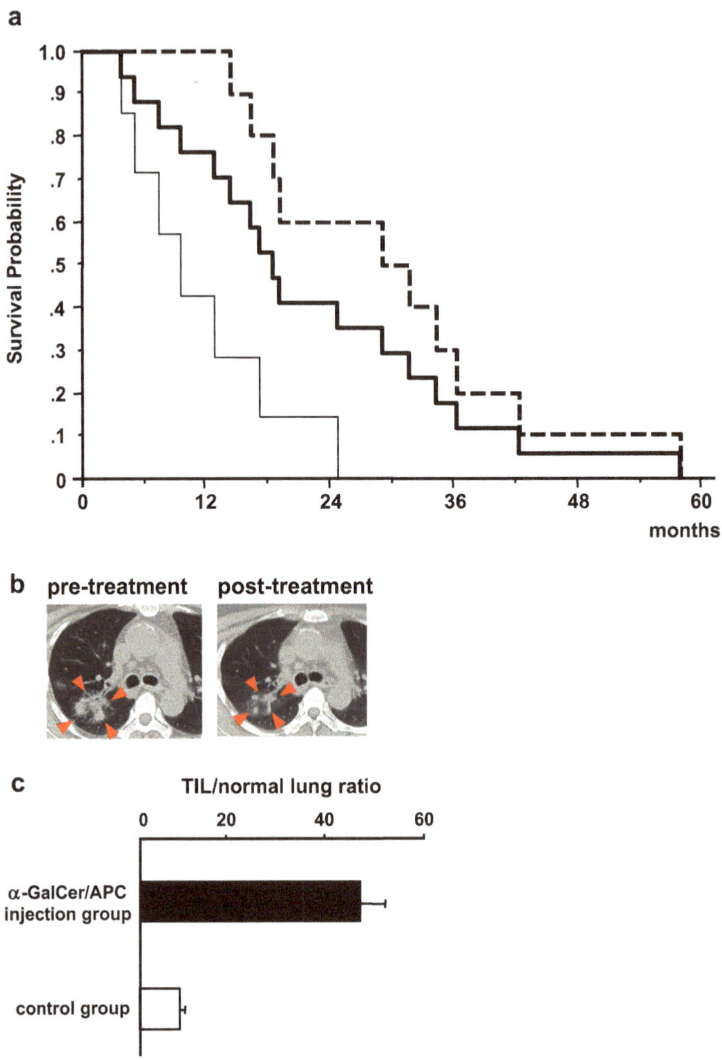


**Fig. 6.2** Clinical trial outcomes in NKT cell-based immunotherapy. (**a**) The overall survival curve of 17 patients who received an intravenous injection of α-GalCer-pulsed APCs four times. *Bold line* overall survival of all 17 cases. *Dashed line* overall survival of good responders ($n = 10$) with increased IFN-γ-producing cells. *Thin line* overall survival of poor responders ($n = 7$) without increased IFN-γ production. (**b**) Chest computed tomography of a NSCLC patient who received four times of α-GalCer-pulsed APCs. An intrapulmonary tumor (*red arrow*) is depicted. (**c**) The ratio of NKT cells in the tumor-infiltrating lymphocytes to NKT cells in the normal lung mononuclear cells

vs. 9.7 months, $p = 0.0011$, log-rank test) (Fig. 6.2a). Based on this result, the number of IFN-γ-producing cells might be useful as a marker to predict the clinical outcome in response to α-GalCer-pulsed APC treatment.

The MST of all enrolled patients was found to be around 17 months (Fig. 6.2a). This raised the possibility that the MST of all patients was superior to that of patients treated with standard chemotherapy and/or radiotherapy. These data are being confirmed by special interim study as "highly advanced medical technology" before the treatment will receive approval from the Japanese pharmaceutical affairs system.

Under this system, we have started a phase II clinical study of NKT cell-targeting immunotherapy, called Chiba-NKT, in patients with NSCLC. The aim of the study is to establish a novel second-line treatment for unresectable NSCLC. We set the investigation of overall survival time as a predefined primary end point. Thirty-five patients who are diagnosed to have advanced or recurrent NSCLC and have already received one regimen of chemotherapy are enrolled (Table 6.1). More than 30 patients have been deemed to meet the inclusion criteria and thus have already been registered. We intravenously injected α-GalCer-pulsed APCs a total of four times and some clinical responses were observed (Fig. 6.2b). This clinical study will be finished within 3 years, including a 2-year observation period.

A pilot study of α-GalCer-pulsed APCs in patients with advanced but resectable NSCLC was performed to explore the NKT cell-specific immune responses more precisely at the tumor site [34]. Four patients received 1 billion cells/$m^2$/injection of α-GalCer-pulsed APCs 1 week before surgical resection (Table 6.1). As a result, tumor-infiltrating lymphocytes spontaneously contained relatively high proportion of NKT cells in the non-injected control group. A dramatic accumulation of NKT cells in the tumor-infiltrating lymphocytes (TIL) was observed in all four patients who received single α-GalCer-pulsed APC injection in comparison to the control group (Fig. 6.2c). Moreover, single injection of α-GalCer-pulsed APCs induced enhanced IFN-γ production by tumor-infiltrating NKT cells. These results clearly indicated that α-GalCer-pulsed APCs provoked the accumulation of activated NKT cells in the tumor microenvironment even though the number of peripheral blood NKT cells seemed to low and to predict a poor response.

### 6.2.3 *Adoptive Transfer of Ex Vivo-Activated NKT Cells*

NKT cells constitute a small population with relatively high variation in human peripheral blood. Numerically and functionally decreased NKT cells have been observed in patients with several malignant diseases [35, 36]. In addition, a decrease in NKT cells was correlated with poor clinical outcome in patients with head and neck carcinoma, and NKT cell accumulation in the tumor microenvironment was correlated with a better survival of colorectal cancer and neuroblastoma, suggesting their important role in the control of tumor growth [37–39]. On the other hand, regardless of the changes in the absolute NKT cell number, the ability of NKT cells to produce IFN-γ was preserved in cancer patients, and even a small number of residual NKT cells might still have the potential to produce enough IFN-γ to antitumor responses [35]. Therefore, an intervention to recover the NKT cell number or function directly with the use of ex vivo-expanded NKT cells could potentiate the antitumor immunity against NSCLC. In addition, it has been shown that treatment with the use of specific ligands, autologous PBMCs and IL-2, can allow for the expansion of large numbers of NKT cells in vitro [40].

A dose escalation study of the adoptive transfer of ex vivo-expanded NKT cells was conducted in patients with recurrent NSCLC [41]. PBMCs from six eligible patients were collected by apheresis and were cultured with α-GalCer and IL-2 and then restimulated with α-GalCer-pulsed autologous PBMCs weekly (Table 6.1). After 2 and 3 weeks of cultivation, the entire collection of cultured cells containing expanded NKT cells was harvested, and they were injected intravenously. The number of NKT cells administered was ten million cells (level 1) or five million cells (level 2) per injection. As a result, the NKT cells originated from advanced cancer-bearing patients could be expanded sufficiently with a 1,290-fold expansion for 2 weeks and 2,380-fold for 3 weeks, and the fold expansion partially depended on the number of NKT cells presented in the pre-cultured PBMCs. The absolute number of circulating NKT cells increased in two of three cases that received a level 2 dose. IFN-γ production (mainly from NKT cells and NK cells) was augmented in all three cases that received a level 2 dose, and two of these patients showed stable disease for 9 and 12 months and survived for 2.8 and 6.3 years, respectively.

## 6.3 Future Perspectives

This chapter summarized the results of NKT cell-based immunotherapy for NSCLC and demonstrated the novel immunological responses and clinical benefits obtained during these studies. Notably, it is quite encouraging that an intravenous injection of α-GalCer-pulsed APCs induced the accumulation of activated NKT cells in the TIL, since the poor effector cell migration into the solid tumor is one of the major obstacles that need to be overcome in cancer immunotherapy. In the trial of preoperative injection of α-GalCer-pulsed APCs in patients with NSCLC, the correlation between clinical effects and immunological responses was not clear at present. Meanwhile, the increased NKT cell number in the TIL was clearly associated with tumor reduction in patients with head and neck cancer who received the combination therapy of ex vivo-activated NKT cells and α-GalCer-pulsed APCs before surgical resection [42]. It is expected that current ongoing clinical study for NSCLC will identify the role of NKT cell-based immunotherapy in prolonging the overall survival, which may also correlate with the NKT cell-specific immune responses.

As a new concept of adoptive cell therapy using NKT cells, Heczey et al. demonstrated that chimeric antigen receptors (CAR)-expressing NKT cells showed potent antitumor activity against a model of GD2-positive neuroblastoma [43]. Chimeric antigen receptors are composed of the single-chain variable fragment of the tumor-recognizing antibody with human T-cell signaling domains, such as

CD3ζ, CD28, or CD137 (4-1BB), to mimic the TCR activation and co-stimulation [5]. Recent clinical studies have demonstrated that the adoptive transfer of conventional T cells engineered to express CARs that target CD19 antigen can be highly effective, as well as toxic, in patients with chronic lymphocytic leukemia or acute lymphoblastic leukemia [44–47]. NKT cells could therefore be a potentially superior CAR carrier against some solid cancers, since NKT cells could infiltrate into some tumors, including lung cancer, as our pilot study showed, in addition to colon cancer and neuroblastoma as has been previously reported. In addition, CAR-transduced invariant NKT cells might also provide some advantages, such as posing a lower risk of graft vs. host disease induction, and these aspects must be investigated more precisely.

Another aspect of future immunotherapy is combination therapy. Immune checkpoint inhibitors have a potential to suppress the immunosuppressive environment [48, 10]. Anti-CTLA4 or anti-PD-1 therapy strongly enhances the amplitude of the antitumor responses in many poorly immunogenic tumor models. On the other hand, PD-L1 expression on tumor cells has been shown to increase in response to a strong endogenous antitumor immune response, such as IFN-γ production [10]. This phenomenon suggests that immunotherapy fails to show any clinical benefit if a simple PD1-pathway blockade is performed without preexistence of an antitumor immune response in the patient. Clinically meaningful efficacy might therefore only be achieved when a PD1-pathway blockade is applied with another therapy that could primarily provoke novel antitumor immune responses. From this point of view, NKT cell-based immunotherapy might be a good approach to provoke the immune responses against tumors, since the NKT cells could be a powerful IFN-γ producer in the tumor microenvironment [29]. To successfully induce NKT cell-based immunotherapy, overcoming the immunosuppressive tumor environment, a combination therapy with immune checkpoint inhibitors is thus considered to be an optimal candidate and we have now found sufficient concrete evidence to plan the performance of clinical trials in the near future.

**Acknowledgments** This work was supported by the Grants-in-Aid for Scientific Research (C) #24592083, MEXT (Japan), the Ministry of Health, Labor and Welfare (Japan).

## References

1. Palucka K, Banchereau J (2012) Cancer immunotherapy via dendritic cells. Nat Rev Cancer 12:265–277
2. Anguille S, Smits EL, Lion E, van Tendeloo VF, Berneman ZN (2014) Clinical use of dendritic cells for cancer therapy. Lancet Oncol 15:e257–e267
3. Restifo NP, Dudley ME, Rosenberg SA (2012) Adoptive immunotherapy for cancer: harnessing the T cell response. Nat Rev Immunol 12:269–281
4. June CH (2007) Adoptive T, cell therapy for cancer in the clinic. J Clin Invest 117:1466–1476

5. Barrett DM, Singh N, Porter DL, Grupp SA, June CH (2014) Chimeric antigen receptor therapy for cancer. Annu Rev Med 65:333–347
6. Kantoff PW, Higano CS, Shore ND, Berger ER, Small EJ, Penson DF et al (2010) Sipuleucel-T immunotherapy for castration-resistant prostate cancer. N Engl J Med 363:411–422
7. Higano CS, Small EJ, Schellhammer P, Yasothan U, Gubernick S, Kirkpatrick P et al (2010) Sipuleucel-T. Nat Rev Drug Discov 9:513–514
8. Hodi FS, O'Day SJ, McDermott DF, Weber RW, Sosman JA, Haanen JB et al (2010) Improved survival with ipilimumab in patients with metastatic melanoma. N Engl J Med 363:711–723
9. Topalian SL, Hodi FS, Brahmer JR, Gettinger SN, Smith DC, McDermott DF et al (2012) Safety, activity, and immune correlates of anti-PD-1 antibody in cancer. N Engl J Med 366:2443–2454
10. Pardoll DM (2012) The blockade of immune checkpoints in cancer immunotherapy. Nat Rev Cancer 12:252–264
11. Kawano T, Cui J, Koezuka Y, Toura I, Kaneko Y, Motoki K et al (1997) CD1d-restricted and TCR-mediated activation of Vα14 NKT cells by glycosylceramides. Science 278:1626–1629
12. Kobayashi E, Motoki K, Uchida T, Fukushima H, Koezuka Y (1995) KRN7000, a novel immunomodulator, and its antitumor activities. Oncol Res 7:529–534
13. Kawano T, Cui J, Koezuka Y, Toura I, Kaneko Y, Sato H et al (1998) Natural killer-like nonspecific tumor cell lysis mediated by specific ligand-activated Vα14 NKT cells. Proc Natl Acad Sci U S A 95:5690–5693
14. Kawano T, Nakayama T, Kamada N, Kaneko Y, Harada M, Ogura N et al (1999) Antitumor cytotoxicity mediated by ligand-activated human Vα24 NKT cells. Cancer Res 59:5102–5105
15. Metelitsa LS, Weinberg KI, Emanuel PD, Seeger RC (2003) Expression of CD1d by myelomonocytic leukemias provides a target for cytotoxic NKT cells. Leukemia 17:1068–1077
16. Stetson DB, Mohrs M, Reinhardt RL, Baron JL, Wang ZE, Gapin L et al (2003) Constitutive cytokine mRNAs mark natural killer (NK) and NK T cells poised for rapid effector function. J Exp Med 198:1069–1076
17. Smyth MJ, Crowe NY, Pellicci DG, Kyparissoudis K, Kelly JM, Takeda K et al (2002) Sequential production of interferon-gamma by NK1.1(+) T cells and natural killer cells is essential for the antimetastatic effect of α-galactosylceramide. Blood 99:1259–1266
18. Barral P, Eckl-Dorna J, Harwood NE, De Santo C, Salio M, Illarionov P et al (2008) B cell receptor-mediated uptake of CD1d-restricted antigen augments antibody responses by recruiting invariant NKT cell help in vivo. Proc Natl Acad Sci U S A 105:8345–8350
19. Fujii S, Shimizu K, Smith C, Bonifaz L, Steinman RM (2003) Activation of natural killer T cells by α-galactosylceramide rapidly induces the full maturation of dendritic cells in vivo and thereby acts as an adjuvant for combined CD4 and CD8 T cell immunity to a coadministered protein. J Exp Med 198:267–279
20. Taniguchi M, Seino K, Nakayama T (2003) The NKT cell system: bridging innate and acquired immunity. Nat Immunol 4:1164–1165
21. Fujii S, Motohashi S, Shimizu K, Nakayama T, Yoshiga Y, Taniguchi M (2010) Adjuvant activity mediated by iNKT cells. Semin Immunol 22:97–102
22. Schmieg J, Yang G, Franck RW, Tsuji M (2003) Superior protection against malaria and melanoma metastases by a C-glycoside analogue of the natural killer T cell ligand α-Galactosylceramide. J Exp Med 198:1631–1641
23. Fujii S, Shimizu K, Hemmi H, Fukui M, Bonito AJ, Chen G et al (2006) Glycolipid α-C-galactosylceramide is a distinct inducer of dendritic cell function during innate and adaptive immune responses of mice. Proc Natl Acad Sci U S A 103:11252–11257
24. Tupin E, Kinjo Y, Kronenberg M (2007) The unique role of natural killer T cells in the response to microorganisms. Nat Rev Microbiol 5:405–417
25. Fuhshuku K, Hongo N, Tashiro T, Masuda Y, Nakagawa R, Seino K et al (2008) RCAI-8, 9, 18, 19, and 49–52, conformationally restricted analogues of KRN7000 with an azetidine or a

pyrrolidine ring: Their synthesis and bioactivity for mouse natural killer T cells to produce cytokines. Bioorg Med Chem 16:950–964
26. Jemal A, Bray F, Center MM, Ferlay J, Ward E, Forman D (2011) Global cancer statistics. CA Cancer J Clin 61:69–90
27. Non-Small Cell Lung Cancer Collaborative G (2010) Chemotherapy and supportive care versus supportive care alone for advanced non-small cell lung cancer. Cochrane Database Syst Rev 12:CD007309
28. Toura I, Kawano T, Akutsu Y, Nakayama T, Ochiai T, Taniguchi M (1999) Cutting edge: inhibition of experimental tumor metastasis by dendritic cells pulsed with α-galactosylceramide. J Immunol 163:2387–2391
29. Fujii S, Shimizu K, Kronenberg M, Steinman RM (2002) Prolonged IFN-γ-producing NKT response induced with α-galactosylceramide-loaded DCs. Nat Immunol 3:867–874
30. Ishikawa E, Motohashi S, Ishikawa A, Ito T, Uchida T, Kaneko T et al (2005) Dendritic cell maturation by $CD11c^-$ T cells and $V\alpha24^+$ natural killer T-cell activation by α-galactosylceramide. Int J Cancer 117:265–273
31. Ishikawa A, Motohashi S, Ishikawa E, Fuchida H, Higashino K, Otsuji M et al (2005) A phase I study of α-galactosylceramide (KRN7000)-pulsed dendritic cells in patients with advanced and recurrent non-small cell lung cancer. Clin Cancer Res 11:1910–1917
32. Motohashi S, Nagato K, Kunii N, Yamamoto H, Yamasaki K, Okita K et al (2009) A phase I–II study of α-galactosylceramide-pulsed IL-2/GM-CSF-cultured peripheral blood mononuclear cells in patients with advanced and recurrent non-small cell lung cancer. J Immunol 182:2492–2501
33. Motohashi S, Nakayama T (2008) Clinical applications of natural killer T cell-based immunotherapy for cancer. Cancer Sci 99:638–645
34. Nagato K, Motohashi S, Ishibashi F, Okita K, Yamasaki K, Moriya Y et al (2012) Accumulation of activated invariant natural killer T cells in the tumor microenvironment after α-galactosylceramide-pulsed antigen presenting cells. J Clin Immunol 32:1071–1081
35. Motohashi S, Kobayashi S, Ito T, Magara KK, Mikuni O, Kamada N et al (2002) Preserved IFN-γ production of circulating Vα24 NKT cells in primary lung cancer patients. Int J Cancer 102:159–165
36. Molling JW, Kolgen W, van der Vliet HJ, Boomsma MF, Kruizenga H, Smorenburg CH et al (2005) Peripheral blood IFN-g-secreting $V\alpha24^+V\beta11^+$ NKT cell numbers are decreased in cancer patients independent of tumor type or tumor load. Int J Cancer 116:87–93
37. Molling JW, Langius JA, Langendijk JA, Leemans CR, Bontkes HJ, van der Vliet HJ et al (2007) Low levels of circulating invariant natural killer T cells predict poor clinical outcome in patients with head and neck squamous cell carcinoma. J Clin Oncol 25:862–868
38. Tachibana T, Onodera H, Tsuruyama T, Mori A, Nagayama S, Hiai H et al (2005) Increased intratumor Vα24-positive natural killer T cells: a prognostic factor for primary colorectal carcinomas. Clin Cancer Res 11:7322–7327
39. Metelitsa LS, Wu HW, Wang H, Yang Y, Warsi Z, Asgharzadeh S et al (2004) Natural killer T cells infiltrate neuroblastomas expressing the chemokine CCL2. J Exp Med 199:1213–1221
40. Rogers PR, Matsumoto A, Naidenko O, Kronenberg M, Mikayama T, Kato S (2004) Expansion of human $V\alpha24^+$ NKT cells by repeated stimulation with KRN7000. J Immunol Methods 285:197–214
41. Motohashi S, Ishikawa A, Ishikawa E, Otsuji M, Iizasa T, Hanaoka H et al (2006) A phase I study of in vitro expanded natural killer T cells in patients with advanced and recurrent non-small cell lung cancer. Clin Cancer Res 12:6079–6086
42. Yamasaki K, Horiguchi S, Kurosaki M, Kunii N, Nagato K, Hanaoka H et al (2011) Induction of NKT cell-specific immune responses in cancer tissues after NKT cell-targeted adoptive immunotherapy. Clin Immunol 138:255–265
43. Heczey A, Liu D, Tian G, Courtney AN, Wei J, Marinova E et al (2014) Invariant NKT cells with chimeric antigen receptor provide a novel platform for safe and effective cancer immunotherapy. Blood 124:2824–2833

44. Porter DL, Levine BL, Kalos M, Bagg A, June CH (2011) Chimeric antigen receptor-modified T cells in chronic lymphoid leukemia. N Engl J Med 365:725–733
45. Kalos M, Levine BL, Porter DL, Katz S, Grupp SA, Bagg A et al (2011) T cells with chimeric antigen receptors have potent antitumor effects and can establish memory in patients with advanced leukemia. Sci Transl Med 3:95ra73
46. Grupp SA, Kalos M, Barrett D, Aplenc R, Porter DL, Rheingold SR et al (2013) Chimeric antigen receptor-modified T cells for acute lymphoid leukemia. N Engl J Med 368:1509–1518
47. Maude SL, Frey N, Shaw PA, Aplenc R, Barrett DM, Bunin NJ et al (2014) Chimeric antigen receptor T cells for sustained remissions in leukemia. N Engl J Med 371:1507–1517
48. Shiao SL, Ganesan AP, Rugo HS, Coussens LM (2011) Immune microenvironments in solid tumors: new targets for therapy. Genes Dev 25:2559–2572

# Chapter 7
# Natural Killer Cells

**Satoshi Kokura**

**Abstract** In recent years, roles of the immune system in immune surveillance of cancer have been explored. And natural killer (NK) cells are considered to be critical players in anticancer immunity. However, cancers are able to develop mechanisms to escape NK cell attack or to induce defective NK cells.

In this review, I mentioned the role of NK cell receptors, therapeutic NK cells, and NK cell modulation in order to enhance anticancer immunity. Namely, I discuss on some of the implications of the various findings with respect to possible therapeutic approaches.

**Keywords** Natural killer cell • CD56 • NKG2D

## 7.1 Natural Killer (NK) Cells

NK cells are lymphocytes in the innate immune system that are an important component both in early infection control and in the body's defense mechanism against tumors (Fig. 7.1). NK cells lack the antigen-specific receptor characteristic of T and B cells but control the responses of these cells by regulating the balance between activating and inhibitory signaling via a group of receptors belonging to the immunoglobulin (Ig)-like receptor family and C-type lectin receptor family. Recent research has identified important molecular groups involved in the recognition mechanisms of NK cells, as well as ligands of these groups expressed on the surface of target cells. Following activation by these recognition mechanisms, NK cells destroy tumors and virus-infected cells by stimulating cytokine production, cytolytic granule release, and cytotoxic ligand expression as well as other effector functions, thereby contributing to host immune surveillance.

As with other lymphocytes, intricate mechanisms control the production and differentiation of NK cells. NK cell differentiation involves the interplay of stroma cells with IL-15, IL-2, IL-7, and other common gamma-chain cytokines, as well as with certain key transcription factors (id2, E4BP4).

---

S. Kokura, M.D., Ph.D. (✉)
Health and Medical Sciences, Kyoto Gakuen University, 1-1 Nanjo-Otani, Sogabe, Kameoka, Kyoto 621-8555, Japan
e-mail: s-kokura@koto.kpu-m.ac.jp



Y. Yamaguchi (ed.), *Immunotherapy of Cancer*,
DOI 10.1007/978-4-431-55031-0_7

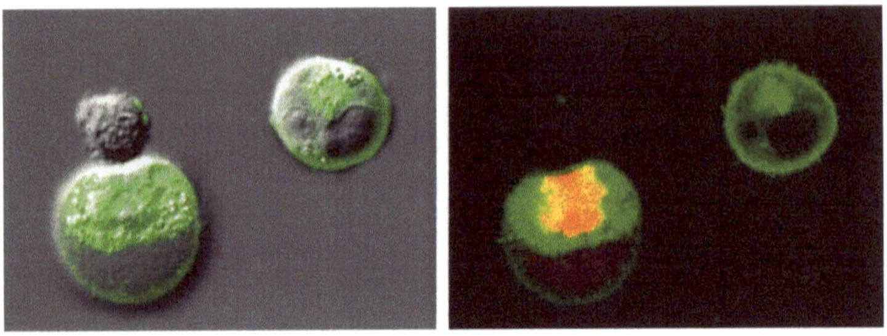

**Fig. 7.1** Supplied by Prof. A Kishi (Louis Pasteur Center for Medical Research), K562 tumor cells destroyed by NK cells were observed by confocal microscopy. K562 tumor cells were stained with 3,3′-dioctadecyloxacarbocyanine perchlorate (DiO). DiO-labeled K562 cells and NK cells were incubated in the medium containing propidium iodide (PI) for 2 h and then observed by confocal microscopy. [*Right panel*] DiO-labeled K562 cells emit a *green fluorescence*, while PI-stained compromised cells emit a *red fluorescence*. *Right cell*, a K562 cell without the attack of NK cell was still alive and stained with a *green fluorescence*. *Left cell*, when K562 cells were destroyed by NK cells, PI could enter through the membrane of K562 cells and conjugated with nucleic acid. A compromised K562 cell was stained with both *green* and *red fluorescence*. *Left panel* shows differential interference contrast (DiC) images of identical cells

## 7.1.1 Functional NK Cell Subsets

As with T and B cells, NK cells have functional subsets. Recent investigations have revealed groups of markers that differentiate these subsets. An early discovery was that subsets of NK cells, called CD56bright and CD56dim NK cells, can be differentiated by their level of CD56 expression. The two cell types function differently. CD56bright NK cells constitute a subset preferentially producing cytokines and are found primarily in lymph nodes and secondary lymph tissues, where they play an immunomodulatory role. CD56dim NK cells have very high cytotoxic activity that makes them ideal as effector cells to destroy tumors and virus-infected cells in the early immune response. In humans, most NK cells in the peripheral circulation are CD56dim NK cells. These two NK subsets can be delineated based on the relative intensity of the CD56 stain when analyzed by flow cytometry. CD56dim cells comprise the majority of circulating NK cells in the blood. These cells are highly cytotoxic but produce fewer cytokines compared with CD56bright NK cells. Furthermore, nearly all CD56dim NK cells express the killer cell immunoglobulin-like receptors (KIRs) as well as the Fcγ receptor, CD16. These receptors contribute to the high cytotoxicity of CD56dim NK cells by making them sensitive to targets with low-MHC expression or to cells bound with antibody. Conversely, CD56 bright NK cells make up a small proportion of circulating NK cells in the blood but are found in greater abundance in the lymph nodes. When stimulated, CD56bright cells are weakly cytotoxic but produce high amount of cytokines, especially IFNγ. These cells also lack expression of CD16 and KIR, which may contribute to their lower cytotoxic potential. Due to their presence in the lymph nodes and their high cytokine production, CDbright cells are believed to play an important role in shaping immune responses by regulating DCs and T cell priming toward Th1.

### 7.1.2 The Role of NK Cells as Effector Cells in the Antitumor Immune Response

Natural killer cells earned their name when researchers discovered they could kill cancer cells without prior sensitization. Many years of focused research, however, were needed to elucidate the recognition mechanism of NK cells that allows them to differentiate cancer cells from normal self cells. The recent discovery of several molecules involved in this recognition mechanism has shown that the response of NK cells to targets depends on the balance between activating and inhibitory receptors. There is a balance between activating signals produced following the recognition by activating receptors of certain ligands in a group of molecules known as stress ligands and inhibitory signals produced following recognition via inhibitory receptors of self-markers of MHC class I. Cancer cells and virus-infected target cells upregulate activating ligand expression and downregulate self-MHC expression, provoking an NK cell response. Activated NK cells destroy cancer cells and virus-infected cells by activating other effector mechanisms with their immunomodulatory ability. Activated NK cells also cause direct damage with perforin, granzyme, and other cytolytic granules; Fas ligand, TRAIL, and other death ligands; and interferons and other cytokines.

### 7.1.3 The Role of NK Cells in Tumor Immunosurveillance and the Importance of Activating Receptors

Research using many experimental models has shown that NK cells are important effector cells in tumor immunosurveillance. Investigations with Rag (-1 or -2)-deficient mice, which lack acquired immunity, experimentally validated the hypothesis that NK cells can control tumorigenesis and the growth and metastasis of established cancer cells. When activated by cytokines or toll-like receptor ligands, NK cells can trigger an antitumor immune response. The previous section noted the identification of many receptor molecules involved in NK cell activation. NKG2D, one such receptor, is expressed on NK and T cells; in the former, NKG2D plays a critical effector role by recognizing stress ligands. The expression of the NKG2D ligand in response to DNA damage and cellular stress related to tumorigenesis, and the presence of this ligand in cancer cell lines, suggest the importance of NKG2D ligand in allowing NK cells to recognize cancer cells. Studies have shown that NKG2D-mediated recognition is important for immunosurveillance for tumors by NK cells.

Cancer appears to be able to progress because certain cancer cells can avoid detection by NK cells and other components of host immunity. The survival of many cancer cells despite the watchful eye of NK cells indicates that these cells can avoid NKG2D-mediated recognition. Researchers have identified various mechanisms used by cancer cells to avoid the antitumor immune response of NK cells. One example is the constant expression of NKG2D ligand, which downregulates NKG2D in NK cells, thereby avoiding recognition. Some cancer cells produce the human NKG2D ligand MIC as soluble MIC (sMIC), made soluble by proteolytic cleavage. As with the constant expression of NKG2D ligand on the cell surface, sMIC downregulates NKG2D, thereby suppressing NK cell activity. Finally, regulatory T cells, which suppress the antitumor immune response, control both the antigen-specific immune response of T and B cells and the activation of NK cells.

### *7.1.4 Inhibitory Receptors*

Human NK cells recognize MHC-I (human HLA-ABC) molecules via the killer cell immunoglobulin-like receptor (KIR) family. Receptors in this family of molecules are stochastically expressed on mature NK cells and bind to HLA in a manner independent of the antigen presented by each MHC-I molecule. Viruses or tumors may decrease HLA expression in order to evade CTL detection; however, NK cells coevolved to become more sensitive to cells in these states. KIR/HLA interactions primarily send an inhibitory signal to the NK cell via intracellular tyrosine-based inhibitory motifs (ITIMs) on the cytoplasmic domain of inhibitory receptors or coreceptors. Therefore, cells which display lower levels of HLA will be more likely to be lysed by the NK cell. Although structurally distinct from the KIR receptors, the CD94/NKG2A receptor binds the MHC-Ib molecule, HLA-E, and sends a similar inhibitory signal via an ITIM pathway.

Overall responsiveness to activation signals is linked to the expression pattern of inhibitory receptors on each NK cell. NK cells expressing inhibitory receptors capable of binding self-MHC become fully responsive, while those not expressing these markers remain hyporesponsive [1]. However, this hyporesponsive state can be overridden upon activation, and therefore, unlicensed NK cells can contribute to antitumor or antiviral responses under certain conditions [2].

For example, KIR3DL1 binds HLA-A or B molecules mimicking the Bw4 epitope, even though a given person may not possess this epitope [3]. Therefore, KIR3DL1-expressing NK cells in an individual lacking the Bw4 epitope may be prone to an autoimmune response since these cells lack an effective "turn off" signal. However, if these cells do not encounter a self-antigen during development, they remain hyporesponsive and thus prevent autoreactivity. This process, termed "licensing" [1], "arming" [4], or "NK education" [5], is believed to be the mechanism through which NK cells achieve self-tolerance, much like the development of T cells in the thymus or B cells in the bone marrow. Licensing has been extensively characterized in the mouse [4].

### 7.1.5 Activation Receptors

While the expression patterns of inhibitory receptors are stochastic, activation receptors are more ubiquitously expressed, especially on CD56dim NK cells. NKG2D and the natural cytotoxicity receptors (NCRs: NKp30, NKp44, NKp46) are believed to be the key receptors involved in sending an activation signal when NK cells encounter a target cell in an immune synapse. However, other activation receptors, such as DNAM-1, NKG2C/CD94, 2B4, and a class of activating KIR receptors, also play a role in the activation of NK cells. In contrast to inhibitory receptors, coreceptors associated with the above proteins express immunoreceptor tyrosine-based activation motifs (ITAMs) to convey an activation signal. The ligands for many NK activation receptors are MHC-Ib molecules which are upregulated during times of cellular stress. For example, the NKG2D ligands MICA/B as well as the UL16-binding protein (ULBP) family can be upregulated during rapid proliferation [6]. The ligands for NKp30, BAT-3, and B7-H6 are expressed on stressed or transformed cells. NKp30 also recognizes the CMV pp65 protein. NKp44 has been shown to bind West Nile and dengue virus envelope glycoproteins [7], and NKp46 has been found to bind vimentin on the surface of mycobacterium tuberculosis-infected cells [8]. Both NKp44 and NKp46 have been shown to bind influenza hemagglutinin (HA); however, further ligands have not been identified. Experiments in which these NCRs are blocked result in a decrease in cytotoxicity against tumor cells not expressing influenza HA, suggesting tumors express yet unidentified NCR ligands [9].

Perhaps the most potent stimulator of NK cells is the CD16 Fc$\gamma$RIIIA. CD16 signals through ITAMs present on the accessory CD3$\zeta$ cytoplasmic accessory protein, which transmits a powerful activation signal [10]. Recognition of IgG antibodies bound to target cells allows NK cells to lyse these antibody-coated cells through a process called antibody-dependent cellular cytotoxicity (ADCC). NK cells, along with the complement system, therefore act as the final mediators to eliminate pathogenic cells recognized by the humoral immune response.

## 7.2 Therapeutic Uses of NK Cells

The therapeutic uses of NK cells fall into four categories:

1. By releasing cytoplasmic granules containing perforin and granzymes that lead to tumor cell apoptosis by caspase-dependent and caspase-independent pathways. Cytotoxic granules reorient toward the tumor cell soon after NK-tumor cell interaction and are released into the intercellular space in a calcium-dependent manner; granzymes enter tumor cells by perforin-induced membrane perforations, leading to apoptosis.
2. By death receptor-mediated apoptosis. Some NK cells express tumor-necrosis factor (TNF) family members, such as FasL, or TNF-related apoptosis-inducing

ligand (TRAIL). These ligands can induce tumor cell apoptosis by interacting with their respective receptors, Fas and TRAIL receptor (TRAILR), on tumor cells. TNF-α produced by activated NK cells can also induce tumor cell apoptosis.

3. By secreting various effector molecules, such as IFNγ, that exert antitumor functions in various ways, including restricting tumor angiogenesis and adaptive immunity. Cytokine activation or exposure to tumor cells is also associated with nitric oxide (NO) production, whereby NK cells kill target tumor cells by NO signaling.
4. Through antibody-dependent cellular cytotoxicity (ADCC) by expressing CD16 to destroy tumor cells. The antitumor activity of NK cells can be further enhanced by cytokine stimulation, such as by IL-2, IL-12, IL-18, and IL-15, or cytokines that induce IFN production.

## 7.3 Therapeutic NK Cells Derived from Several Sources

### *7.3.1 Autologous NK Cells*

Early studies at the National Cancer Institute with lymphokine-activated killer (LAK) cells essentially consisted of infusions of expanded polyclonal T cells only containing a small fraction of NK cells [11]. A number of uncontrolled trials reported the infusion of selected autologous NK cells usually combined with higher doses of IL-2 [12]. Although no side effects (except those expected from IL-2) were seen, no clear benefit of the NK cell infusions was noted. A group at the National Heart, Lung, and Blood Institute treated patients with various malignancies with increasing doses of autologous expanded NK cells (after CD3 depletion and CD56 enrichment) with the use of EBV-transformed feeder cells. After infusion of the NK cells, IL-2 (2 Mill units/$m^2$) was administered twice daily for 1 week. Except for the typical side effects of IL-2 (constitutional symptoms, thyroiditis), the infusions were well tolerated. However, no clear responses were noted in this phase I study.

In a recent study [13], autologous PBMC was depleted of CD3 cells and expanded on a feeder layer of autologous PBMC in the presence of IL-2. Seven patients with progressive, advanced melanoma or renal cancer received the cells after lymphodepleting chemotherapy (cytoxan/fludarabine), followed by administration of a high dose of recombinant IL-2 (720,000 IU/kg every 8 h). No clinical responses were noted, but the adoptively transferred NK cells persisted in the patient's circulation and were still capable of mediating ADCC with rituximab or antiHER2/neu antibody. This study is relevant because it shows that even a fairly elaborate treatment protocol involving lymphodepleting chemotherapy, extensive ex vivo NK cell expansion, and high doses of IL-2 after infusion will not necessarily result in a clinically meaningful response to infusion of unmanipulated autologous NK cells. Also, detecting NK cells in the blood circulation after infusion does not necessarily mean that they provide antitumor activity.

### 7.3.2 *Allogeneic NK Cells*

Alloreactive NK cells with KIR mismatch have been shown to demonstrate greater tumor-killing activity and the ability to better control AML relapse [14, 15]. Based on the effectiveness of NK cell alloreactivity in this and other studies, specific criteria for selecting mismatched donors have been established. Indeed, strategies using adoptively transferred human-mismatched (haploidentical) allogeneic NK cells have been more successful for cancer immunotherapy, including against leukemia and solid cancers, and have been shown to be a safe therapy causing minimal toxicity. Adoptively transferred human-mismatched allogeneic NK cells have also been shown effective in patients with various malignancies, including metastatic melanoma, renal cell carcinoma, Hodgkin's disease, and poor-prognosis AML [16]. Adoptive transfer of allogeneic NK cells that were activated and expanded with IL-15/HC in vitro has been demonstrated to be safe and potentially effective in a phase I clinical trial when used in combination with standard chemotherapy in patients with advanced non-small cell lung cancer [17]. A disadvantage to this approach is that using KIR mismatched allogeneic NK cells eventually led to immune-mediated rejection due to MHC mismatch.

### 7.3.3 *NK Cell Lines (NK-92 Cell Line)*

This cell line was established in 1994 from the peripheral blood of a 50-year-old male patient with rapidly progressive non-Hodgkin's lymphoma and has a CD56 +CD2+CD57+CD3- phenotype [18, 19]. The growth of NK-92 cells is dependent on the presence of recombinant IL-2. NK-92 cells express a large number of activating receptors including NKp30, NKp46, 2B4, NKGD/E, and CD28 and high levels of molecules associated with cytotoxicity such as perforin, granzyme, FasL, TRAIL, TWEAK, and TNF-α, while expressing few inhibitory receptors and lacking almost all of the inhibitory KIRs [20]. Therefore, NK-92 cells exhibit the characteristics of activated NK cells and are cytolytic toward a wide array of malignant cells [21].

Studies of NK-92 cells for tumor immunotherapy were carried out in mouse models and clinical trials. Immunotherapy treatment of malignant melanoma with NK-92 cells was first demonstrated in an SCID mouse model. NK-92 cells were highly cytotoxic to human melanoma cells, including MEWO melanoma cells and the WM1341 cell line, both in vitro and in vivo. NK-92 cells reduced the WM1341 primary tumor size by 40–90 % and the MEWO tumors by 30–75 % in xenografted SCID mice. Following mouse studies and ex vivo applications such as purging of leukemia, lymphoma, and CML, the NK-92 cell line has been directly infused into patients [22]. NK-92 cells are FDA approved for testing in patients with advanced malignant melanoma and renal cell carcinoma in the United States [23, 24]. This therapy is safe and has demonstrated antitumor effects toward advanced renal cell carcinoma and malignant melanoma. Irradiation of NK-92 cells with 5 Gy [16] prevents further cell division, and substantial tumor cytotoxicity can be maintained with up to 10 Gy irradiation for 48 h in vitro. No toxicity against nonmalignant allogeneic cells has been reported. Data from these trials suggest that infusion with NK-92 cells may be safe and potentially beneficial, making these cells an excellent candidate for adoptive cellular immunotherapy. To date, NK-92 is the only NK cell line that has entered clinical trials. The NK-92 cell line will serve as a platform for the future study of NK cell-based tumor immunotherapy.

## 7.4 ADCC

Antibody-targeting agents for cancer have been used in the clinic for many years and have a well-respected pedigree. Two common examples are trastuzumab for HER2 breast cancer and rituximab for CD20 lymphoma and leukemia. These therapies use both compliment-mediated cytotoxicity and ADCC to lyse antibody-coated cells. The contribution of NK cells to antitumor effects has been clearly demonstrated in trials where IL-2 was combined with rituximab in tumors previously resistant to rituximab. Therapies combining NK cells and antibody targeting have the added advantage of locally activated NK cells at the tumor site via CD16 activation. Interestingly, unlicensed NK cells were shown to be the predominant subset of NK cells responsible for potent ADCC due to their lack of inhibitory receptors for self. Recent studies further attempted to locally activate NK cells by conjugating NK-activating cytokines to the Fc region of humanized antibodies. For example, conjugations of both IL-2 and IL-12 to an anti-CD30 antibody for Hodgkin's lymphoma have shown efficacy in mouse models. These therapies may also expand NK cells at the tumor site, which may be particularly important in solid tumors where NK infiltrates are rare.

## 7.5 Indirect NK-Mediated Antitumor Immunity

NK cells act as regulatory cells when reciprocally interacted with DCs, macrophages, T cells, and endothelial cells by producing various cytokines (IFN-γ, TNF-α, and IL-10), as well as chemokines and growth factors. By producing IFN-γ, activated NK cells induce CD8+ T cells to become cytotoxic T lymphocytes (CTLs) and also help to differentiate CD4+ T cells toward a Th1 response to promote CTL differentiation [25]. NK cell-derived cytokines might also regulate antitumor antibody (Ab) production by B cells [26]. In addition, cancer cells killed by NK cells could provide tumor antigens for DCs, inducing them to mature and present antigen. By lysing surrounding DCs that have phagocytosed and processed foreign antigens, activated NK cells also could provide additional antigenic cellular debris for other DCs. Thus, activated NK cells promote antitumor immunity by regulating DC activation and maturation, as these DCs can facilitate the generation of antigen-specific CTL responses through their ability to cross-present tumor-specific antigens (derived from NK cell-mediated tumor lysis) to CD8+ T cells.

## 7.6 NK Cell Modulation

As mentioned previously, the use of cytokines alone has a potent effect on the cytolytic ability of NK cells. As such, many NK cell-activating cytokines have been administered clinically with the hopes of improving endogenous NK cell recognition and lysis of malignant cell types. IL-2 has been FDA approved to treat renal cell carcinoma and melanoma and has been shown to increase NK cell numbers in the periphery, NK cell cytotoxicity, and overall survival [27]. Although IL-2 as a single agent has provided encouraging responses, it presents several issues. First, repeated administration of high doses of IL-2 leads to a number of morbidities, including vascular leak syndrome, which severely limit the duration of IL-2 administrations and thus the longevity of the transferred NK cells [11, 28]. Second, IL-2 selectively expands the less cytotoxic CD56bright population of NK cells since these cells, rather than CD56dim NK cells, more highly express the CD25 high-affinity IL-2 receptor [29]. Third, IL-2 is known to expand and activate T regulatory cells (Tregs) which also constitutively express high-affinity IL-2Rα and can outcompete NK cells for IL-2. This Treg expansion can nullify any enhanced antitumor effects from NK cells since NK cells are highly sensitive to Treg-produced inhibitory cytokines, namely, TGF-β and IL-10. Thus, a likely therapeutic strategy involves depleting Treg cells prior to the administration of IL-2 to prevent Treg expansion and thus maximize antitumor effects. In mouse models, we showed that this approach led to a greater expansion of NK cells and greater cytotoxicity when compared with IL-2 administration alone.

IL-15 is an attractive candidate for activating NK cells in vivo as it apparently does not expand Tregs but can potently activate NK cells and expand memory CD8 T cells. Also, unlike IL-2, IL-15 equally activates CD56dim and CD56bright NK cells and leads to the expansion of both populations. Primate models have not reported severe toxicities with IL-15, and Phase I clinical trials are well underway.

Lastly, several immunomodulators have been shown to increase the sensitivity of tumor cells to NK therapies. Bortezomib, a proteasome inhibitor, is FDA approved for use against multiple myeloma and mantle cell lymphoma. Bortezomib prevents the degradation of IκB from NF-κB and thus prevents the translocation of NF-κB into the nucleus to initiate transcription. This nonspecific regulation of NF-κB has direct effects on tumor proliferation and survival [30]. However, bortezomib is also associated with an upregulation of the death receptors Fas and DR5, both of which may be triggered by an NK cell to initiate an apoptotic cascade. Furthermore, disrupting the proteasome limits the availability of peptides which may be presented on MHC-I molecules. This effectively decreases the amount of MHC-I expressed on the tumor cell and further increases its susceptibility to NK cell attack. However, bortezomib is highly toxic to NK cells, which necessitates careful timing when administering it along with an NK-based therapy. Also, there are several reports that NK cell numbers and their function in vivo can be affected by certain drugs. Aside from requiring confirmation in clinical trials, these observations alert us to several possible interactions: Dasatinib can increase NK cell numbers in vitro and in vivo [31], and imatinib can activate NK cell function through dendritic cells [32]. Furthermore, NK cells expanded in the presence of the histone deacetylase inhibitor depsipeptide display enhanced expression of the activating receptor NKG2D as well as TRAIL receptor [33], which, in addition to the perforin/granzyme system, can cause tumor cell apoptosis. Trail receptors on NK cells can also be upregulated by bortezomib [34]. Inhibition of JAK1 and JAK2 can increase the susceptibility of tumors to being killed by NK cells [35]. Lenalidomide also increases NK cell function, an effect that is abrogated by concurrent dexamethasone treatment [36]. Several studies have focused on making cancer cells more susceptible to being killed by improving synapse formation between NK cells and tumor cells. On the other hand, NK cell function is inhibited by sorafenib as a consequence of impaired phosphorylation of PI3K and ERK, which directly control NK cell reactivity [37].

## References

1. Kim S, Poursine-Laurent J, Truscott SM, Lybarger L, Song YJ, Yang L et al (2005) Licensing of natural killer cells by host major histocompatibility complex class I molecules. Nature 436 (7051):709–713
2. Sun K, Alvarez M, Ames E, Barao I, Chen M, Longo DL et al (2012) Mouse NK cell-mediated rejection of bone marrow allografts exhibits patterns consistent with Ly49 subset licensing. Blood. doi:10.1182/blood-2011-08-374314
3. Tarek N, Le Luduec JB, Gallagher MM, Zheng J, Venstrom JM, Chamberlain E et al (2012) Unlicensed NK cells target neuroblastoma following anti-GD2 antibody treatment. J Clin Invest. doi:10.1172/JCI62749
4. Raulet DH, Vance RE (2006) Self-tolerance of natural killer cells. Nat Rev Immunol 6 (7):520–531
5. Orr MT, Lanier LL (2010) Natural killer cell education and tolerance. Cell 142(6):847–856. doi:10.1016/j.cell.2010.08.031
6. Jung H, Hsiung B, Pestal K, Procyk E, Raulet DH (2012) RAE-1 ligands for the NKG2D receptor are regulated by E2F transcription factors, which control cell cycle entry. J Exp Med 209(13):2409–2422. doi:10.1084/jem.20120565
7. Hershkovitz O, Rosental B, Rosenberg LA, Navarro-Sanchez ME, Jivov S, Zilka A et al (2009) NKp44 receptor mediates interaction of the envelope glycoproteins from the West Nile and dengue viruses with NK cells. J Immunol 183(4):2610–2621. doi:10.4049/jimmunol.0802806
8. Garg A, Barnes PF, Porgador A, Roy S, Wu S, Nanda JS et al (2006) Vimentin expressed on mycobacterium tuberculosis-infected human monocytes is involved in binding to the NKp46 receptor. J Immunol 177(9):6192–6198
9. Lakshmikanth T, Burke S, Ali TH, Kimpfler S, Ursini F, Ruggeri L et al (2009) NCRs and DNAM-1 mediate NK cell recognition and lysis of human and mouse melanoma cell lines in vitro and in vivo. J Clin Invest 119(5):1251–1263. doi:10.1172/JCI36022

10. Hallett WH, Murphy WJ (2006) Positive and negative regulation of natural killer cells: therapeutic implications. Semin Cancer Biol 16(5):367–382
11. Rosenberg SA, Lotze MT, Muul LM, Leitman S, Chang AE, Ettinghausen SE et al (1985) Observations on the systemic administration of autologous lymphokine-activated killer cells and recombinant interleukin-2 to patients with metastatic cancer. N Engl J Med 313 (23):1485–1492
12. Krause SW, Gastpar R, Andreesen R, Gross C, Ullrich H, Thonigs G et al (2004) Treatment of colon and lung cancer patients with ex vivo heat shock protein 70-peptide-activated, autologous natural killer cells: a clinical phase i trial. Clin Cancer Res 10(11):3699–3707
13. Parkhurst MR, Riley JP, Dudley ME, Rosenberg SA (2011) Adoptive transfer of autologous natural killer cells leads to high levels of circulating natural killer cells but does not mediate tumor regression. Clin Cancer Res 17(19):6287–6297. doi:10.1158/1078-0432.CCR-11-134
14. Stern M, Passweg JR, Meyer-Monard S, Esser R, Tonn T, Soerensen J et al (2013) Pre-emptive immunotherapy with purified natural killer cells after haploidentical SCT: a prospective phase II study in two centers. Bone Marrow Transplant 48(3):433–438. doi:10.1038/bmt.2012.162
15. Rizzieri DA, Storms R, Chen DF, Long G, Yang Y, Nikcevich DA et al (2010) Natural killer cell-enriched donor lymphocyte infusions from A 3–6/6 HLA matched family member following nonmyeloablative allogeneic stem cell transplantation. Biol Blood Marrow Transplant 16(8):1107–1114. doi:10.1016/j.bbmt.2010.02.018
16. Tam YK, Maki G, Miyagawa B, Hennemann B, Tonn T, Klingemann HG et al (1999) Characterization of genetically altered, interleukin 2-independent natural killer cell lines suitable for adoptive cellular immunotherapy. Hum Gene Ther 10(8):1359–1373
17. Iliopoulou EG, Kountourakis P, Karamouzis MV, Doufexis D, Ardavanis A, Baxevanis CN et al (2010) A phase I trial of adoptive transfer of allogeneic natural killer cells in patients with advanced non-small cell lung cancer. Cancer Immunol Immunother 59(12):1781–1789. doi:10.1007/s00262-010-0904-3
18. Gong JH, Maki G, Klingemann HG et al (1994) Characterization of a human cell line (NK-92) with phenotypical and functional characteristics of activated natural killer cells. Leukemia 8 (4):652–658
19. Yan Y, Steinherz P, Klingemann HG, Dennig D, Childs BH, McGuirk J et al (1998) Antileukemia activity of a natural killer cell line against human leukemias. Clin Cancer Res 4(11):2859–2868
20. Tam YK, Miyagawa B, Ho VC, Klingemann HG (1999) Immunotherapy of malignant melanoma in a SCID mouse model using the highly cytotoxic natural killer cell line NK-92. J Hematother 8(3):281–290
21. Maki G, Klingemann HG, Martinson JA, Tam YK et al (2001) Factors regulating the cytotoxic activity of the human natural killer cell line, NK-92. J Hematother Stem Cell Res 10 (3):369–383
22. Klingemann HG, Wong E, Maki GA (1996) A cytotoxic NK-cell line (NK-92) for ex vivo purging of leukemia from blood. Biol Blood Marrow Transplant 2(2):68–75
23. Semino C, Martini L, Queirolo P, Cangemi G, Costa R, Alloisio A et al (1999) Adoptive immunotherapy of advanced solid tumors: an eight year clinical experience. Anticancer Res 19 (6C):5645–5649
24. Arai S, Meagher R, Swearingen M, Myint H, Rich E, Martinson J et al (2008) Infusion of the allogeneic cell line NK-92 in patients with advanced renal cell cancer or melanoma: a phase I trial. Cytotherapy 10(6):625–632. doi:10.1080/14653240802301872
25. Klingemann HG (2005) Natural killer cell-based immunotherapeutic strategies. Cytotherapy 7 (1):16–22
26. Sutlu T, Alici E (2009) Natural killer cell-based immunotherapy in cancer: current insights and future prospects. J Intern Med 266(2):154–181. doi:10.1111/j.1365-2796.2009.02121.x
27. Rosenstein M, Ettinghausen SE, Rosenberg SA et al (1986) Extravasation of intravascular fluid mediated by the systemic administration of recombinant interleukin 2. J Immunol 137 (5):1735–1742

28. Meropol NJ, Porter M, Blumenson LE, Lindemann MJ, Perez RP, Vaickus L et al (1996) Daily subcutaneous injection of low-dose interleukin 2 expands natural killer cells in vivo without significant toxicity. Clin Cancer Res 2(4):669–677
29. Hallett WH, Ames E, Alvarez M, Barao I, Taylor PA, Blazar BR et al (2008) Combination therapy using IL-2 and anti-CD25 results in augmented natural killer cell-mediated antitumor responses. Biol Blood Marrow Transplant 14(10):1088–1099. doi:10.1016/j.bbmt.2008.08.001
30. Ames E, Hallett WH, Murphy WJ (2009) Sensitization of human breast cancer cells to natural killer cell-mediated cytotoxicity by proteasome inhibition. Clin Exp Immunol 155(3):504–513. doi:10.1111/j.1365-2249.2008.03818.x
31. Tanaka J, Sugita J, Shiratori S, Shigematsu A, Imamura M (2012) Dasatinib enhances the expansion of CD56+CD3- NK cells from cord blood. Blood 119(25):6175–6176. doi:10.1182/blood-2012-03-416800
32. Borg C, Terme M, Taïeb J, Ménard C, Flament C, Robert C (2004) Novel mode of action of c-kit tyrosine kinase inhibitors leading to NK cell-dependent antitumor effects. J Clin Invest 114(3):379–388
33. Skov S, Pedersen MT, Andresen L, Straten PT, Woetmann A, Odum N (2005) Cancer cells become susceptible to natural killer cell killing after exposure to histone deacetylase inhibitors due to glycogen synthase kinase-3-dependent expression of MHC class I-related chain A and B. Cancer Res 65(23):11136–11145
34. Khuu H, Bettera DM, Cook L (2010) Adoptive transfer of escalating doses of ex vivo expanded autologous natural killer (NK) dells in patients with advanced malignancies following bortezomib treatment to sensitize to NK-TRAIL cytotoxicity. Blood 116:4296
35. Bellucci R, Nguyen HN, Martin A, Heinrichs S, Schinzel AC, Hahn WC et al (2012) Tyrosine kinase pathways modulate tumor susceptibility to natural killer cells. J Clin Invest 122(7):2369–2383. doi:10.1172/JCI58457. Epub 2012 Jun 11
36. Hsu AK, Quach H, Tai T, Prince HM, Harrison SJ, Trapani JA et al (2011) The immunostimulatory effect of lenalidomide on NK-cell function is profoundly inhibited by concurrent dexamethasone therapy. Blood 117(5):1605–1613. doi:10.1182/blood-2010-04-278432. Epub 2010 Oct 26
37. Krusch M, Salih J, Schlicke M, Baessler T, Kampa KM, Mayer F et al (2009) The kinase inhibitors sunitinib and sorafenib differentially affect NK cell antitumor reactivity in vitro. J Immunol 183(12):8286–8294. doi:10.4049/jimmunol.0902404

# Chapter 8
# γδ T Cell-Based Cancer Immunotherapy

**Hirokazu Matsushita and Kazuhiro Kakimi**

**Abstract** γδ T cell-based cancer immunotherapy is attracting attention for the treatment of various malignancies because these cells secrete Th1-type cytokines, exert potent cytotoxicity against a variety of cancer cells irrespective of MHC class I expression, and bridge innate and adaptive immunity. They comprise 1–5 % of peripheral blood mononuclear cell (PBMC); the majority of them express the Vγ9Vδ2 T cell receptor that recognizes phosphoantigens. There are two strategies to develop γδ T cell-based cancer immunotherapy. One is in vivo direct activation/expansion of γδ T cells in cancer patients; the other is adoptive transfer of ex vivo-expanded γδ T cells. Both strategies have been tested in several clinical trials. We have established a large-scale in vitro expansion method for Vγ9Vδ2 T cells using zoledronate and interleukin-2. We found that Vγ9Vδ2 T cells from patients with advanced cancer underwent extensive proliferation under these conditions. Such cultured Vγ9Vδ2 T cells retained cytokine secretion capacity and mediated cytotoxicity against a variety of cancer cell lines. Recently, we conducted phase I clinical studies to evaluate safety and potential antitumor effects of intravenous injection of Vγ9Vδ2 T cells in patients with non-small cell lung cancer (NSCLC) and intraperitoneal injection of Vγ9Vδ2 T cells for the treatment of gastric cancer with malignant ascites. γδ T cells produced IFN-γ immediately upon recognition of cancer cells in ascites. Measuring IFN-γ in patients' sera might be a good prognostic marker in lung cancer patients receiving γδ T cells. γδ T cell therapy trials are being conducted at present with safety and response results already reported for selected cases. Despite the limited number of patients in the phase I studies, the clinical response is thus far promising and warrants further study.

**Keywords** γδ T cells • IPP • Zoledronate • Adoptive transfer

---

H. Matsushita, M.D., Ph.D. • K. Kakimi, M.D., Ph.D. (✉)
Department of Immunotherapeutics, The University of Tokyo Hospital, 7-3-1 Hongo, Bunkyo-Ku, Tokyo 113-8655, Japan
e-mail: kakimi@m.u-tokyo.ac.jp



Y. Yamaguchi (ed.), *Immunotherapy of Cancer*,
DOI 10.1007/978-4-431-55031-0_8

# 8.1 γδ T Cells

## 8.1.1 Characteristics

While most human peripheral blood T lymphocytes are αβ T cells expressing T cell receptors (TCR) composed of α and β chains, 1–5 % are γδ T cells with TCR γ and δ chains. Like αβ T cells, γδ T cells are derived from bone marrow double-negative (DN) precursor cells; αβ/γδ lineage commitment occurs during the development of thymocytes. While αβ T cells express either CD4 or CD8, γδ T cells generally express neither. According to their TCR δ chain expression, human γδ T cells are divided into two subsets, Vδ1 and Vδ2. Vδ2 T cells, usually paired with Vγ9, constitute the majority of peripheral blood γδ T lymphocytes. The others, $V\delta1^+$ T cells, are found mainly within epithelia, where they function as a first line of defense against pathogens and malignancies [1, 2]. It has been reported that the gene expression profiles of human γδ T cells show a mixture of αβ T and NK cell signatures [3]. Therefore, γδ T cells are "transitional" T cells sharing features of both innate and adaptive immune systems and considered to bridge their responses. In that respect, γδ T cells are close to natural killer T (NKT) cells expressing TCR invariant chains (Vα24, Vβ11). The characteristics of these three types of lymphocytes are summarized in Table 8.1.

γδ T cells play a role in the rapid lymphoid stress-surveillance system for mycobacteria, tissue perturbation, and transformed cells. They express not only γδ TCR but also natural killer group 2 member D (NKG2D), DNAM-1, and toll-like receptors (TLRs) and recognize many stress-induced ligands on the cell surface via those receptors (Fig. 8.1). Bacteria-derived 4-hydroxy-3-methyl-but-2-enyl pyrophosphate (HMB-PP) [4] and host-derived isopentenyl pyrophosphate (IPP) or triphosphoric acid 1-adenosin-5′-yl ester 3-(3-methylbu-3-enyl) ester (ApppI) are recognized by Vγ9Vδ2 TCR (Fig. 8.1) [5, 6]. IPP is an intermediate metabolite of the mevalonate/cholesterol pathway in mammalian cells. Aminobisphosphonates such as pamidronate and zoledronate, which are clinically used to treat osteoporosis or bone metastasis of malignant tumors, inhibit farnesyl pyrophosphate (FPP) synthase that mediates the conversion of IPP and its isomer dimethylallyl pyrophosphate (DMAPP) to FPP. Thus, inhibition of FPP synthase results in increased accumulation of endogenous IPP and DMAPP [7]. Therefore, bisphosphonate is used to sensitize tumor cells to γδ T cell recognition.

The issue of how phosphoantigens are presented to Vγ9Vδ2 T cells has long been a mystery. Recently, it was discovered that phosphoantigens such as HMB-PP and IPP bind to butyrophilin 3A1 (BTN3A1) on the cell surface [8], analogous to MHC class I/peptide complex generation, and stimulate human γδ TCR in a BTN3A1-restricted manner. In addition, γδ T cells can recognize stress-induced MHC class I-related molecules A and B (MICA/B), UL16-binding proteins (ULBPs) 1–6, and retinoic acid early transcript 1 (RAET1) on the cell surface via NKG2D receptors. Nectin-2 (CD112) and PVR (CD155) are detected by γδ T cells via DNAM-1 (CD226) [9]. Danger-associated molecular patterns (DAMPs) or

Table 8.1 Comparison of αβ T cells, γδ T cells, and NKT cells

| | αβ T cell | γδ T cell | NKT cell |
|---|---|---|---|
| PBMC (%) | 65–75 | 1–5 | <1 |
| Distribution | Blood, lymphoid organ | Blood, epithelium, lymphoid organ | Blood, bone marrow, liver, lung |
| Cell surface molecule | αβ TCR, CD3, CD4/CD8 | γδ TCR, CD3, $CD4^-CD8^-$/$CD8\alpha\alpha^+$, NKG2D | Invariant TCR (Vα24, Vβ11), CD3, CD4/CD8, NK receptors |
| Antigen | MHC/peptide complex | BTN3A1/IPP, MICA/B | CD1d/glycolipid |
| MHC restriction | Yes | No | No |
| TCR diversity | Very diverse | Relatively restricted, expression variance dictated by tissue localization | Restricted |
| Cytotoxicity | Yes | Yes | Yes |
| Function | Adaptive immunity | Immune regulation, surveillance, homeostasis | Immune regulation |

*TCR* T cell receptor, *MICA/B* MHC class I-related molecules A and B, *BTN3A1* butyrophilin 3A1, *IPP* isopentenyl pyrophosphate, *PBMC* peripheral blood mononuclear cell

pathogen-associated molecular patterns (PAMPs) are also recognized by γδ T cells via pattern recognition receptors such as the TLRs [10]. γδ T cells produce cytokines such as IFN-γ, IL-17, IL-5, IL-13, IL-10, IL-4, and LT-β and chemokines like MIP-1α/β and RANTES immediately after they recognize these ligands. They also display cytotoxicity and antibody-dependent cellular cytotoxicity (ADCC) depending on antigen recognition. A rapid production of cytokines, chemokines, and other factors contributes to the recruitment of other immune cells and affects subsequent adaptive immune responses.

### 8.1.2 Immunosurveillance of Cancer by γδ T Cells

Lymphoid stress-surveillance responses of γδ T cells appear to be an initiation step in cancer immunosurveillance. γδ T cells efficiently recognize transformation-induced changes. It has been shown that mutant p53, often detected in human cancers, transcriptionally regulates the expression of mevalonate pathway genes and upregulates this pathway in tumor cells [11]. IPP and DMAPP accumulate in tumor cells with mutant p53 and are thus well recognized by Vγ9Vδ2 T cells [12]. In addition, F1-ATPase expressed on the surface of tumor cells is recognized by Vγ9Vδ2 TCRs; MICA/B as well as ULBP 1–6 expressed by different types of epithelial tumor cells are recognized by γδ T cells through NKG2D receptors [13]. Thus, γδ T cells can directly recognize stress-induced molecules on cancer

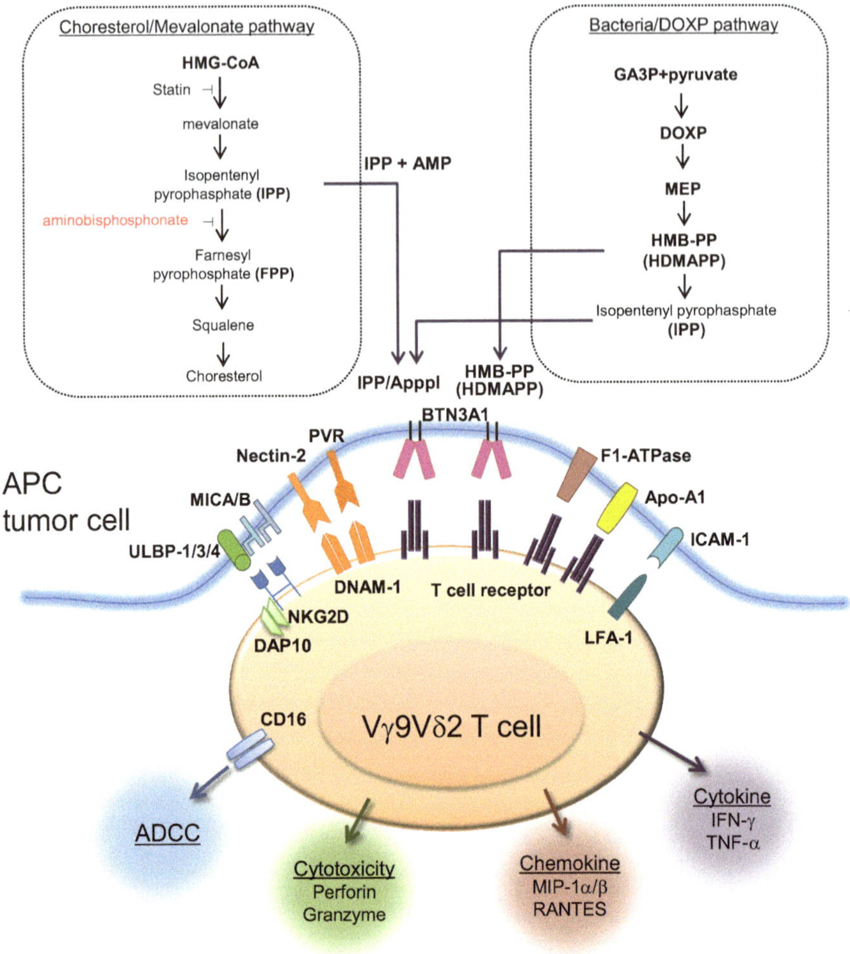


**Fig. 8.1** Ligands recognized by human γδ T cells. *Left panel*, IPP is an intermediate metabolite of the cholesterol/mevalonate pathway in mammalian cells. Pharmacological agents such as aminobisphosphonate block farnesyl pyrophosphate (FPP) synthesis and lead to increased intracellular IPP levels. Endogenous IPP accumulation is observed in various cancer cells; IPP metabolites can be converted into ApppI, which could then be presented at the cell surface with much higher affinity to γδ TCR than IPP. *Right panel*, in pathogen-infected cells (e.g., mycobacterial infection), bacterial (E)-4-hydroxy-3-methyl-but-2-enyl pyrophosphate (HMB-PP) or 4-hydroxy-3-dimethylallyl pyrophosphate (HDMAPP) in bacterial DOXP pathway could be presented. The IPP-BTN3A1 and HMB-PP-BTN3A1 complexes bind to the TCR of γδ T cells

cells and exert antitumor responses even on target cells with reduced or absent expression of MHC class I.

Tumor-infiltrating lymphocytes (TILs) often include γδ T cells. It has been reported that γδ T cells represent a sizable fraction of the TILs in approximately one fourth of lung cancers [14]. The recruitment and retention of γδ T cells in esophageal cancer are associated with their expression of adhesion molecules [15]. γδ T cell clones have been isolated from malignant ascites of colon cancer patients [16]. Cordova et al. showed that γδ T cells represent the major lymphocyte population infiltrating melanoma, and both Vδ2 and Vδ1 T cells are involved [17]. Furthermore, a higher rate of γδ T cell infiltration and percentages of Vδ2 cells correlate with early stage development of melanoma and esophageal tumors [18], and both $V\delta1^+$ and $V\delta2^+$ TILs in lung cancer killed the N592 lung cancer cell line [14]. Furthermore, Vγ9Vδ2 T cells stimulated by the synthetic phosphoantigen BrHPP lysed tumor cell lines [19]. These reports imply that γδ T cells may contribute to immunosurveillance against different cancers.

### 8.1.3 *γδ T Cells as Antigen Presenting Cells (APCs)*

In addition to the features of γδ T cells as effector cells, they are known to function as antigen-presenting cells (APCs) to cross-present microbial or tumor antigens to $CD8^+$ T cells [20]. Like dendritic cells (DCs), γδ T-APCs can take up and process soluble proteins and induce proliferation, cytotoxic activity, and cytokine production of antigen-experienced and naive $CD8^+$ T cells. Moreover, γδ T-APCs were shown to be more efficient than monocyte-derived DCs in antigen cross-presentation, which was accompanied by the upregulation of costimulatory and MHC class I molecules. Recently, it has been reported that γδ T-APCs can also present antigens to iNKT cells, which critically depends on trogocytosis of CD1d-containing membrane fragments from phosphoantigen-expressing cells [21]. Further studies will be needed to explore the utilization of such properties of human γδ T cells as APCs in cancer immunotherapy research.

## 8.2 γδ T Cell-Based Cancer Immunotherapy

### 8.2.1 *Expansion of γδ T Cells In Vivo*

Two different approaches are currently applied in γδ T cell immunotherapy (Fig. 8.2): in vivo activation and expansion of γδ T cells (Table 8.2) and adoptive transfer of ex vivo-expanded γδ T cells (Table 8.3) [22]. Fever that developed in aminobisphosphonate-treated patients was an important indicator that γδ T cells had probably been activated [23]. Four of ten patients given pamidronate who had an acute-phase reaction (fever) displayed a substantial increase in the percentage of γδ T cells in their PBMCs. Since then, strategies to activate γδ T cells by administering aminobisphosphonates such as pamidronate or zoledronate, together with interleukin-2 (IL-2), have been developed as promising cancer immunotherapies.

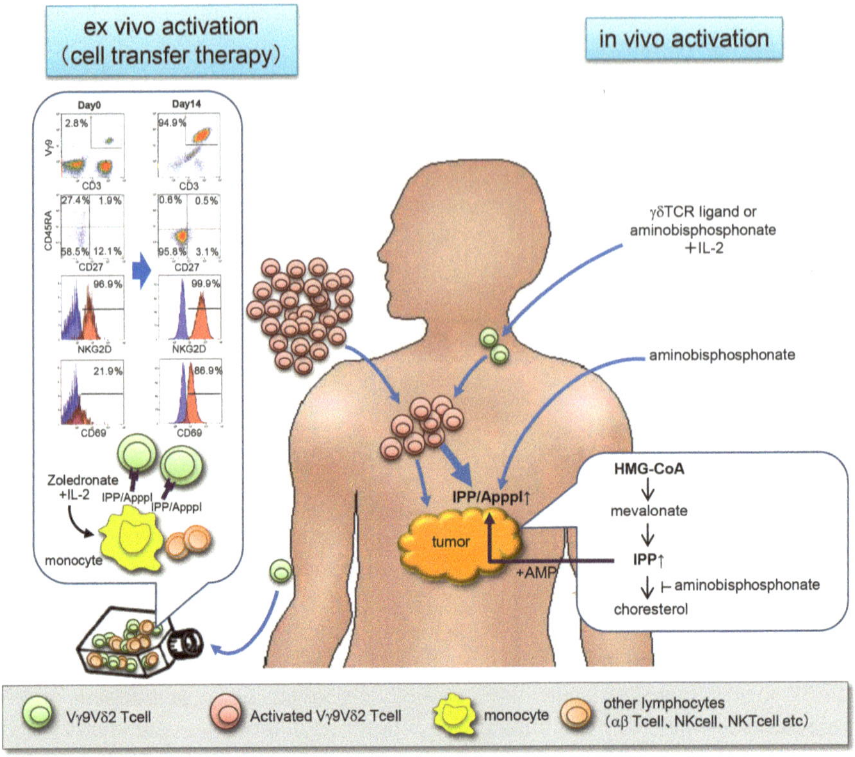


**Fig. 8.2** Strategies for γδ T cell-based immunotherapy. *Left panel*, adoptive cell transfer of in vitro-expanded γδ T cells. *Right panel*, in vivo activation of γδ T cells by phosphoantigens (e.g., BrHPP) or aminobisphosphonates and low-dose IL-2. The concomitant injection of aminobisphosphonate leads to intracellular accumulation of IPP/ApppI in tumor cells by blocking the mevalonate pathway, resulting in the sensitization of tumor cells to γδ T cells

The first clinical study of intravenous infusion of pamidronate and low-dose IL-2 was performed in patients with relapsed and/or refractory low-grade non-Hodgkin lymphoma or multiple myeloma. The activation and proliferation of γδ T cells in vivo was observed in five (55 %), and partial responses (PRs) were observed in three (33 %) of the nine patients for which expansion of γδ T cells was observed in vitro [24]. Hormone-refractory prostate cancer was treated with either zoledronate alone ($n=9$) or zoledronate in combination with IL-2 ($n=9$) [25]. No severe adverse events were reported. The response rate was 22 % in the first group and 67 % in the second group. Actual responses depended on the expansion, number, and phenotype of stimulated γδ T cells. Furthermore, this kind of therapy using zoledronate and IL-2 has been tested in other types of cancers including metastatic breast cancer, renal cell carcinoma (RCC), malignant melanoma, and acute myeloid leukemia (AML), and some clinical benefits were observed in patients with increased γδ T cells in peripheral blood [26–28].

**Table 8.2** Immunotherapy with in vivo activation of γδ T cells

| Cancer type | γδ T cell activation | Treatment | No. of patients | Results | Remarks | Ref. |
|---|---|---|---|---|---|---|
| Non-Hodgkin lymphoma multiple myeloma | Aminobisphosphonate | Pamidronate (90 mg) + IL-2 ($0.25–3 \times 10^6$ IU/m$^2$) on days 3–8 | 10 | SD 1<br>PD 8<br>NE 1 | Increased γδ T cell in those whose γδ T cells expanded well in vitro | [24] |
| | | Pamidronate (90 mg) + IL-2 ($0.25–2 \times 10^6$ IU/m$^2$) on days 1–6 (only patients whose γδ T cells proliferated in vitro) | 9 | PR 3<br>SD 2<br>PD 4 | | |
| Hormone-refractory, metastatic prostate cancer | | Zoledronate (4 mg) every 21 days | 9 | PR 1<br>SD 1<br>PD 7 | No therapy-related severe adverse events, clinical responses in patients who received both zoledronate and IL-2 | [25] |
| | | Zoledronate (4 mg) + IL-2 ($0.6 \times 10^6$ IU) every 21 days | 9 | PR 2<br>SD 4<br>PD 3 | | |
| Therapy-refractory, metastatic breast cancer (stage IV) | | Zoledronate (4 mg) + IL-2 ($1 \times 10^6$ IU) every 21 days | 10 | PR 1<br>SD 2<br>PD 7 | Correlation between increased peripheral γδ T cells and clinical outcome | [26] |
| Metastatic RCC | | Zoledronate (4 mg) on day 1+ IL-2 ($1–7 \times 10^6$ IU/m$^2$/day) on days 1–5, 8–12, and 15–19 of a 28-day course | 12 | SD 7<br>PD 1<br>N/A 4 | Diminished γδ Tcell response | [27] |
| RCC<br>Metastatic malignant melanoma<br>AML | | Zoledronate (4 mg) on day 1 + IL-2 ($2 \times 10^6$ IU/m$^2$) on days 1–6, maximum 6 cycles | 21 | PR 2<br>SD 6<br>PD 12<br>NE 1 | Increased γδ Tcell in all patients evaluated | [28] |

(continued)

**Table 8.2** (continued)

| Cancer type | γδ T cell activation | Treatment | No. of patients | Results | Remarks | Ref. |
|---|---|---|---|---|---|---|
| RCC | Ligand | BrHPP (IPH1101) (200, 600, 1,200, 1,800, and 2,400 mg/m$^2$, dose-escalating regimen) every 21 days + IL-2 ($1 \times 10^6$ IU/m$^2$/day) on days 1–7 | 28 | No description | Exploratory research, safe and feasible, γδ T cell expanded in the body | [29] |
| Colorectal cancer | | | | | | |
| Esophageal cancer | | | | | | |
| Gastric cancer | | | | | | |
| Ovarian cancer | | | | | | |
| Breast cancer | | | | | | |
| Non-Hodgkin lymphoma | | Rituximab (375 mg/m$^2$) on days 0, 7, 14, and 21 (total 4 times) + BrHPP (IPH1101) (750 mg/m$^2$) on days 8, 29, and 50 (total 3 times) +IL-2 ($8 \times 10^6$ IU/m$^2$/day) for 5 days after BrHPP injection | 38 | CR 10<br>(CR+PR 17, 45 %) | Multi-institutional phase II clinical study combined with antibody therapy, strong ADCC activity induced on second and third injections of BrHPP | [30] |

*RCC* renal cell carcinoma, *AML* acute myeloid leukemia, *CR* complete response, *PR* partial response, *SD* stable disease, *PD* progressive disease
*NE* not evaluated, *N/A* not applicable

**Table 8.3** Immunotherapy with ex vivo-activated γδ T cells

| Cancer type | Expansion conditions | Treatment | No. of patients | Results | Remarks | Ref. |
|---|---|---|---|---|---|---|
| Metastatic RCC | BrHPP (IPH1101) (3 μM) | Innacell γδ ™ (autologous γδ T cells) 1, 4, and 8 × $10^9$ cells (1,6, and 3 cases, respectively), IL-2 (2 × $10^6$ IU/$m^2$/day) for 7 days, every 21 days (total 3 times) | 10 | SD 6 | IL-2 related adverse events | [32] |
| | | | | PD 4 | | |
| RCC (after nephrectomy) | 2-methyl-3-butenyl-1-pyrophosphate (2M3B1-PP) (100 μM) | Autologous γδ T cells + IL-2 (70JRU) every 14 days, 6–12 times | 7 | No description | Exploratory research, no therapy-related severe adverse events | [33] |
| RCC with lung metastasis (after nephrectomy) | 2-methyl-3-butenyl-1-pyrophosphate (2M3B1PP) (100 μM) | Zoledronate (4 mg) + autologous γδ T cells + IL-2(5 days) every 28 days, total 6 times | 11 | CR 1 | Doubling time of tumor extended in all cases | [34] |
| | | | | SD 5 | | |
| | | | | PD 5 | | |
| Therapy-refractory, metastatic solid cancers | Zoledronate(1 μM)+ IL-2 (700 IU/ml) | Zoledronate (1 mg) + γδT cells (0.5 × $10^7$–500 × $10^7$ cells), 6–8 times injection | 15 | SD 3 | Transferred γδ T cells detected in lung, liver, spleen, and bone metastatic site | [35] |
| Melanoma | | | | PD 12 | | |
| Ovarian cancer | | | | | | |
| Colorectal cancer | | | | | | |
| Adenocarcinoma | | | | | | |
| Bile duct cancer | | | | | | |
| Duodenal carcinoma | | | | | | |
| Breast cancer | | Zoledronate (1 mg) + γδ T cells (0.5 × $10^7$–500 × $10^7$ cells) combined with hormone therapy (breast cancer) or chemotherapy | 3 | Hormone therapy: CR 1 | | |
| Cervical cancer | | | | Chemotherapy, SD 2 | | |

(continued)

**Table 8.3** (continued)

| Cancer type | Expansion conditions | Treatment | No. of patients | Results | Remarks | Ref. |
|---|---|---|---|---|---|---|
| Multiple myeloma | Zoledronate (5 μM) + IL-2 (1,000 IU/ml) | γδ T cells | 6 | No description | Exploratory research, no therapy-related severe adverse events | [36] |
| Solid cancers | Zoledronate(5 μM) + IL-2 (1,000 IU/ml) | γδ T cells | 5 | No description | Transferred γδ T cell accumulated in the body | [37] |
| | | γδ T cells combined with chemotherapy | 20 | No description | | |
| NSCLC | Zoledronate(5 μM) + IL-2 (1,000 IU/ml) | γδ T cells | 15 | SD 6 | Safe and feasible, IFN-γ detected in the sera | [38] |
| | | | | PD 6 | | |

*RCC* renal cell carcinoma, *CR* complete response, *SD* stable disease, *PD* progressive disease

While aminobisphosphonates indirectly activate γδ T lymphocytes by inhibiting FPP synthesis (a key enzyme of the mevalonate pathway) and increasing the accumulation of endogenous phosphoantigens, synthetic ligands for γδ TCR that directly activate γδ T cells have also been tested in clinical trials. The synthetic ligand, bromohydrin pyrophosphate (BrHPP), was administered together with IL-2 [29, 30] and found to induce potent γδ T cell expansion in patients. However, the antitumor activity of this approach was not clear. One of the disadvantages of in vivo activation of γδ T cells is that the response to BrHPP and IL-2 is transient and limited probably because activation-induced cell death or exhaustion of the response is caused by repeated stimulation of γδ T cells [31].

### 8.2.2 *Adoptive Transfer of Ex Vivo-Activated γδ T Cells*

The other approach is adoptive transfer of γδ T cells expanded ex vivo with IL-2 and phosphoantigen or aminobisphosphonate. Vγ9Vδ2 T cells can be expanded efficiently by coculturing PBMCs with γδ TCR ligands, such as 2-methyl-3-butenyl-1-pyrophosphate (2M3B1-PP) and BrHPP. Ex vivo-expanded γδ T cells (more than $1 \times 10^9$) have been transferred to patients with metastatic renal cell carcinoma, multiple myeloma, or non-small cell lung cancer [32–38]. Administration of γδ T cells was well tolerated, and objective clinical responses in a subset of patients were reported. The injection of zoledronate preceding the infusion of expanded γδ T cells might be a desirable strategy in patients with cancer, since zoledronate accumulates intracellular IPP/ApppI in tumor cells by blocking the mevalonate pathway, and these cells can then be recognized by Vγ9Vδ2 T cells. However, a quite high concentration of zoledronate was required to achieve optimum inhibition of FPP synthase activity in tumor cells [39]. According to the pharmacokinetic data, the serum concentration declines rapidly after infusion and might not be sufficient for the inhibition of FPP synthase activity after intravenous administration of zoledronate [40].

We have established a large-scale in vitro expansion method for Vγ9Vδ2 T cells using zoledronate and IL-2 [41, 42]. PBMC were stimulated with 5 μM zoledronate and 1,000 IU/mL IL-2. Fourteen days later, ex vivo-expanded γδ T cells were harvested and controlled for their sterility and purity. The percentage of $CD3^+TCRV\gamma9^+$ T cells in PBMC was generally 1–5 % on day 0. The dominant populations were $CD27^+CD45RA^+$ naive or $CD27^+CD45RA^-$ central memory phenotypes. When successfully stimulated, the frequency of γδ T cells can exceed 90 % of the cultured cells on day 14 (Fig. 8.2). The cultured γδ T cells upregulated NKG2D and CD69 expression and displayed a $CD27^-CD45RA^-$ effector memory phenotype (Fig. 8.2). We have shown that Vγ9Vδ2 T cells from patients with advanced cancer as well as from healthy donors undergo extensive proliferation under these conditions, and such cultured Vγ9Vδ2 T cells produce cytokines such as IFN-γ or TNF-α, while exerting cytotoxicity against a variety of cancer cell lines (Fig. 8.3).

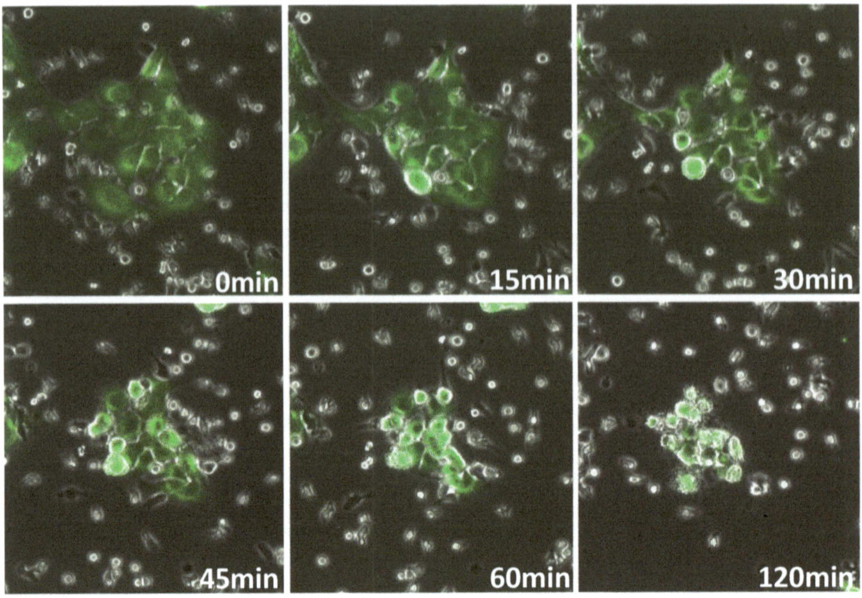


**Fig. 8.3** γδ T cell cytotoxicity. γδ T cells kill the esophageal cancer cell line, OE-21. OE-21 cells were treated with 50 mM zoledronate overnight, stained with calcein (*green*), and cultured with γδ T cells for the indicated time periods (0, 15, 30, 45, 60, and 120 min)

## 8.3 Clinical Trials of γδ T Cell Immunotherapy

### *8.3.1 γδ T Cell Therapy for the Treatment of NSCLC*

A phase I clinical trial was conducted to evaluate safety and potential antitumor effects of adoptive γδ T cell immunotherapy in patients with recurrent or advanced NSCLC [38]. Patients' PBMCs were stimulated with zoledronate and IL-2 for 14 days. γδ T cells were given intravenously every 2 weeks without additional IL-2, a total of six times. If some clinical benefit was observed, the treatment was repeated until disease progression. Fifteen patients received ex vivo-expanded γδ T cells. Adverse events were observed in five, such as influenza-like symptoms, dyspnea, weight loss, tumor pain, elevated liver enzymes, bacterial pneumonia, and radiation pneumonitis. However, there were no severe adverse events related to the adoptive γδ T cell therapy.

The number of intravenous γδ T cell infusions ranged from 3 to 12. Twelve patients completed a course of 6 injections, 3 of whom received additional infusions. According to the response evaluation criteria in solid tumors, 6 patients had stable disease (SD), whereas the remaining 6 evaluable patients experienced progressive disease (PD) 4 weeks after the sixth transfer. All patients remained alive during the study period; median survival time was 589 days, and median progression-free survival (PFS) was 126 days. We concluded that γδ T cell transfer therapy is safe and feasible in patients with NSCLC refractory to other treatment. It has been reported that median PFS was 2 months in gefitinib (250 mg/d)- or docetaxel (60 mg/m$^2$)-treated patients with advanced/metastatic NSCLC who had failed 1 or 2 chemotherapy regimens [43]. Considering that the study population receiving γδ T cell therapy for NSCLC was quite comparable to that chemotherapy study, we conclude that the former approach is promising, although the number of study subjects was small.

The peripheral γδ T cells gradually accumulated in patients' circulation with increasing numbers of infusions and maintained their function (Fig. 8.4). However, there were no associations between increases of γδ T cells in PBMC after transfer therapy and clinical responses. Whether γδ T cells infiltrated the tumor and exerted any antitumor effector activity remains to be elucidated. In this clinical trial, we found two possible biomarkers related to prognosis. An increased level of plasma IFN-γ was a potential indicator of better prognosis in the patient, although this association did not reach statistical significance. IFN-γ is well recognized to be a critical cytokine in cancer immunosurveillance. In contrast, soluble MICA in patients' plasma was related to poor prognosis. It has been reported that MICA is expressed by a variety of cancers including primary lung cancers, and its recognition by NKG2D contributes to cancer immunosurveillance. However, tumor cells escape destruction by shedding MICA molecules into the serum, which are no longer recognized by immune cells. Furthermore, soluble MICA is known to downregulate NKG2D expression on CD8 T cells, NK cells, and γδ T cells [44].

We are currently conducting a phase II clinical trial to determine the efficacy of adoptive γδ T cell therapy for the treatment of NSCLC in a larger population. We are also verifying whether IFN-γ and soluble MICA can be applied as biomarkers for better or poorer prognosis of patients under γδ T cell therapy. This will help to determine in advance which patients would be likely to benefit from this treatment in the future.

### 8.3.2 *γδ T Cell Therapy for the Treatment of Malignant Ascites from Gastric Cancer*

It is difficult to evaluate whether intravenously transferred γδ T cells can infiltrate into the tumor site and function as effector T cells, unless the tumor tissues can be obtained by surgery or biopsy. To investigate more directly whether ex vivo-expanded γδ T cells recognize and kill cancer cells in vivo, we conducted a phase I clinical trial in patients with malignant ascites due to gastric cancer [40]. Recurrent and/or advanced gastric cancers with malignant ascites are characterized by rapid progression, resistance to chemotherapy, and a poor prognosis. Expanded γδ T cells were administered intraperitoneally in four weekly infusions. The day before γδ T cell injection, patients received an intraperitoneal injection of zoledronate (1 mg) to sensitize their tumor cells to γδ T cell recognition. Seven patients were enrolled in

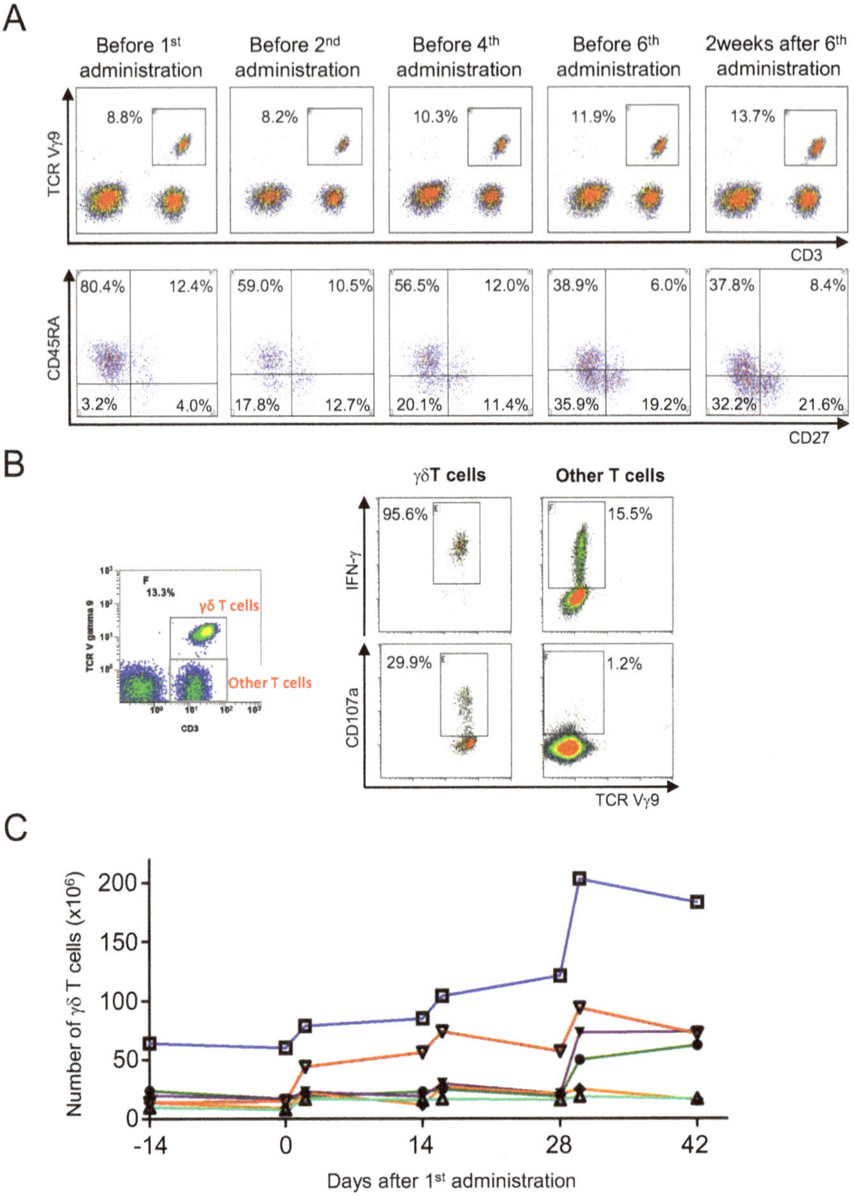


**Fig. 8.4** Accumulation of γδ T cells in peripheral blood mononuclear cells (PBMCs) during the course of treatment. PBMCs were harvested before each administration and 2 weeks after the sixth administration and were stained with anti-CD3, Vγ9, CD27, and CD45RA mAb. (**a**) Representative data showing the frequency and phenotype of γδ T cells in PBMC at the indicated time points. (**b**) Effector function of γδ T cells ($CD3^+V\gamma9^+$) and other T cells ($CD3^+V\gamma9^-$) in PBMC was evaluated in terms of IFN-γ secretion and CD107a translocation (cytotoxic granule release). (**c**) The number of γδ T cells in PBMCs of patients who received γδ T cell therapy at the indicated time points

this study. The number of γδ T cells in each injection ranged from 0.6 to 69.8 × $10^8$ (median 59.0 × $10^8$). There were no severe adverse events related to the therapy.

Intraperitoneal injection of γδ T cells allows them access to the tumor cells in the peritoneal cavity. Fluorescence microscopy revealed that many of the injected γδ T cells attached to the $EpCAM^+$ cancer cells in the ascites fluid (Fig. 8.5a). Increased IFN-γ production was detected at each γδ T cell injection, suggesting that the transferred γδ T cells recognized cancer cells and exerted antitumor effector activity. By flow cytometry, the number of cancer cells in the ascites was significantly reduced even after the first round of therapy and remained substantially lower over the course of treatment. Computed tomography revealed a significant reduction in the volume of ascites in two of seven patients (Fig. 8.5b). In one individual patient, the appearance of the ascites was initially bloody but became clear after repeated γδ T cell injections (Fig. 8.5c). Thus, injection of γδ T cells could control local malignant ascites in patients for whom no standard therapy apart from paracentesis is available. Of note, these observations indicated that adoptively transferred γδ T cells did indeed recognize cancer cells and display antitumor effector activity in vivo, when they can gain access to the cancer cells.

In this clinical trial, we found that Vγ9Vδ2 T cell injection and zoledronate treatment showed a clear clinical benefit for the local control of malignant ascites. However, this therapy is unlikely to impact on overall survival in such advanced disease, especially with metastasis, probably because γδ T cells administered into the peritoneal cavity did not migrate into the systemic circulation. Therefore, systemic therapy should be combined with intraperitoneal γδ T cell injections to obtain survival benefit. Combinations of this therapy with newly emerging molecular-targeted therapy or antibody therapy targeting immune checkpoint as well as established surgical, radiotherapy, and chemotherapy treatments are expected to improve the survival of cancer patients in future.

## 8.4 Future Directions

### *8.4.1 Enhancement of the Effector Role of γδ T Cells*

γδ TCR binding to phosphoantigen/BTN3A1 complex on tumor cells appears not to be strong enough for efficient recognition of their presence on tumor cells and exertion of antitumor effector functions. One strategy to overcome this problem is to increase the accumulation of pyrophosphate antigen IPP in cancer cells by properly timed aminobisphosphonate treatment via an appropriate injection route to enhance binding avidity [40].

Another strategy is to transduce high-affinity TCR or chimeric antigen receptors (CARs) specific for tumor antigens into γδ T cells. Transfer strategies for TCR or CAR specific for tumor antigens are now being tested and are emerging as promising approaches for adoptive immunotherapy. So far, activated $CD4^+$ and $CD8^+$ αβ

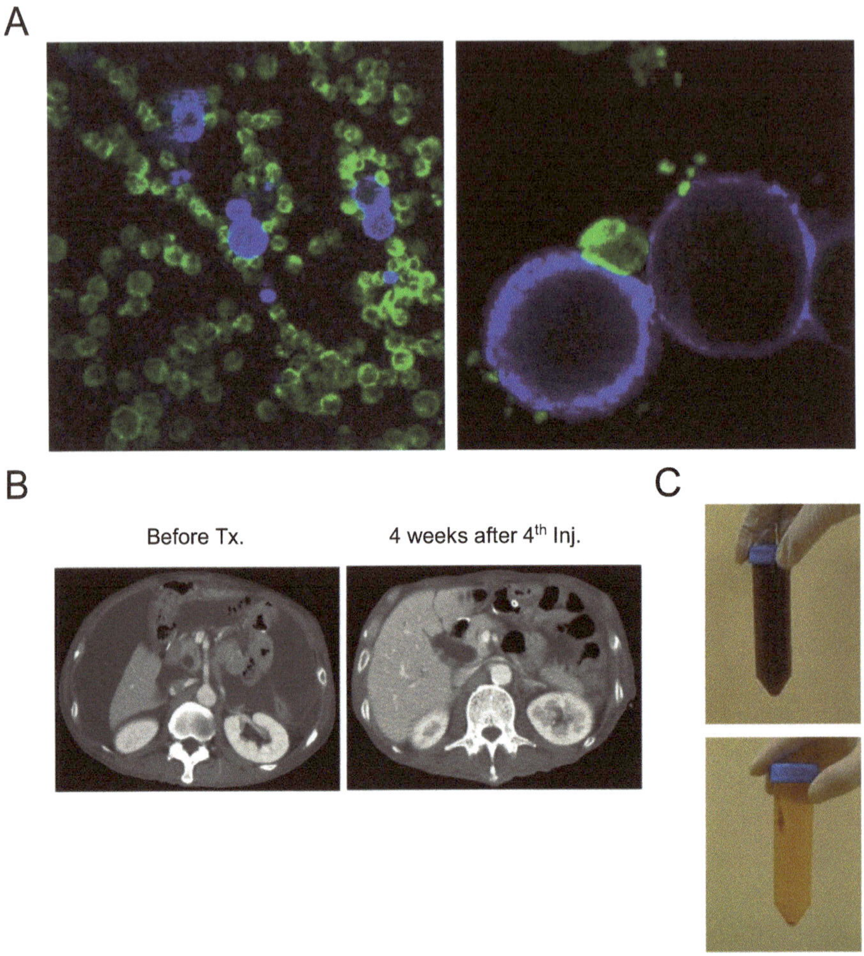


**Fig. 8.5** Clinical responses in ascites fluid and computed tomography findings on γδ T cell therapy for the treatment of gastric cancer. (**a**) The ascites fluid was harvested 24 h after Vγ9Vδ2 T cell injection; the cells were stained with anti-TCRVγ9-FITC and anti-EpCAM-APC mAbs and examined by confocal fluorescence microscopy. The EpCAM$^+$ tumor cells (*blue*) are attached to and surrounded by Vγ9Vδ2 T cells (*green*) in ascites after Vγ9Vδ2 T cell injections. Magnification is 50× on the *left* and 600× on the *right*. (**b**) Computed tomography findings demonstrating retention of a large amount of ascites before treatment (*left panels*). The amount of ascites was reduced 4 weeks (*right panels*) after four courses of Vγ9Vδ2 T cell injections. (**c**) The appearance of ascites before and after four courses of Vγ9Vδ2 T cell injections (Modified from Ref. Wada et al. [40])

T cells have generally been used for gene transfer studies. However, those T cells may produce suppressive cytokines such as IL-10 or TGF-β because activated CD4$^+$ and CD8$^+$ T cells consist of heterogeneous populations, resulting in immunosuppression as well as antitumor effects. On the other hand, expanded γδ T cells have features of a homogeneous population producing IFN-γ and TNF-α Th1 cytokines. Thus, γδ T cells may be promising effector cells for TCR or CAR gene transfer adoptive immunotherapy. Further preclinical studies should be conducted.

### *8.4.2 Regulation of Immune Suppressive Mechanisms*

It is clear that immune suppression is induced in the tumor microenvironment. Immune suppressive cells such as regulatory T cells (Tregs) and myeloid-derived suppressor cells (MDSCs) infiltrate the tumor suppressor antitumor immune responses. Furthermore, immune checkpoint molecules such as CTLA-4, PD-1, TIM-3, LAG-3, etc. are induced or expressed in the tumor microenvironment and inhibit antitumor immune responses. Therefore, to achieve effective immune responses against cancers, such immune suppressive cells and immune checkpoint molecules should be regulated, allowing infiltrating T cells to continue to survive, proliferate, produce cytokines, and mediate tumor rejection [45].

In γδ T cells, immune checkpoint molecules and expression of their ligands are not fully investigated. Dynamic changes of PD-1 and Tim-3 expression were observed in ex vivo-expanded γδ T cells (Fig. 8.6). To develop more effective γδ

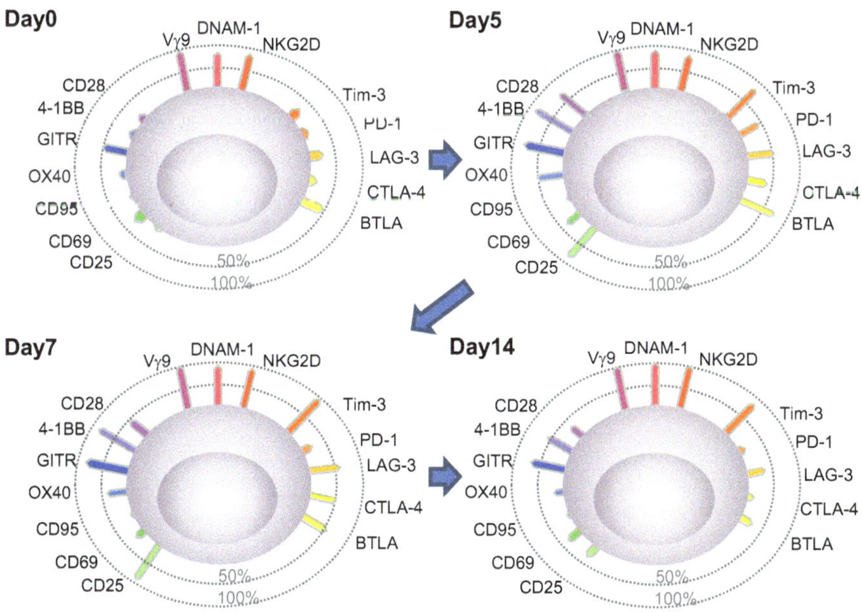


**Fig. 8.6** Dynamic changes of surface receptors and stimulatory/inhibitory molecules on γδ T cells. γδ T cells were expanded from PBMC with zoledronate and IL-2. They express TCR Vγ9, DNAM-1, and NKG2D receptors to recognize their cognate antigens or ligands. They also express both stimulatory and inhibitory molecules on their surface. Their expression changes over time

T cell-based therapy, the expression of these molecules and the corresponding ligands should be investigated so that interactions between γδ T cells and tumor cells or other immunosuppressive cells can be modulated. It is widely accepted that surgery, chemotherapies, and molecularly targeted agents can remove immune suppressive cells. Monoclonal antibodies that block immune checkpoint molecules enhance antitumor immunity. These treatments work synergistically with γδ T cell-based immunotherapy, making combinatorial strategies a key area of future clinical research.

## 8.5 Conclusions

γδ T cells can be efficiently expanded from patients' PBMC and infused back into the same patient for the treatment of cancer. Some clinical benefit was demonstrated following adoptive transfer of ex vivo-expanded γδ T cells into NSCLC patients and those with malignant ascites. The clinical efficacy of γδ T cell transfer therapy should be further evaluated in prospective clinical trials; however, combinations with established treatments and genetically engineered γδ T cells will augment their antitumor potential and contribute to future cancer therapies.

**Acknowledgments** We thank Manami Miyai, Takamichi Izumi, Takuya Takahashi, Yukari Kobayashi, Kosuke Odaira, Kaori Kambara, Nao Fujieda, and Akiko Fukuzawa for preparing the manuscript.
**Disclosure** Dr. Kazuhiro Kakimi received research support from Medinet Co. Ltd. (Yokohama, Japan). The costs of the entire γδ T cell culture production and some of the immunological assays for the phase I study performed in our institution were covered by Medinet Co. Ltd. The study sponsors had no involvement in study design; collection, analysis, and interpretation of data; writing the report; or the decision to submit the report for publication.

## References

1. Ferrarini M, Ferrero E, Dagna L, Poggi A, Zocchi MR (2002) Human gammadelta T cells: a nonredundant system in the immune-surveillance against cancer. Trends Immunol 23 (1):14–18. doi:10.1016/S1471-4906(01)02110-X
2. Narayan K, Sylvia KE, Malhotra N, Yin CC, Martens G, Vallerskog T et al (2012) Intrathymic programming of effector fates in three molecularly distinct gammadelta T cell subtypes. Nat Immunol 13(5):511–518. doi:10.1038/ni.2247
3. Pont F, Familiades J, Dejean S, Fruchon S, Cendron D, Poupot M et al (2012) The gene expression profile of phosphoantigen-specific human gammadelta T lymphocytes is a blend of alphabeta T-cell and NK-cell signatures. Eur J Immunol 42(1):228–240. doi:10.1002/eji.201141870

4. Modlin RL, Pirmez C, Hofman FM, Torigian V, Uyemura K, Rea TH et al (1989) Lymphocytes bearing antigen-specific gamma delta T-cell receptors accumulate in human infectious disease lesions. Nature 339(6225):544–548. doi:10.1038/339544a0
5. Tanaka Y, Morita CT, Tanaka Y, Nieves E, Brenner MB, Bloom BR (1995) Natural and synthetic non-peptide antigens recognized by human gamma delta T cells. Nature 375 (6527):155–158. doi:10.1038/375155a0
6. Champagne E (2011) Gammadelta T cell receptor ligands and modes of antigen recognition. Arch Immunol Ther Exp (Warsz) 59(2):117–137. doi:10.1007/s00005-011-0118-1
7. Riganti C, Massaia M, Davey MS, Eberl M (2012) Human gammadelta T-cell responses in infection and immunotherapy: common mechanisms, common mediators? Eur J Immunol 42 (7):1668–1676. doi:10.1002/eji.201242492
8. Vavassori S, Kumar A, Wan GS, Ramanjaneyulu GS, Cavallari M, El Daker S et al (2013) Butyrophilin 3A1 binds phosphorylated antigens and stimulates human gammadelta T cells. Nat Immunol 14(9):908–916. doi:10.1038/ni.2665
9. Toutirais O, Cabillic F, Le Friec G, Salot S, Loyer P, Le Gallo M et al (2009) DNAX accessory molecule-1 (CD226) promotes human hepatocellular carcinoma cell lysis by Vgamma9Vdelta2 T cells. Eur J Immunol 39(5):1361–1368. doi:10.1002/eji.200838409
10. Hayday AC (2009) Gammadelta T, cells and the lymphoid stress-surveillance response. Immunity 31(2):184–196. doi:10.1016/j.immuni.2009.08.006
11. Freed-Pastor WA, Mizuno H, Zhao X, Langerod A, Moon SH, Rodriguez-Barrueco R et al (2012) Mutant p53 disrupts mammary tissue architecture via the mevalonate pathway. Cell 148(1–2):244–258. doi:10.1016/j.cell.2011.12.017
12. Thurnher M, Nussbaumer O, Gruenbacher G (2012) Novel aspects of mevalonate pathway inhibitors as antitumor agents. Clin Cancer Res 18(13):3524–3531. doi:10.1158/1078-0432. CCR-12-0489
13. Raulet DH, Gasser S, Gowen BG, Deng W, Jung H (2013) Regulation of ligands for the NKG2D activating receptor. Annu Rev Immunol 31:413–441. doi:10.1146/annurev-immunol-032712-095951
14. Ferrarini M, Heltai S, Pupa SM, Mernard S, Zocchi R (1996) Killing of laminin receptor-positive human lung cancers by tumor infiltrating lymphocytes bearing gammadelta(+) t-cell receptors. J Natl Cancer Inst 88(7):436–441
15. Thomas ML, Badwe RA, Deshpande RK, Samant UC, Chiplunkar SV (2001) Role of adhesion molecules in recruitment of Vdelta1 T cells from the peripheral blood to the tumor tissue of esophageal cancer patients. Cancer Immunol Immunother 50(4):218–225
16. Corvaisier M, Moreau-Aubry A, Diez E, Bennouna J, Mosnier JF, Scotet E et al (2005) V gamma 9V delta 2 T cell response to colon carcinoma cells. J Immunol 175(8):5481–5488. doi:10.4049/jimmunol.175.8.5481
17. Cordova A, Toia F, La Mendola C, Orlando V, Meraviglia S, Rinaldi G et al (2012) Characterization of human gammadelta T lymphocytes infiltrating primary malignant melanomas. PLoS One 7(11), e49878. doi:10.1371/journal.pone.0049878
18. Thomas ML, Samant UC, Deshpande RK, Chiplunkar SV (2000) Gammadelta T cells lyse autologous and allogenic oesophageal tumours: involvement of heat-shock proteins in the tumour cell lysis. Cancer Immunol Immunother 48(11):653–659. doi:00480653.262 [pii]
19. Shojaei H, Oberg HH, Juricke M, Marischen L, Kunz M, Mundhenke C et al (2009) Toll-like receptors 3 and 7 agonists enhance tumor cell lysis by human gammadelta T cells. Cancer Res 69(22):8710–8717. doi:10.1158/0008-5472.CAN-09-1602
20. Brandes M, Willimann K, Moser B (2005) Professional antigen-presentation function by human gammadelta T cells. Science 309(5732):264–268. doi:10.1126/science.1110267
21. Schneiders FL, Prodohl J, Ruben JM, O'Toole T, Scheper RJ, Bonneville M et al (2014) CD1d-restricted antigen presentation by Vgamma9Vdelta2-T cells requires trogocytosis. Cancer Immunol Res 2(8):732–740. doi:10.1158/2326-6066.CIR-13-0167

22. Gomes AQ, Martins DS, Silva-Santos B (2010) Targeting gammadelta T lymphocytes for cancer immunotherapy: from novel mechanistic insight to clinical application. Cancer Res 70 (24):10024–10027. doi:10.1158/0008-5472.CAN-10-3236
23. Kunzmann V, Bauer E, Wilhelm M (1999) Gamma/delta T-cell stimulation by pamidronate. N Engl J Med 340(9):737–738. doi:10.1056/NEJM199903043400914
24. Wilhelm M, Kunzmann V, Eckstein S, Reimer P, Weissinger F, Ruediger T et al (2003) Gammadelta T cells for immune therapy of patients with lymphoid malignancies. Blood 102 (1):200–206. doi:10.1182/blood-2002-12-3665
25. Dieli F, Vermijlen D, Fulfaro F, Caccamo N, Meraviglia S, Cicero G et al (2007) Targeting human {gamma}delta} T cells with zoledronate and interleukin-2 for immunotherapy of hormone-refractory prostate cancer. Cancer Res 67(15):7450–7457. doi:10.1158/0008-5472. CAN-07-0199
26. Meraviglia S, Eberl M, Vermijlen D, Todaro M, Buccheri S, Cicero G et al (2010) In vivo manipulation of Vgamma9Vdelta2 T cells with zoledronate and low-dose interleukin-2 for immunotherapy of advanced breast cancer patients. Clin Exp Immunol 161(2):290–297. doi:10.1111/j.1365-2249.2010.04167.x
27. Lang JM, Kaikobad MR, Wallace M, Staab MJ, Horvath DL, Wilding G et al (2011) Pilot trial of interleukin-2 and zoledronic acid to augment gammadelta T cells as treatment for patients with refractory renal cell carcinoma. Cancer Immunol Immunother 60(10):1447–1460. doi:10. 1007/s00262-011-1049-8
28. Kunzmann V, Smetak M, Kimmel B, Weigang-Koehler K, Goebeler M, Birkmann J et al (2012) Tumor-promoting versus tumor-antagonizing roles of gammadelta T cells in cancer immunotherapy: results from a prospective phase I/II trial. J Immunother 35 (2):205–213. doi:10.1097/CJI.0b013e318245bb1e
29. Bennouna J, Levy V, Sicard H, Senellart H, Audrain M, Hiret S et al (2010) Phase I study of bromohydrin pyrophosphate (BrHPP, IPH 1101), a Vgamma9Vdelta2 T lymphocyte agonist in patients with solid tumors. Cancer Immunol Immunother 59(10):1521–1530. doi:10.1007/ s00262-010-0879-0
30. Fournie JJ, Sicard H, Poupot M, Bezombes C, Blanc A, Romagne F et al (2013) What lessons can be learned from gammadelta T cell-based cancer immunotherapy trials? Cell Mol Immunol 10(1):35–41. doi:10.1038/cmi.2012.39
31. Sicard H, Ingoure S, Luciani B, Serraz C, Fournie JJ, Bonneville M et al (2005) In vivo immunomanipulation of V gamma 9V delta 2 T cells with a synthetic phosphoantigen in a preclinical nonhuman primate model. J Immunol 175(8):5471–5480. doi:175/8/5471 [pii]
32. Bennouna J, Bompas E, Neidhardt EM, Rolland F, Philip I, Galea C et al (2008) Phase-I study of Innacell gammadelta, an autologous cell-therapy product highly enriched in gamma9delta2 T lymphocytes, in combination with IL-2, in patients with metastatic renal cell carcinoma. Cancer Immunol Immunother 57(11):1599–1609. doi:10.1007/s00262-008-0491-8
33. Kobayashi H, Tanaka Y, Yagi J, Osaka Y, Nakazawa H, Uchiyama T et al (2007) Safety profile and anti-tumor effects of adoptive immunotherapy using gamma-delta T cells against advanced renal cell carcinoma: a pilot study. Cancer Immunol Immunother 56(4):469–476. doi:10.1007/s00262-006-0199-6
34. Kobayashi H, Tanaka Y, Yagi J, Minato N, Tanabe K (2011) Phase I/II study of adoptive transfer of gammadelta T cells in combination with zoledronic acid and IL-2 to patients with advanced renal cell carcinoma. Cancer Immunol Immunother 60(8):1075–1084. doi:10.1007/ s00262-011-1021-7
35. Nicol AJ, Tokuyama H, Mattarollo SR, Hagi T, Suzuki K, Yokokawa K et al (2011) Clinical evaluation of autologous gamma delta T cell-based immunotherapy for metastatic solid tumours. Br J Cancer 105(6):778–786. doi:10.1038/bjc.2011.293
36. Abe Y, Muto M, Nieda M, Nakagawa Y, Nicol A, Kaneko T et al (2009) Clinical and immunological evaluation of zoledronate-activated Vgamma9gammadelta T-cell-based immunotherapy for patients with multiple myeloma. Exp Hematol 37(8):956–968. doi:10. 1016/j.exphem.2009.04.008

37. Noguchi A, Kaneko T, Kamigaki T, Fujimoto K, Ozawa M, Saito M et al (2011) Zoledronate-activated Vgamma9gammadelta T cell-based immunotherapy is feasible and restores the impairment of gammadelta T cells in patients with solid tumors. Cytotherapy 13(1):92–97. doi:10.3109/14653249.2010.515581
38. Sakamoto M, Nakajima J, Murakawa T, Fukami T, Yoshida Y, Murayama T et al (2011) Adoptive immunotherapy for advanced non-small cell lung cancer using zoledronate-expanded gammadelta Tcells: a phase I clinical study. J Immunother 34(2):202–211. doi:10.1097/CJI.0b013e318207ecfb
39. Idrees AS, Sugie T, Inoue C, Murata-Hirai K, Okamura H, Morita CT et al (2013) Comparison of gammadelta T cell responses and farnesyl diphosphate synthase inhibition in tumor cells pretreated with zoledronic acid. Cancer Sci 104(5):536–542. doi:10.1111/cas.12124
40. Wada I, Matsushita H, Noji S, Mori K, Yamashita H, Nomura S et al (2014) Intraperitoneal injection of in vitro expanded Vgamma9Vdelta2 T cells together with zoledronate for the treatment of malignant ascites due to gastric cancer. Cancer Med 3(2):362–375. doi:10.1002/cam4.196
41. Kondo M, Sakuta K, Noguchi A, Ariyoshi N, Sato K, Sato S et al (2008) Zoledronate facilitates large-scale ex vivo expansion of functional gammadelta T cells from cancer patients for use in adoptive immunotherapy. Cytotherapy 10(8):842–856. doi:10.1080/14653240802419328
42. Kondo M, Izumi T, Fujieda N, Kondo A, Morishita T, Matsushita H, et al (2011) Expansion of human peripheral blood gammadelta T cells using zoledronate. J Vis Exp (55):3182. doi:10.3791/3182
43. Maruyama R, Nishiwaki Y, Tamura T, Yamamoto N, Tsuboi M, Nakagawa K et al (2008) Phase III study, V-15-32, of gefitinib versus docetaxel in previously treated Japanese patients with non-small-cell lung cancer. J Clin Oncol 26(26):4244–4252. doi:10.1200/JCO.2007.15.0185
44. Groh V, Wu J, Yee C, Spies T (2002) Tumour-derived soluble MIC ligands impair expression of NKG2D and T-cell activation. Nature 419(6908):734–738. doi:10.1038/nature01112
45. Curran MA, Montalvo W, Yagita H, Allison JP (2010) PD-1 and CTLA-4 combination blockade expands infiltrating T cells and reduces regulatory T and myeloid cells within B16 melanoma tumors. Proc Natl Acad Sci U S A 107(9):4275–4280. doi:10.1073/pnas.0915174107

# Chapter 9
# Genetically Engineered T Cells

**Hiroaki Ikeda**

**Abstract** Despite the long-standing expectations for the potential of the cancer immunotherapy, it had been difficult to offer an efficient therapy for cancer patients until recently. However, the clinical trials of immunotherapy such as immune checkpoint inhibitor therapy or adoptive cell therapy with genetically engineered T cells have reported their significant efficacies. Lately, immunotherapy is expected not only to control tumor progression but even cure cancer in some patients. On the other hand, severe adverse events associated with efficacy have frequently been reported in clinical trials, suggesting that the assessment and control of safety will be indispensable in the future development of the therapy. Current and near-future challenges for the development of adoptive cell therapy of cancer using genetically engineered T cells will include prediction and minimization of adverse events; identification of new targets, including patient-specific mutations; improvement of T cell persistence, memory-formation capacity, and functionality; and utilization of allogeneic T cells.

**Keywords** CAR-T cell therapy • TCR-T cell therapy • Adverse events • New targets • Allogeneic cells

## Abbreviations

| | |
|---|---|
| ALL | Acute lymphoid leukemia |
| CAR | Chimeric antigen receptor |
| CR | Complete response |
| CTL | Cytotoxic T lymphocytes |
| DLI | Donor lymphocyte infusion |
| GvHD | Graft-versus-host disease |
| HSCT | Hematopoietic stem cell transplantation |
| PR | Partial response |
| RECIST | Response evaluation criteria in solid tumors |

H. Ikeda (✉)
Department of Immuno-Gene Therapy, Mie University Graduate School of Medicine,
2-174 Edobashi, Tsu, Mie 514-8507, Japan
e-mail: hikeda@clin.medic.mie-u.ac.jp



Y. Yamaguchi (ed.), *Immunotherapy of Cancer*,
DOI 10.1007/978-4-431-55031-0_9

siRNA Short inhibitory RNA
TCR T cell receptor
TIL Tumor-infiltrating lymphocytes

## 9.1 Introduction

After the proposal of cancer immunosurveillance concept by Burnet and Thomas in the late 1950s [1], people have interest in the potential of immune system to recognize and eradicate cancer and expected the application of the power of immunity to the therapy of cancer patients. However, it took more than a half century to see the expectation come true. In the recent clinical trials, immune checkpoint inhibitor therapy has shown its efficacy in the treatment of patients with various types of malignancy including melanoma, non-small cell lung carcinoma, ovarian cancer, or renal cell carcinoma. Chimeric antigen receptor (CAR)-T cell therapy has been reported to be significantly effective in the treatment of several types of hematopoietic malignancy. Reports of successful treatments of cancer patients with genetically engineered lymphocytes encouraged the academia and industry to rapidly introduce such treatments into clinical use. However, it is becoming evident that this approach holds promise, but not without severe adverse events. Particularly, the artificially engineered receptor needs high caution on the unexpected cross-reactivity to normal tissue because such receptor has never gone through the physiological checking system that excludes self-reactive T cells.

## 9.2 Chimeric Antigen Receptor (CAR)-T Cell Therapy

CAR-T cell therapy is a unique approach to confer T cells with tumor reactivity by transducing an artificial receptor gene CAR that recognizes tumor cells with high affinity [2, 3]. CAR consists of the antigen-binding region of an antibody fused with the signal-transduction domains of CD3ζ and co-stimulatory molecules such as CD28 or 4-1BB (Fig. 9.1). The signals through co-stimulatory molecules were found to be indispensable for the sufficient activation and long-term in vivo persistence of CAR-T cells. However, the selection and combination of co-stimulatory molecules for the best CAR construct remains controversial. CAR-T cell therapy aims to generate large number of tumor-reactive T cells with high affinity in relatively short period by transducing a CAR gene into patients' peripheral blood-derived T cells followed by in vitro culture before infusing the resulting tumor-reactive T cells into the patient. This approach has tested several target molecules in clinical trials [4–17].

CD19-CAR-T cell therapy that targets CD19 molecule expressed on B cells for the treatment of patients with B cell malignancy has been achieved and is one of the most successful clinical responses among the tested adoptive T cell therapy.

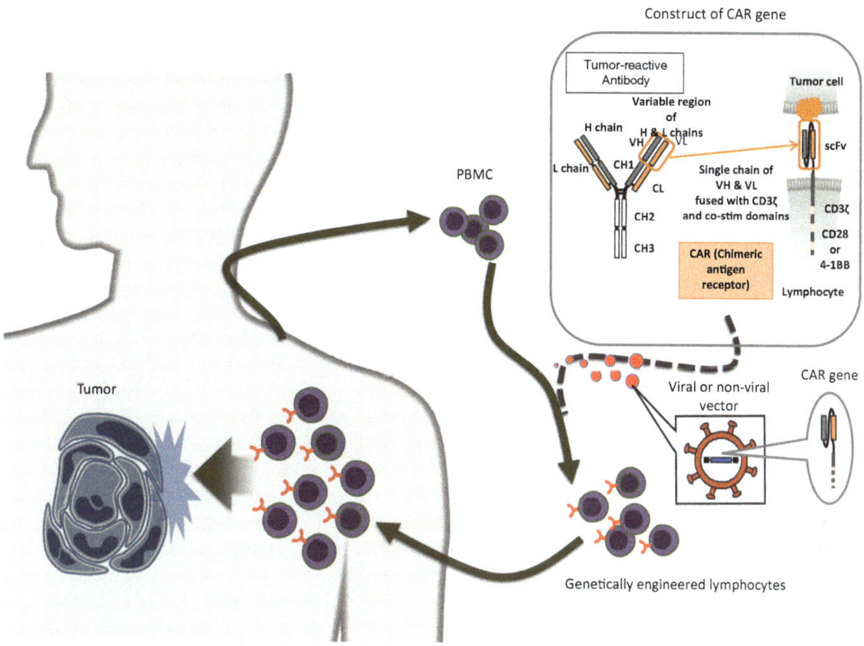


**Fig. 9.1** Chimeric antigen receptor (CAR)-T cell therapy. Patients receive the T cells that are genetically engineered to express CAR gene that consists of the antigen-binding region of an antibody fused with the signal-transduction domains of CD3ζ and co-stimulatory molecules

Specifically, a complete response (CR) rate around 90 % and sustained remission with 6-month event-free survival rate of 67 % (95 % confidence interval [CI], 51–88) and an overall survival rate of 78 % (95 % CI, 65–95) in relapsed or refractory acute lymphocytic leukemia (ALL) in children and young adults were reported [16]. The persistence of infused cells was observed in the patients with response, suggesting that the infused CAR-T cells contributed to the surveillance and control of the tumor for long period [16]. FDA recently designated this approach as a "breakthrough therapy." In clinical trials for patients with chronic lymphocytic leukemia or B cell lymphoma, the reported CR rate of CD19-CAR-T cell therapy were lower than those in ALL, but were still highly impressive [13, 14].

The success of CD19-CAR-T cell therapy for hematological malignancy encourages the development of an effective CAR-T in the treatment of solid tumors. However, there is a critical question which target (tumor-specific molecules or molecules on the dispensable cell types for survival of patients) can be useful in the CAR-T cell therapy for solid tumors. The improvement of infiltration of CAR-T cells into solid tumor is an important issue. Recent report suggested the superiority of CAR-T cells engineered to express heparanase that degrades an extracellular matrix, heparan sulfate proteoglycan, in the capacity to promote tumor T cell infiltration and antitumor activity [17]. An interesting approach to improve in vivo survival of infused CAR-T cells was reported in the clinical trial to treat patients with brain tumor using the CAR-T cells generated by the transduction of GD2-specific CAR into Epstein-Barr virus (EBV)-specific T cells [15]. By the EBV vaccination after the infusion of the CAR-T cells, the CAR-T cells received physiological stimulation through endogenous T cell receptor (TCR) and were reported to gain improved in vivo survival.

CAR-T cell therapy takes advantage of reactivity of an antibody, and therefore, the target is limited to the cell surface molecules in general. On the other hand, CAR-T cell therapy has its advantage in (1) the possibility to endow tumor reactivity not only in $CD8^+$ T cells but also in $CD4^+$ T cells and non-T cells, (2) the MHC-independent recognition, and (3) high binding affinity originated from interaction between an antibody and its ligand.

## 9.3 T Cell Receptor (TCR)-T Cell Therapy

Another approach to create tumor-reactive T cells by genetic engineering has been achieved by transducing patients' lymphocytes with TCR genes derived from tumor-specific T cell clones [18, 19] (Fig. 9.2). Rosenberg et al. in National Cancer Institute treated metastatic melanoma patients with lymphocytes genetically engineered to express a MART-1-specific TCR by retroviral vector and reported tumor regression in 2 out of 17 patients according to the Response Evaluation Criteria in Solid Tumors (RECIST) criteria in 2006 [20]. A subsequent study, in which patients were treated with lymphocytes engineered to express a MART-1-specific TCR of higher affinity, reported long-term persistence of infused cells in patients and tumor regression in 6 (30 %) of 20 patients [21]. They also observed tumor regression in 3 (19 %) of 16 patients who received mouse-derived, high-affinity gp100-specific TCR. Another study using artificially modified, high-affinity TCR recognizing NY-ESO-1 antigen demonstrated objective clinical responses in 4 (60 %) of 6 patients with synovial cell sarcomas and 5 (45 %) of 11 patients with melanoma [22]. Regarding the patients with epithelial cancers, a clinical trial with CEA (carcinoembryonic antigen)-specific TCR for the treatment of colorectal cancer [23] and a trial with MAGE-A4-specific TCR for the treatment of esophageal cancer [24] have been reported.

The existence of endogenous TCR in lymphocytes has been reported to reduce the expression of transduced TCR and cause the assembly of mispaired TCR between endogenous and transduced TCR $\alpha$ and $\beta$ subunits that produces TCR with unexpected specificity including self-reactive TCR [25]. To solve this issue, introduction of an additional disulfate bond in TCR constant region [26], replacement of human $C\alpha$ and $C\beta$ domains with corresponding murine C domains [27], or introduction of short inhibitory RNA (siRNA) specific for endogenous TCR in retrovirus vector have been proposed [28]. The genome-editing technology such as zinc finger nucleases was reported to work for the same purpose [29].

TCR-T cell therapy has an advantage being able to target intracellular antigens. On the other hand, it depends on the expression of restricted MHC molecule on the

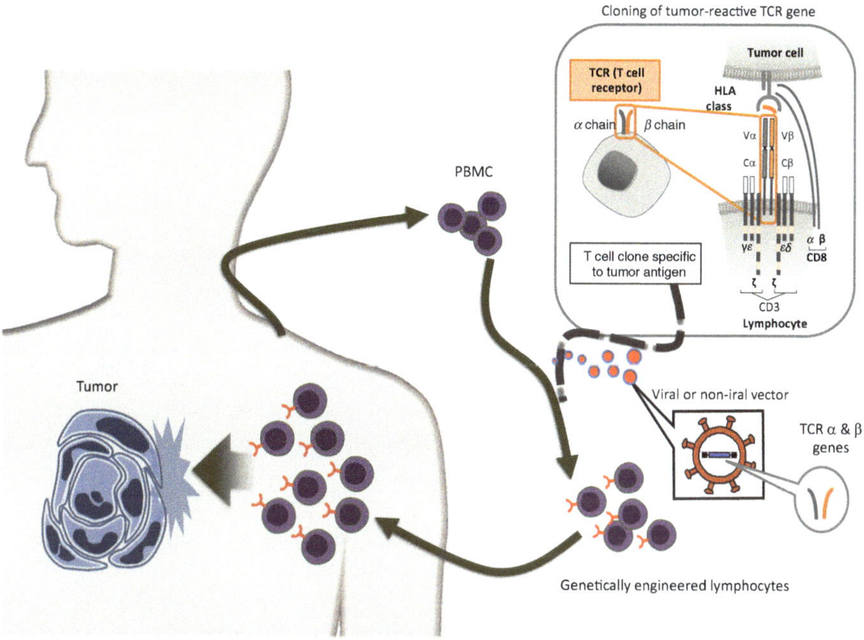


**Fig. 9.2** T cell receptor (TCR)-T cell therapy. Patients receive the T cells that are genetically engineered to express TCR α and β genes derived form a T cell clone that specifically recognizes a tumor-associated antigen

target cells. In addition, it may be critical to use a TCR with appropriate affinity. The low-affinity TCR (such as the majority of the reported TCRs for self-antigen) may not be strong enough to eradicate tumor cells. However, very high-affinity TCR is suggested to induce activation-induced cell death or anergy in T cells. Moreover, artificially generated, high-affinity TCR needs high caution on the possibility of cross-reactivity to self-tissues as discussed below.

## 9.4 Tumor-Infiltrating Lymphocytes (TIL) Therapy

Long before the development of CAR-T cell therapy or TCR-T cell therapy, there has been an attempt to isolate tumor-infiltrating lymphocytes (TIL) from tumor sample followed by the stimulation by tumor cells or tumor antigen in vitro to generate large number of tumor-reactive T cells to be infused into cancer patients [18, 19]. Identification of human tumor antigens recognized by lymphocytes started in the early 1990s and accelerated the development of adoptive immunotherapy using tumor-reactive lymphocytes [30]. Rosenberg et al. treated metastatic melanoma patients with patient's TIL and reported a 49–72 % response (CR+PR) ratio according to the RECIST criteria [18, 19, 31]. Adoptive immunotherapy with TIL has almost exclusively treated patients with malignant melanoma, with very few exceptions, because of the difficulty of isolating and expanding preexisting tumor-reacting T cells from patients with most tumor types.

## 9.5 Issues on the T Cell Persistence, Memory-Formation Capacity, and Functionality

In the process to develop an effective adoptive cell therapy with TIL, the procedure was improved to incorporate the pretreatment of patients with lymphodepleting chemotherapy and/or total body irradiation [18, 19]. These pretreatments are considered to reprogram the immunosuppressive environment of cancer patients and can induce homeostatic proliferation in infused lymphocytes. The in vitro culture became shorter to avoid the exhausted and senile phenotypes of the cultured T cells [18, 19]. These tips in developing an effective TIL therapy have been applied to the recent cell therapy with genetically engineered T cells. The improvement of T cell surviving and memory-formation capacities of the engineered T cells was reported by the addition of IL-21 or IL-15 in the in vitro culture [32, 33]. It will be important in the future development of genetically engineered T cells to find the methods to avoid T cell exhaustion by the combination with checkpoint inhibitors.

Intensive genetic engineering may offer an effective means to enhance T cell functionality and persistence in the future adoptive cell therapy. Introduction of cytokines or chemokines to enhance cytotoxic T cell function, differentiation, or tumor-homing capacity are the typical examples of this challenge [34, 35]. Introduction of molecules that cancel negative signals such as co-inhibitory signals including PD-1/PD-L1 axis has been proposed [36]. Enforced expression of heparanase that degrades an extracellular matrix was proposed to promote T cell infiltration into solid tumor as discussed above [17].

## 9.6 Adverse Events with Genetically Engineered Lymphocytes

Although significant clinical responses have been frequently observed in therapies using adoptive cell therapy with tumor-specific T cells, adverse events have observed with a high frequency in many trials. The vitiligo observed in the TIL therapy targeting melanocyte-differentiating antigens is one typical example. This is a type of adverse event caused by the antigen reactivity of the infused cells. This type of the adverse event was reported with higher severity and frequency when artificially modified high-affinity TCR or animal-derived high-affinity TCR were used. Specifically, patients treated with lymphocytes with MART-1- or gp100-specific, high-affinity TCR exhibited severe histological destruction in normal tissues where melanocytic cells were present, such as skin, eyes, and inner ears [21]. Patients with metastatic colorectal carcinoma treated with CEA-specific high-affinity TCR showed severe inflammatory colitis [23]. In these cases, the adverse events could be attributed to T cell reactivity against normal tissue where the target protein was expressed. In a trial where melanoma patients were treated with HLA-A2-restricted, MAGE-A3-specific, high-affinity TCR, three out of nine patients exhibited mental disturbance and two of them died of leukoencephalopathy [37]. In this trial, cross-reactivity of the MAGE-A3-specific TCR to MAGE-A12, which contains the same epitope sequence, was considered to be responsible. In a trial using another MAGE-A3-specific, high-affinity TCR (HLA-A1-restricted), two patients died from cardiac shock [38]. A peptide derived from titin, expressed in cardiac muscle, was found to cross-react with the TCR. Surprisingly, the titin-derived peptide possessed limited sequence similarity (five out of nine amino acids) to the MAGE-A3-derived epitope peptide.

In CD19 CAR trials, nearly all patients with response experienced adverse events that were largely mediated by cytokine release syndrome, macrophage activation syndrome, and/or tumor lysis syndrome [4–10, 12–14, 16]. In most cases, the adverse events were controllable; however, deleterious outcomes (including death) have been reported. Effectiveness seems to correlate with appearance of adverse events. In addition, long-term depletion of normal B cells has been observed in many patients with response.

When high-affinity TCRs were established by genetic modification of TCR sequences or by immunizing HLA transgenic mice, the resultant TCRs have never experienced thymic negative selection in human bodies and therefore have not gone through "inspection" for cross-reactivity to normal tissues. These receptors need high caution on the cross reactivity to normal tissues. To reduce the risk in utilizing these receptors, it is critical to develop a preclinical study strategy for predicting the adverse effects. To predict cross-reactivity, it would be informative to combine database search, core sequence analysis based on amino acid substitutions, reactivity screening of a panel of normal cells, and use of complex tissue-organ cultures. It is also important to select appropriate antigens. A strategy for monitoring patients, early detection, and treatment such as administration of anti-interleukin-6 receptor antibody should be established. Development of the technology that controls the fate of the infused cells including the incorporation of a suicide gene will be useful [39].

## 9.7 Search for New Targets

Although CAR-T cell therapy targeting CD19 has achieving a remarkable success, the search for new targets for effective cell therapy is a critical challenge. It has been difficult to find cell surface molecules that are strictly tumor specific. A surface molecule expressed in dispensable cell/tissue that represents another category for candidate targets has not been easy to find either. As discussed above, it is a critical challenge to select targets that can be used in the CAR-T cell therapy for solid tumors. It will be useful to develop a CAR-T cell therapy that can target intracellular antigens by establishing antibodies that selectively bind to MHC molecule complexed with peptide from intracellular proteins, similar to the binding manner of TCR.

The clinical responses of TIL therapy for melanoma patients were comparable to, or sometimes even higher than, those of immunotherapy with lymphocytes transduced with tumor-reacting, high-affinity TCRs [18, 19]. Moreover, far fewer adverse events have been observed in TIL therapy compared to TCR gene therapy. It has been discussed that the observation might be explained by the presence of T cells in TIL that specifically recognizes mutated proteins unique to individual tumor [40, 41]. Because the mutated antigens are nonself neo-antigens, the T cells that are reactive to them can sustain high avidity. Moreover, non-engineered native TCRs against neo-antigen are less likely to possess the cross-reactivity to normal self-tissues. Tran et al. reported that adoptive transfer of neo-antigen-specific $CD4^+$ T cells that were generated from TIL induced regression of lung and liver metastasis in a patient with cholangiocarcinoma [41]. Supported with advancing technology in next-generation sequencing, future development of adoptive cell therapy using T cells specific to unique mutations may open a new door to effective and safe cancer immunotherapy.

## 9.8 Development of Adoptive Cell Therapy with Allogeneic T Cells

If we can utilize allogeneic lymphocytes for the adoptive T cell therapy, it will offer an off-the-shelf cell product that can be applied to the patients timely when required to be infused with quality-controlled manner. Recent significant progress in genome-editing technology has suggested the possibility of reducing the induction of Graft-versus-host disease (GvHD) that is caused by the alloreactivity of the infused lymphocytes against host tissues and inhibiting the rejection of the infused cells by host immune system, by the deletion of the molecules critical to the immunological recognition of allogeneic targets [29]. Induced pluripotent stem cells (iPS cells) will also be useful to generate allogeneic T cell products [42], although several critical issues including the risk of tumorigenicity need to be controlled. We utilized the siTCR vector that silences the expression of endogenous TCR in the genetically engineered T cells by siRNA sequences to develop TCR gene therapy using allogeneic T cells because it might reduce the capacity of allogeneic cells to induce GvHD [43]. These T cells will be applicable to donor lymphocyte infusion (DLI) therapy following allogeneic hematopoietic stem cell transplantation (HSCT) for the treatment of hematological malignancy (Fig. 9.3).

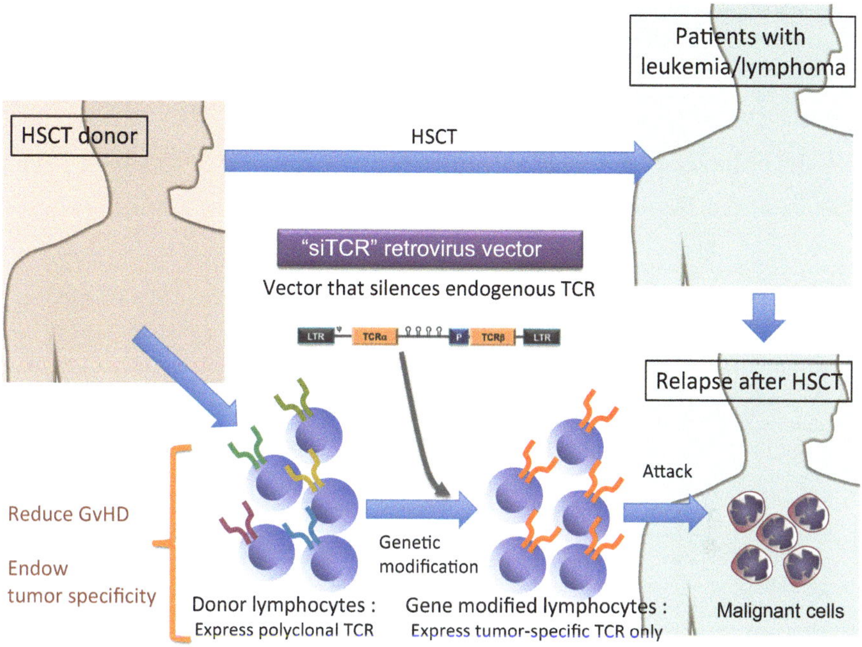


**Fig. 9.3** Efficient and safe donor lymphocyte infusion by the transduction of tumor-specific TCR with siTCR vector. A siTCR vector encodes α and β chains of TCR genes of interest and siRNA sequences targeting the constant regions of endogenous TCR. TCR genes for transduction are codon optimized to avoid the influence of the siRNA. The leukemia/lymphoma patient who relapsed after HSCT will receive donor lymphocyte infusion therapy with reduced capacity to induce GvHD and enhanced specificity to tumor antigen by the use of genetically engineered T cells with siTCR vector

## 9.9 Conclusion

After a long controversy regarding the existence of immunosurveillance of tumors, we can now confidently discuss the efficient and safe application of tumor immunity to control and even cure the cancer. Future subjects for scientific and regulatory challenges include minimization and prediction of adverse events; the regulatory harmonization in handling of personalized cell products; identification of the new target molecules for effective and safe CARs and TCRs (including T cells against patients' unique mutation-derived neo-antigen); strategies for enhancing surviving capacity, memory formation, and functionality of the infused T cell products; and the development of allogeneic or cell line-based T cell therapy. When these challenges are overcome, we envisage that genetically engineered lymphocytes will become an indispensable tool for the effective treatment of multiple types of cancer.

**Acknowledgments** This work was supported by the Project for Development of Innovative Research on Cancer Therapeutics (P-DIRECT); the Grant-in-Aid for Scientific Research from the Ministry of Education, Culture, Sports, Science and Technology of Japan; the Grant-in-Aid for Scientific Research from the Ministry of Health, Labour and Welfare of Japan; and Japan Agency for Medical Research and Development (AMED).

**Conflict of Interest** Hiroaki Ikeda is provided with research funding from Takara Bio Inc.

## References

1. Dunn GP, Bruce AT, Ikeda H et al (2002) Cancer immunoediting: from immunosurveillance to tumor escape. Nat Immunol 3:991–998
2. Sadelain M, Brentjens R, Riviere I (2009) The promise and potential pitfalls of chimeric antigen receptors. Curr Opin Immunol 21:215–223
3. Gill S, June CH (2015) Going viral: chimeric antigen receptor T-cell therapy for hematological malignancies. Immunol Rev 263(1):68–89
4. Savoldo B, Ramos CA, Liu E et al (2011) CD28 costimulation improves expansion and persistence of chimeric antigen receptor-modified T cells in lymphoma patients. J Clin Invest 121:1822–1826
5. Porter DL, Levine BL, Kalos M et al (2011) Chimeric antigen receptor-modified T cells in chronic lymphoid leukemia. N Engl J Med 365:725–733
6. Kalos M, Levine BL, Porter DL et al (2011) T cells with chimeric antigen receptors have potent antitumor effects and can establish memory in patients with advanced leukemia. Sci Trans Med 3:95ra73
7. Kochenderfer JN, Dudley ME, Feldman SA et al (2012) B-cell depletion and remissions of malignancy along with cytokine-associated toxicity in a clinical trial of anti-CD19 chimeric-antigen-receptor-transduced T cells. Blood 119:2709–2720
8. Brentjents RJ, Riviere I, Park JH et al (2011) Safety and persistence of adoptively transferred autologous CD19-targeted T cells in patients with relapsed or chemotherapy refractory B-cell leukemias. Blood 118(18):4817–4828
9. Till BG, Jensen MC, Wang J et al (2012) CD20-specific adoptive immunotherapy for lymphoma using a chimeric antigen receptor with both CD28 and 4-1BB domains: pilot clinical trial results. Blood 119:3940–3950
10. Brentjens R, Yeh R, Bernal Y et al (2010) Treatment of chronic lymphocytic leukemia with genetically targeted autologous T cells: case report of an unforeseen adverse event in a phase I clinical trial. Mol Ther 18:666–668
11. Morgan RA, Yang JC, Kitano M et al (2010) Case report of a serious adverse event following the administration of T cells transduced with a chimeric antigen receptor recognizing ERBB2. Mol Ther 18:843–851
12. Brentjens R, Davila ML, Riviere I et al (2013) CD19-targeted T cells rapidly induce molecular remissions in adults with chemotherapy-refractory acute lymphoblastic leukemia. Sci Transl Med 5(177):177ra38
13. Kochenderfer JN, Dudley ME, Carpenter RO et al (2013) Donor-derived CD19-targeted T cells cause regression of malignancy persisting after allogeneic hematopoietic stem cell transplantation. Blood 122:4129–4139
14. Kochenderfer JN, Dudley ME, Kassim SH et al (2015) Chemotherapy-refractory diffuse large B-cell lymphoma and indolent B-cell malignancies can be effectively treated with autologous T cells expressing an anti-CD19 chimeric antigen receptor. J Clin Oncol 33(6):540–549

15. Louis CU, Savoldo B, Dotti G et al (2011) Antitumor activity and long-term fate of chimeric antigen receptor-positive T cells in patients with neuroblastoma. Blood 18(23):6050–6056
16. Maude SL, Frey N, Shaw PA et al (2014) Chimeric antigen receptor T cells for sustained remissions in leukemia. N Engl J Med 371(16):1507–1517
17. Caruana I, Savoldo B, Hoyos V et al (2015) Heparanase promotes tumor infiltration and antitumor activity of CAR-redirected T lymphocytes. Nat Med 21:524–529
18. Restifo NP, Dudley ME, Rosenberg SA (2012) Adoptive immunotherapy for cancer: harnessing the T cell response. Nat Rev Immunol 12(4):269–281
19. Resenberg SA, Restifo NP (2015) Adoptive cell transfer as personalized immunotherapy for human cancer. Science 348(6230):62–68
20. Morgan RA, Dudley ME, Wunderlich JR et al (2006) Cancer regression in patients after transfer of genetically engineered lymphocytes. Science 314:126–129
21. Johnson LA, Morgan RA, Dudley ME et al (2009) Gene therapy with human and mouse T-cell receptors mediates cancer regression and targets normal tissues expressing cognate antigen. Blood 114:535–546
22. Robbins PF, Morgan RA, Feldman SA et al (2011) Tumor regression in patients with metastatic synovial cell sarcoma and melanoma using genetically engineered lymphocytes reactive with NY-ESO-1. J Clin Oncol 29:917–924
23. Parkhurst MR et al (2011) T cells targeting carcinoembryonic antigen can mediate regression of metastatic colorectal cancer but induce severe transient colitis. Mol Ther 19:620–626
24. Kageyama S, Ikeda H, Miyahara Y et al (2015) Adoptive transfer of MAGE-A4 T-cell receptor gene-transduced lymphocytes in patients with recurrent esophageal cancer. Clin Cancer Res 21(10):2268–2277
25. Bendle GM, Linnemann C, Hooijkaas AI et al (2010) Lethal graft-versus-host disease in mouse models of T cell receptor gene therapy. Nat Med 6(5):565–570
26. Cohen CJ, Li YF, El-Gamil M et al (2007) Enhanced antitumor activity of T cells engineered to express T-cell receptors with a second disulfide bond. Cancer Res 67(8):3898–3903
27. Cohen CJ, Zhao Y, Zheng Z et al (2006) Enhanced antitumor activity of murine-human hybrid T-cell receptor (TCR) in human lymphocytes is associated with improved pairing and TCR/CD3 stability. Cancer Res 66(17):8878–8886
28. Okamoto S, Mineno J, Ikeda H et al (2009) Improved expression and reactivity of transduced tumor-specific TCRs in human lymphocytes by specific silencing of endogenous TCR. Cancer Res 69(23):9003–9011
29. Provasi E, Genovese P, Lombardo A et al (2012) Editing T cell specificity towards leukemia by zinc finger nucleases and lentiviral gene transfer. Nat Med 18(5):807–815
30. Boon T, Coulie PG, Van den Eynde BJ et al (2006) Human T cell responses against melanoma. Annu Rev Immunol 24:175–208
31. Rosenberg SA (2011) Cell transfer immunotherapy for metastatic solid cancer–what clinicians need to know. Nat Rev Clin Oncol 8:577–585
32. Chapuis AG, Ragnarsson GB, Nguyen HN et al (2013) Transferred WT1-reactive CD8+ T cells can mediate antileukemic activity and persist in post-transplant patients. Sci Transl Med 5(174):174ra27
33. Butler MO, Friedlander P, Milstein MI et al (2011) Establishment of antitumor memory in humans using in vitro-educated CD8+ T cells. Sci Transl Med 3(80):80ra34
34. Karkar SP, Muranski P, Kaiser A et al (2010) Tumor-specific CD8+ T cells expressing interleukin-12 eradicate established cancers in lymphodepleted hosts. Cancer Res 70(17): 6725–6734
35. Asai H, Fujiwara H, An J et al (2013) Co-introduced functional CCR2 potentiates in vivo anti-lung cancer functionality mediated by T cells double gene-modified to express WT1-specific T-cell receptor. PLoS One 8(2):e56820
36. Prosser ME, Brown CE, Shami AF et al (2012) Tumor PD-L1 co-stimulates primary human CD8(+) cytotoxic T cells modified to express a PD1:CD28 chimeric receptor. Mol Immunol 51(3–4):263–272

37. Morgan RA, Chinnasamy N, Abate-Daga D et al (2013) Cancer regression and neurological toxicity following anti-MAGE-A3 TCR gene therapy. J Immunother 36(2):133–151
38. Linette GP, Stadtmauer EA, Maus MV et al (2013) Cardiovascular toxicity and titin cross-reactivity of affinity-enhanced T cells in myeloma and melanoma. Blood 122(6):863–871
39. Di Stasi A, Tey SK, Dotti G et al (2011) Inducible apoptosis as a safety switch for adoptive cell therapy. N Engl J Med 365(18):1673–1683
40. Robbins PF, Lu YC, El-Gami M et al (2013) Mining exomic sequencing data to identify mutated antigens recognized by adoptively transferred tumor-reactive T cells. Nat Med 19(6): 747–752
41. Tran E, Turcotte S, Gros A et al (2014) Cancer immunotherapy based on mutation-specific CD4+ T cells in a patient with epithelial cancer. Science 344(6184):641–645
42. Themeli M, Kloss CC, Ciriello G et al (2013) Generation of tumor-targeted human T lymphocytes from induced pluripotent stem cells for cancer therapy. Nat Biotechnol 31(10): 928–933
43. Ikeda H, Ueno H, Tawara I et al (2014) Tumor-specific TCR-engineered donor lymphocyte infusion therapy with reduced GVHD induction utilizing novel retrovirus vector silencing endogenous TCR expression American Society of Hematology 56th Annual Meeting, San Francisco, 2014

# Part IV
# Vaccine Therapy

# Chapter 10
# Peptide Vaccine

**Koji Kono**

**Abstract** Although induction of antitumor immune responses through cancer vaccine is theoretically promising and would be straightforward, it is currently difficult to prove the clinical benefits of cancer vaccine except for one phase III trial that has documented improved overall survival with the vaccine, Sipuleucel-T. In contrast, immune checkpoint blockade with anti-CTLA4 mAb and anti-PD-1 mAb has demonstrated clear evidence of objective responses including improved overall survival and tumor shrinkage, driving renewed enthusiasm for cancer immunotherapy in multiple cancer types. We are now facing new era of cancer immunotherapy with a great hope for the anticancer therapy.

## 10.1 Introduction

Recent approval of Sipuleucel-T, which is cancer vaccine consisting of PSA-based antigens with activated antigen presenting cells (APCs) and lymphocyte mixture for hormone-refractory prostate cancer, paved the way to antigen-specific cancer immunotherapy [1]. Moreover, immune checkpoint blockade with therapeutic mAbs such as anti-CTLA4 mAb and anti-PD-1 mAb for melanoma implicates a new era of the immunotherapy in the anticancer strategy [2, 3]. Due to recent advances in molecular and cellular immunology, it has been reported that several immunogenic tumor antigens expressed by tumor cells are identified, and the characterization of tumor-specific cytotoxic T lymphocytes (CTLs) in cancer patients was successfully performed [4, 5]. These observations have attracted the interest of researchers and clinicians in the use of vaccines as one of antitumor interventions. In this chapter, recent advances in cancer vaccine with peptides will be discussed.

K. Kono, Ph.D., M.D. (✉)
Department of Surgery, National University of Singapore, Level 8, NUHS Tower Block, 1E Kent Ridge Road, Singapore 119228, Singapore

Cancer Science Institute of Singapore, National University of Singapore, Singapore, Singapore
e-mail: surkoji@nus.edu.sg



Y. Yamaguchi (ed.), *Immunotherapy of Cancer*,
DOI 10.1007/978-4-431-55031-0_10

## 10.2 Current Status of Cancer Vaccine

A number of investigations have generated in-depth insights into the molecular and cellular mechanisms to induce antitumor immune responses. Cancer vaccines are attractive approach to control cancer through activation of patient's antitumor immunity. The recent FDA approval of Sipuleucel-T, which is cancer vaccine consisting of PSA-based antigen with activated APCs for hormone-refractory prostate cancer, heralds a new era of immunotherapy as anticancer treatment [1]. Therefore, if one could identify the specific peptides that are presented in the context of HLA molecules expressed by tumor cells and recognized by the immune system, it could be possible to activate the cognate cytotoxic T lymphocytes (CTLs) by peptide vaccination, leading to anticancer killing (Fig. 10.1). Identification of immunogenic tumor antigens and the characterization of tumor-specific CTLs in cancer patients [4, 5] could attract an enormous interest in translational research, which leads to several clinical trials of cancer vaccine. Although this field is progressing quickly and several clinical trials using cancer vaccines have been performed in various types of cancer, clinical success has so far been limited. Currently, a panel of preparations for cancer vaccine has been tested for their ability to elicit tumor-specific immune responses and induce antitumor effects in vivo. There are a number of possibilities of cancer vaccine preparations [6–9]: (1) synthetic tumor-associated antigens (TAAs), in the form of either short peptides or full-length proteins, which can bind MHC molecules on the surface of APCs or rely on the uptake and processing by APCs; (2) tumor lysates, containing TAAs

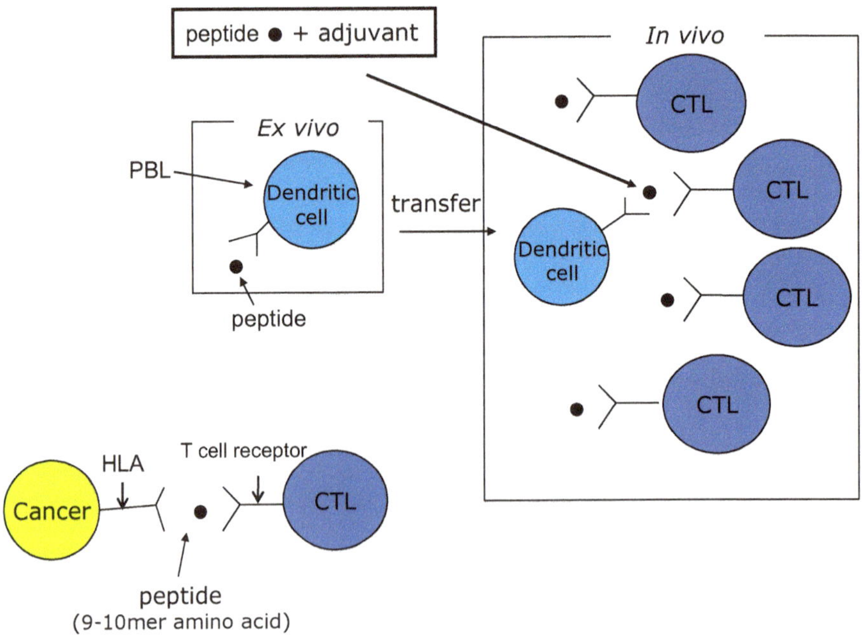


**Fig. 10.1** Scheme of cancer vaccine. HLA, human leukocyte antigens

Table 10.1 Difficulties in cancer vaccine

| | |
|---|---|
| 1. | Poor antigenicity of tumor antigen |
| 2. | Heterogenic expression of tumor antigen |
| 3. | No optimal way of administration (schedule, route, and type of adjuvants) |
| 4. | Immunosuppression at both local and systemic levels |

alone or complexed with chaperones; (3) TAA-encoding vectors, in the form of naked DNA or RNA; and (4) DC-based vaccines, including DCs loaded with TAAs ex vivo as well as fusion proteins that allow the selective delivery of TAAs to DCs in vivo.

Among them, only one cell-based vaccine, Sipuleucel-T (Provenge®), has been clinically approved for the treatment of patients with metastatic hormone-refractory prostate cancer in 2010 [1]. No other vaccines based on synthetic TAAs or DNA-based preparation are currently approved for clinical use for malignant tumors, with exceptions of Cervarix® and Gardasil®, two multivalent vaccines that have been approved as prophylactic measures against HPV-infection-related cervical cancer [10, 11]. Thus, cancer vaccine has been straggling to show a clinical evidence in terms of improvement of patient's survival. There are several reasons to explain the difficulties in the development of effective cancer vaccines [12, 13] (Table 10.1): (1) poor antigenicity of tumor antigen, (2) heterogenic expression of tumor antigen, (3) no optimal way of vaccine administration schedule and route as well as the presence and type of adjuvants, and (4) immunosuppressive status at both local and systemic levels.

Thus, in order to prove the safety and feasibility as well as immunogenicity and clinical benefits of cancer vaccine, several clinical trials with different antigens as well as different preparations are ongoing (Table 10.2).

## 10.2.1 Multi-peptide Vaccine

Several phase II and III clinical trials have recently demonstrated the promising and the therapeutic potentials of cancer vaccination [1, 14–17]. However, most of them are performed with single antigen-based vaccination with several modifications, and the clinical benefit seems to be very limited. In order to further improve the clinical responses of cancer vaccine, it is necessary to consider the application of a combination of multiple vaccines derived from the different target molecules, because it may overcome the issue of heterogeneity of tumor cells and also avoid the escape of tumor cells from peptide-specific immune response by loss of antigen expression [18, 19]. In general, the preferable characteristic of the target molecules for development of cancer vaccines are (1) high immunogenicity, (2) common expression in cancer cells, (3) specific expression in cancer cells, (4) homogeneous expression in cancer cells, and (5) essential molecules for cell survival to avoid loss of expression (Table 10.3).

**Table 10.2** Recent clinical trials of cancer vaccine with processed TAAs or peptides

| Indications | Phase | Antigen preparation | Antigens |
|---|---|---|---|
| Melanoma | I | Full-length TAAs, peptides | NY-ESO-1 |
| | I | HSP-TAA complexes | gp100 |
| | I | Phosphopeptides | BCAR3, IRS2 |
| | I/II | Peptides | MAGE-A3.A1 NA17.A2 |
| NSCLC | I/II | Peptides | MUC1 |
| | I/II | Peptides | TERT |
| | III | Protein | MAGE-A3 |
| Prostate cancer | I/II | Peptides | TERT |
| Beast | II | Peptides | HER2 |
| CIN | I | Fusion proteins | E7 |
| GBM | I/II | Peptides | Multiple |
| | II | HSP-TAA complexes | Multiple |
| MPM | II | Peptides | WT1 |
| Multiple myeloma | I | Peptides | Multiple |
| Hematological malignancy (AML, CML, etc.) | I | Fusion proteins | NY-ESO-1 |
| Hematological malignancy (AML, CML, etc.) | I/II | Fusion proteins | MAGE-A10, WT1 |

*TAA* tumor-associated antigen, *NSCLC* non-small cell lung carcinoma, *CIN* cervical intraepithelial neoplasia, *GBM* glioblastoma multiforme, *HSP* heat-shock protein, *MPM* malignant pleural mesothelioma, *AML* acute myeloid leukemia, *CML* chronic myeloid leukemia

**Table 10.3** Ideal targets for cancer vaccine

| | |
|---|---|
| 1. | High immunogenicity |
| 2. | Frequent expression in cancer cells |
| 3. | Specific expression in cancer cells |
| 4. | Homogeneous expression in cancer cells |
| 5. | Essential molecules for cell survival (to avoid loss of expression) |

We have been shown that three novel HLA-A24-restricted immunodominant peptides, which are derived from three different cancer-testis antigens, TTK protein kinase (TTK), lymphocyte antigen 6 complex locus K (LY6K), and insulin-like growth factor (IGF)-II mRNA-binding protein 3 (IMP-3), are promising targets for cancer vaccination for esophageal squamous cell carcinoma (ESCC) patients [15, 20, 21]. This is due to the findings: limited expression in tumor tissue and highly frequent expression (>95 %) of ESCC, homogenous expression within ESCC, and essential molecules for survival and proliferation of tumor cells. Moreover, it has shown that these peptides could stimulate CTL that recognized and killed ESCC cells endogenously expressing these antigens in vitro. Therefore, we had performed a phase I clinical cancer vaccination trials with a combination of multiple peptides that were derived from TTK, LY6K, and IMP3 for the *HLA-*

*A*2402* (+) patients with advanced ESCC, and the evidence in the phase I trial supported a recommendation moving forward to the phase II trial [21]. In the following phase II trial, 60 ESCC patients who failed the standard therapy were enrolled [15]. All enrolled patients had received the vaccination without knowing HLA-A type, and the HLA type were key-opened at analysis point, and then, the endpoints were evaluated between HLA-A*2402 positive (24(+)) and HLA-A*2402 negative (24(−)) group in subgroup analysis. As a result, the OS in the 24 (+) group tended to be better than that in the 24(−) group. The PFS in the 24 (+) group was significantly better than that in the 24(−) group. The patients having LY6K-, TTK-, and KOC1-specific CTL responses revealed the better OS in comparison to those not having CTL responses, respectively. We reported that the phase II clinical trial of cancer vaccination demonstrated the immune response induced by the vaccination could induce the better prognosis in advanced ESCC.

Another promising phase I/II trial of cancer vaccine with multiple antigenic peptides, which consist of HLA class I- and II-binding peptides, is reported [22]. A total of 96 renal cell cancer patients were treated with multi-peptide vaccine in combination with cyclophosphamide. The trial showed the combination of multi-peptide vaccine with cyclophosphamide could provide clinical survival benefits and better induction rates of antigen-specific T cell responses. Therefore, a randomized phase III trial is currently ongoing in Germany. In the report, authors concluded that there was a significant role of cyclophosphamide to reduce a number of regulatory T cells, leading to appropriate levels of antigen-specific T cell responses, and that vaccination with multiple antigenic peptides with HLA class I- and II-binding capacities played an important role in inducing clinical benefits.

### *10.2.2 MAGRIT Trial (MAGE-A3 Vaccine)*

It is generally believed that MAGRIT trial (the phase III trial of cancer vaccine with MAGE-A3 against non-small cell lung cancer) is a promising clinical trial to show the clinical benefit of cancer vaccine. The reasons are (1) the trial is performed as an adjuvant setting for patients with curatively resected tumors, (2) MAGE-A3 is a well- characterized tumor antigen, and (3) the preceding phase II trial was shown to have a promising result.

MAGE-A3 is a well-characterized cancer-testis antigen [23] that is selectively expressed on tumor cells, but not expressed in normal cells except for the testes, where MHC molecules are not expressed. Immunogenicity of MAGE-A3 was extensively evaluated at both peptide and cellular levels in vivo as well as in vitro. In lung cancer, MAGE-A3 expression increases with tumor stage; the antigen is expressed in approximately 35 % of lung tumors [24]. The pharmaceutical company, GlaxoSmithKline (GSK), has been developing a cancer vaccine strategy using MAGE-A3 protein with several combinations of adjuvants, which can stimulate DCs and enhance antigen uptake by DCs. In the phase II study of the MAGE-A3 vaccine, 182 patients with curatively resected, MAGE-A3-positive

NSCLC tumors (stages IB and II) were randomly assigned to receive MAGE-A3 vaccine or placebo at 2:1 ratio. Although the primary end point of the trial, disease-free survival, was not significantly different between the two groups (HR 0.74, 95 % CI 0.44–1.2, $P = 0.107$), there was a promising tendency of better disease-free survival in the vaccine group (data not published and available in the meeting proceeding). Of note, a tumor gene-expression profile was investigated in this phase II clinical trial and revealed a 43 % relative risk reduction for recurrence in the vaccine-treated group in patients with a favorable gene-signature profile (HR 0.57, 95 % CI 0.25–1.34, $P = 0.99$). These data supported the design and initiation of a large phase III trial, called MAGRIT.

In the MAGRIT trial, 2,270 patients with curatively resected tumors expressing MAGE-A3 were randomly assigned to receive either vaccine or placebo setting as same as the previous phase II trial, but with some modification of adjuvant. Notably, this trial is the largest interventional study of cancer vaccine, attracting a huge interest in immunotherapy all over the world. Disappointedly, the preliminary results from the MAGRIT trial has just been released (March 2014), where cancer vaccine did not significantly extend the disease-free survival compared to the placebo group (only available in the press release). More detail analysis relating to the favorable gene-signature profile is waiting.

## 10.3 Combination Therapy of Peptide Vaccine with Immune Checkpoint Blockade

Modern engineering technologies enabled to generate mAbs specific for certain target molecules, and recent breakthrough results from therapeutic mAbs inhibiting immune checkpoints such a CTLA4 and PD-1 could pave the way to a new field of cancer immunotherapy. Of note, animal and preclinical data suggested that there was a strong synergy between tumor vaccines and inhibition of immune checkpoints [25]. Anti-CTLA4 and anti-PD-1 mAbs strongly enhance the amplitude of vaccine-induced antitumor responses in many poorly immunogenic tumor models [25, 26]. However, in contrast to animal models, there was no synergistic effect between cancer vaccine and anti-CTLA4 mAb in a pivotal phase III RCT, in which combination of gp100 peptide vaccine with anti-CTLA4 mAb did not show any survival benefits compared to the group with anti-CTLA4 mAb alone [27]. Optimal strategies to enhance the synergistic effect between antigen-specific immunotherapy and immune checkpoint blockade are desirable in clinical settings.

## 10.4 Conclusion and Future Prospective

To prove clinical benefits of cancer vaccine is currently difficult, except for one phase III trial that has documented improved overall survival with the vaccine, Sipuleucel-T, although induction of antitumor immune responses through cancer vaccine is theoretically promising. In contrast, immune checkpoint blockade with anti-CTLA4 mAb and anti-PD-1 mAb has demonstrated clear evidence of objective responses, driving renewed enthusiasm for cancer immunotherapy in multiple cancer types. It would be ideal to combine antigen-specific immunotherapy such as cancer vaccine with immune checkpoint blockade.

## References

1. Kantoff PW, Higano CS, Shore ND, Berger ER, Small EJ, Penson DF et al (2010) Sipuleucel-T immunotherapy for castration-resistant prostate cancer. N Engl J Med 363:411–422
2. Bachy E, Coiffier B (2014) Anti-PD1 antibody: a new approach to treatment of lymphomas. Lancet Oncol 15:7–8
3. Freeman GJ, Long AJ, Iwai Y, Bourque K, Chernova T, Nishimura H et al (2000) Engagement of the PD-1 immunoinhibitory receptor by a novel B7 family member leads to negative regulation of lymphocyte activation. J Exp Med 192:1027–1034
4. Huppa JB, Davis MM (2003) T-cell-antigen recognition and the immunological synapse. Nat Rev Immunol 3:973–983
5. Masopust D, Schenkel JM (2013) The integration of T cell migration, differentiation and function. Nat Rev Immunol 13:309–320
6. Tacken PJ, de Vries IJ, Torensma R, Figdor CG (2007) Dendritic-cell immunotherapy: from ex vivo loading to in vivo targeting. Nat Rev Immunol 7:790–802
7. Bonifaz LC, Bonnyay DP, Charalambous A, Darguste DI, Fujii S, Soares H et al (2004) In vivo targeting of antigens to maturing dendritic cells via the DEC-205 receptor improves T cell vaccination. J Exp Med 199:815–824
8. Aranda F, Vacchelli E, Eggermont A, Galon J, Sautes-Fridman C, Tartour E et al (2013) Trial watch: peptide vaccines in cancer therapy. Oncoimmunology 2:e26621
9. Drake CG, Lipson EJ, Brahmer JR (2014) Breathing new life into immunotherapy: review of melanoma, lung and kidney cancer. Nat Rev Clin Oncol 11:24–37
10. Agosti JM, Goldie SJ (2007) Introducing HPV vaccine in developing countries – key challenges and issues. N Engl J Med 356:1908–1910
11. Paavonen J, Naud P, Salmeron J, Wheeler CM, Chow SN, Apter D et al (2009) Efficacy of human papillomavirus (HPV)-16/18 AS04-adjuvanted vaccine against cervical infection and precancer caused by oncogenic HPV types (PATRICIA): final analysis of a double-blind, randomised study in young women. Lancet 374:301–314
12. Keir ME, Butte MJ, Freeman GJ, Sharpe AH (2008) PD-1 and its ligands in tolerance and immunity. Annu Rev Immunol 26:677–704
13. Drake CG, Jaffee E, Pardoll DM (2006) Mechanisms of immune evasion by tumors. Adv Immunol 90:51–81
14. Schwartzentruber DJ, Lawson DH, Richards JM, Conry RM, Miller DM, Treisman J et al (2011) gp100 peptide vaccine and interleukin-2 in patients with advanced melanoma. N Engl J Med 364:2119–2127

15. Kono K, Iinuma H, Akutsu Y, Tanaka H, Hayashi N, Uchikado Y et al (2012) Multicenter, phase II clinical trial of cancer vaccination for advanced esophageal cancer with three peptides derived from novel cancer-testis antigens. J Transl Med 10:141
16. Okada H, Kalinski P, Ueda R, Hoji A, Kohanbash G, Donegan TE et al (2011) Induction of CD8+ T-cell responses against novel glioma-associated antigen peptides and clinical activity by vaccinations with {alpha}-type 1 polarized dendritic cells and polyinosinic-polycytidylic acid stabilized by lysine and carboxymethylcellulose in patients with recurrent malignant glioma. J Clin Oncol 29:330–336
17. Slingluff CL Jr, Petroni GR, Chianese-Bullock KA, Smolkin ME, Ross MI, Haas NB et al (2011) Randomized multicenter trial of the effects of melanoma-associated helper peptides and cyclophosphamide on the immunogenicity of a multipeptide melanoma vaccine. J Clin Oncol 29:2924–2932
18. Cecco S, Muraro E, Giacomin E, Martorelli D, Lazzarini R, Baldo P et al (2011) Cancer vaccines in phase II/III clinical trials: state of the art and future perspectives. Curr Cancer Drug Targets 11:85–102
19. Lesterhuis WJ, Haanen JB, Punt CJ (2011) Cancer immunotherapy – revisited. Nat Rev Drug Discov 10:591–600
20. Mizukami Y, Kono K, Daigo Y, Takano A, Tsunoda T, Kawaguchi Y et al (2008) Detection of novel cancer-testis antigen-specific T-cell responses in TIL, regional lymph nodes, and PBL in patients with esophageal squamous cell carcinoma. Cancer Sci 99:1448–1454
21. Kono K, Mizukami Y, Daigo Y, Takano A, Masuda K, Yoshida K et al (2009) Vaccination with multiple peptides derived from novel cancer-testis antigens can induce specific T-cell responses and clinical responses in advanced esophageal cancer. Cancer Sci 100:1502–1509
22. Walter S, Weinschenk T, Stenzl A, Zdrojowy R, Pluzanska A, Szczylik C et al (2012) Multipeptide immune response to cancer vaccine IMA901 after single-dose cyclophosphamide associates with longer patient survival. Nat Med 18:1254–1261
23. Simpson AJ, Caballero OL, Jungbluth A, Chen YT, Old LJ (2005) Cancer/testis antigens, gametogenesis and cancer. Nat Rev Cancer 5:615–625
24. Brichard VG, Lejeune D (2007) GSK's antigen-specific cancer immunotherapy programme: pilot results leading to phase III clinical development. Vaccine 27(25 Suppl 2):B61–B71
25. van Elsas A, Hurwitz AA, Allison JP (1999) Combination immunotherapy of B16 melanoma using anti-cytotoxic T lymphocyte-associated antigen 4 (CTLA-4) and granulocyte/macrophage colony-stimulating factor (GM-CSF)-producing vaccines induces rejection of subcutaneous and metastatic tumors accompanied by autoimmune depigmentation. J Exp Med 190:355–366
26. Li B, VanRoey M, Wang C, Chen TH, Korman A, Jooss K (2009) Anti-programmed death-1 synergizes with granulocyte macrophage colony-stimulating factor – secreting tumor cell immunotherapy providing therapeutic benefit to mice with established tumors. Clin Cancer Res 15:1623–1634
27. Hodi FS, O'Day SJ, McDermott DF, Weber RW, Sosman JA, Haanen JB et al (2010) Improved survival with ipilimumab in patients with metastatic melanoma. N Engl J Med 363:711–723

# Chapter 11
# Personalized Peptide Vaccine

**Masanori Noguchi**

**Abstract** Selection of suitable peptide vaccines for individual patients based on the preexisting host immunity before vaccination could induce potent antitumor responses that provide clinical benefit to cancer patients. We have developed a novel immunotherapeutic approach of personalized peptide vaccination (PPV) in which a maximum of four human leukocyte antigen (HLA) class IA-matched peptides are selected for vaccination among pooled peptides on the basis of both HLA class IA type and the preexisting host immunity before vaccination. We conducted a series of phase I and phase II clinical trials of PPV, which have shown better antigen-specific immune responses and promising clinical outcomes in patients with various types of advanced cancers. Further randomized phase III trials would be recommended to prove the clinical benefits of PPV. In addition, novel biomarkers for selecting patients who would benefit most from PPV remain to be identified.

**Keywords** Immunotherapy • Personalized peptide vaccine • Cancer vaccine • Advanced cancer • Biomarker • Clinical trial

## 11.1 Introduction

Since the identification of tumor-associated antigens (TAA) in different tumor histological types, many cancer vaccination strategies have been investigated, including peptide-based vaccines, recombinant DNA- or protein-based vaccines, and cell-based vaccines. Results from early trials, although demonstrating the feasibility and the good toxicity profile of this approach, provided evidence of clinical activity in only a minority of patients [1]. However, there have recently been noteworthy advances in the clinical application of immunotherapy. In 2010, sipuleucel-T (Provenge; Dendreon Corporation, Seattle, WA), an autologous cellular immunotherapy product designed to stimulate T-cell immune responses against human prostatic acid phosphatase (PAP), was first approved for patients

M. Noguchi, M.D., Ph.D. (✉)
Clinical Research Division of Research Center for Innovative Cancer Therapy, Kurume University School of Medicine, 67 Asahi-machi, Kurume, Fukuoka 830-0011, Japan
e-mail: noguchi@med.kurume-u.ac.jp



Y. Yamaguchi (ed.), *Immunotherapy of Cancer*,
DOI 10.1007/978-4-431-55031-0_11

with castration-resistant prostate cancer (CRPC) by the US Food and Drug Administration (FDA) [2]. In addition, another immunotherapeutic agent, ipilimumab, an anti-cytotoxic T-lymphocyte antigen (CTLA)-4 monoclonal antibody, was also approved for melanoma patients by the FDA in 2011 [3]. Despite these significant advances, however, most other randomized clinical trials of immunotherapies have so far failed to show beneficial therapeutic effects in patients compared to existing treatments [4]. The failure of recent clinical trials has raised several issues that need to be addressed for the successful development of cancer vaccines. We describe here a novel immunotherapeutic approach, "personalized peptide vaccination (PPV)," in which a maximum of four human leukocyte antigen (HLA) class IA-matched peptides are selected for vaccination from a pool of peptides on the basis of both HLA class IA type and the preexisting host immunity before vaccination. This strategy may confer several advantages, such as the possibility of bypassing both immunological diversity and tumor heterogeneity. For example, "personalized" antigens with preexisting immunity, which are designed to stimulate antigen-specific memory T cells, could be expected to induce rapid and strong secondary immune responses. For example, we previously reported that PPV quickly induced infiltration of CD45RO+ memory T cells, rather than naïve T cells or B cells, into cancer tissues [5]. In addition, selection of multiple epitopes for PPV could reduce the risk of tumor escape through existence and/or induction of antigen-negative clones escaping peptide-specific immune responses. Indeed, it would be relatively rare that tumor cells escape from peptide-specific immune responses by simultaneously losing all of multiple antigens selected for vaccination.

## 11.2 Personalized Peptide Vaccine (PPV)

A large number of tumor-associated antigens (TAA) have been identified by several different approaches, including complementary DNA (cDNA) expression cloning [6], serologic analysis of recombinant cDNA expression libraries (SEREX) [7], and a reverse immunological approach. Since 1995, when Hu et al. reported the first clinical trial of the vaccination of a peptide derived from melanoma antigen gene-1 (MAGE-1) [8], many clinical trials of peptide vaccines have been reported [9, 10]. In earlier stages of clinical trials of peptide vaccines, one to several HLA class I-restricted peptides emulsified with Montanide ISA51, a clinical grade of Freund's incomplete adjuvant, were employed. Although the early-phase clinical trials demonstrated the feasibility and good toxicity profile of this approach, most of the late-phase randomized trials, other than few exceptions [11], failed to show beneficial therapeutic effects in patients compared to existing treatments [9, 10]. Therefore, a variety of new types of peptide-based vaccines, including PPV, multiple-peptide vaccine, hybrid peptide vaccine, and long peptide vaccine, have been developed [12, 13].

Cancer patients possess antitumor immunity, which may depend strongly on both the tumor cell characteristics and the immunological status of the host [14–17]. The antitumor immunity might differ widely among individuals, since the tumor cell characteristics and the host immune cell repertoires are quite diverse and heterogeneous among patients, even among those with identical HLA types and the same pathological types of cancer. Nevertheless, before patients are enrolled in clinical trials of cancer vaccines, the expressions of vaccine antigens in tumor cells are sometimes confirmed, but the immunological statuses of the hosts are rarely evaluated. Considering the complexity and diversity of the host immune cell repertoires, it is likely that vaccine antigens that are selected and administered without considering the host immunological status might not efficiently induce beneficial antitumor immune responses [17]. Since, in most clinical trials of therapeutic cancer vaccines, common antigens are employed for vaccination independently of the immunological status of patients [9, 10], the low clinical efficacies might be explained at least in part by mismatches between the vaccine antigens and the host immune cell repertoires. To evaluate the host immune cell repertoires, we examine patients' preexisting immunity to a panel of vaccine candidates before vaccination and select appropriate vaccine antigens with immunological memory in each patient [18]. Vaccine antigens, to which patients already possess antigen-specific immunological memory, are expected to cause quick and strong secondary immune responses after vaccination (Fig. 11.1). In contrast, vaccinations with inadequate antigens without immunological memory could not easily provide clinical benefits, especially in advanced cancer patients who show higher disease progression [19]. In light of this, it would be quite reasonable to select vaccine antigens on the basis of the preexisting immune cell repertoires in each patient.

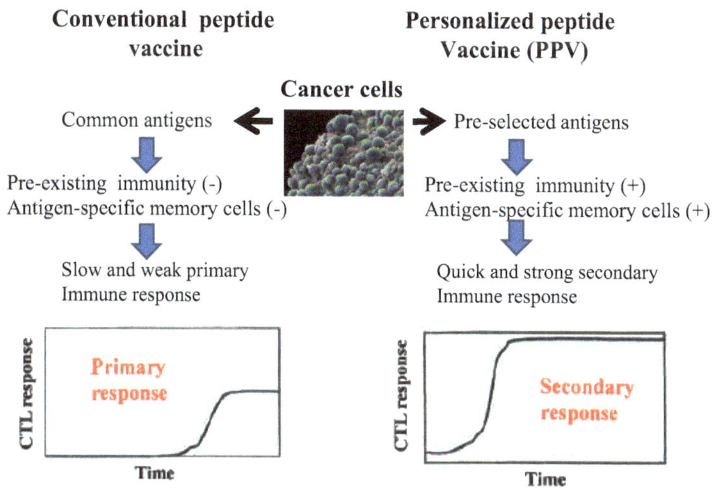


**Fig. 11.1** Concept of personalized peptide vaccination. Patients who have an immunological memory to vaccine antigens are expected to show quick and strong immune responses to them. In contrast, patients with no immunological memory against vaccine antigens would take more time to develop effective antitumor immune responses because several rounds of repeated vaccinations might be required to prime antigen-specific naïve T cells to functional effector cells

### 11.2.1 Rationale for PPV

Cancer cells can develop various mechanisms to accelerate malignant behavior [14]. For example, it has been well recognized that cancer cells might escape the host's immunological surveillance. After the interaction/competition between tumor cells and host immune cells, tumor cell variants resistant to the immunological pressure often emerge through the selection of mutants with reduced antigenicity [14]. Therefore, the selection and administration of multiple vaccine antigens could reduce the risk of tumor escape through the existence and/or induction of antigen-negative variants escaping antigen-specific immune responses [15, 20], since it would be rare for tumor cells to simultaneously lose all of the multiple antigens selected for vaccination.

Collectively, our new concept of "personalized" cancer vaccine formulation, where multiple peptide antigens are selected for vaccination by the preexisting host immunity from a list of vaccine candidates, may confer several advantages, including the possibility of bypassing both immunological diversity and tumor heterogeneity.

### 11.2.2 PPV Procedures

For PPV, a maximum of four peptides are selected based on the results of HLA typing and the preexisting immune responses specific to each of the 31 HLA class I-restricted cytotoxic T lymphocyte (CTL) epitope peptides with minimal optimal lengths (9-mer or 10-mer): 12 peptides for HLA-A2, 14 peptides for HLA-A24, 9 peptides for HLA-A3 supertype (A3, A11, A31, or A33), and 4 peptides for HLA-A26 (Table 11.1). These peptides were identified mainly through the cDNA expression cloning method with tumor-infiltrating T-lymphocyte lines [18, 21–27]. The safety and potential immunological effects of these vaccine candidates have been demonstrated in clinical studies [18, 28, 29]. It should be noted that we currently employ these 31 CTL epitopes, which are also shown to induce antigen-specific B-cell immune responses, as vaccine antigen candidates for PPV, since it has been suggested that a CTL peptide with the ability to induce antigen-specific B-cell responses could provide more effective immune responses than a CTL peptide without it [30, 31].

Although short peptide epitopes with minimal optimal lengths have been reported to bear the potential to induce immune tolerance rather than activate antigen-specific immune responses [32–34], our PPV formulation with short epitopes has been demonstrated to efficiently induce antigen-specific IFN-$\gamma$-producing $CD8^+$ T cells but not tolerance to them, possibly because only immunogenic epitopes are selected in each patient by screening before vaccination. Although long synthetic peptides have shown excellent immune responses and promising

**Table 11.1** Peptide candidates used for personalized peptide vaccines (PPV)

| Original protein | Peptide name | Position of peptide | Amino acid sequence | HLA restriction |
|---|---|---|---|---|
| Cyclophilin B | CypB-129 | 129–138 | KLKHYGPGWV | A2, A3sup |
| p56 lck | Lck-246 | 246–254 | KLVERLGAA | A2 |
| p56 lck | Lck-422 | 422–430 | DVWSFGILL | A2, A3sup |
| ppMAPkkk | MAP-432 | 432–440 | DLLSHAFFA | A2, A26 |
| WHSC2 | WHSC2-103 | 103–111 | ASLDSDPWV | A2, A3sup, A26 |
| HNRPL | HNRPL-501 | 501–510 | NVLHFFNAPL | A2, A26 |
| UBE2V | UBE-43 | 43–51 | RLQEWCSVI | A2 |
| UBE2V | UBE-85 | 85–93 | LIADFLSGL | A2 |
| WHSC2 | WHSC2-141 | 141–149 | ILGELREKV | A2 |
| HNRPL | HNRPL-140 | 140–148 | ALVEFEDVL | A2 |
| SART3 | SART3-302 | 302–310 | LLQAEAPRL | A2 |
| SART3 | SART3-309 | 309–317 | RLAEYQAYI | A2 |
| SART2 | SART2-93 | 93–101 | DYSARWNEI | A24 |
| SART3 | SART3-109 | 109–118 | VYDYNCHVDL | A24, A3sup, A26 |
| p56 lck | Lck-208 | 208–216 | HYTNASDGL | A24 |
| PAP | PAP-213 | 213–221 | LYCESVHNF | A24 |
| PSA | PSA-248 | 248–257 | HYRKWIKDTI | A24 |
| EGFR | EGFR-800 | 800–809 | DYVREHKDNI | A24 |
| MRP3 | MRP3-503 | 503–511 | LYAWEPSFL | A24 |
| MRP3 | MRP3-1,293 | 1,293–1,302 | NYSVRYRPGL | A24 |
| SART2 | SART2-161 | 161–169 | AYDFLYNYL | A24 |
| p56 lck | Lck-486 | 486–494 | TFDYLRSVL | A24 |
| p56 lck | Lck-488 | 488–497 | DYLRSVLEDF | A24 |
| PSMA | PSMA-624 | 624–632 | TYSVSFDSL | A24 |
| EZH2 | EZH2-735 | 735–743 | KYVGIEREM | A24 |
| PTHrP | PTHrP-102 | 102–111 | RYLTQETNKV | A24 |
| SART3 | SART3-511 | 511–519 | WLEYYNLER | A3sup |
| SART3 | SART3-734 | 734–742 | QIRPIFSNR | A3sup |
| p56 lck | Lck-90 | 90–99 | ILEQSGEWWK | A3sup |
| p56 lck | Lck-449 | 449–458 | VIQNLERGYR | A3sup |
| PAP | PAP-248 | 248–257 | GIHKQKEKSR | A3sup |

*A3sup* HLA-A3 supertype (A3, A11, A31, or A33), *EGFR* epidermal growth factor receptor, *EZH2* enhancer of zeste homolog 2, *HNRPL* heterogeneous nuclear ribonucleoprotein L, *ppMAPkkk* partial putative mitogen-activated protein kinase kinase kinase, *MRP3* multidrug resistance-associated protein 3, *PAP* prostatic acid phosphatase, *PSA* prostate-specific antigen, *PSMA* prostate-specific membrane antigen, *PTHrP* parathyroid hormone-related peptide, *SART2* squamous cell carcinoma antigen recognized by T cells 2, *SART3* squamous cell carcinoma antigen recognized by T cells 3, *UBE2V* ubiquitin-conjugated enzyme variant Kua, *WHSC2* Wolf-Hirschhorn syndrome candidate 2

clinical results in some clinical trials [35, 36], we do not currently use long peptides for PPV, since they may contain undesirable T-cell epitopes that activate other immune cells, such as T helper two cells and/or regulatory T cells [37, 38], which could negatively affect beneficial antigen-specific immune responses.

## 11.3 Clinical Trials of PPV for Advanced Cancers

To date, a series of phase I, I/II, and II clinical trials of PPV have been conducted in the past several years for various types of advanced cancer patients. We have summarized the observed immune and clinical responses in advanced cancer patients induced by the PPV (Table 11.2). In the following sections, we provide a more detailed account of these studies, categorized by the different cancer types.

### *11.3.1 Castration-Resistant Prostate Cancer (CRPC)*

Most prostate cancer-related deaths occur in patients with advanced CRPC. Chemotherapy plays only a palliative role in the treatment of prostate cancer, although two docetaxel-based randomized clinical trials demonstrated a survival benefit of only 2.4 months compared with those with mitoxantrone and prednisone in CRPC patients. A large number of agents and treatment strategies including immunotherapy are currently under investigation for various stages of CRPC. Indeed, several immunotherapy strategies for advanced CRPC, such as single-peptide-based vaccine, multiple-peptide-based vaccine, cell-based vaccine, viral vaccine, antibody-based therapy, and their combination with other therapies, have been evaluated. In phase I studies of PPV for advanced CRPC, we have reported the increase in cellular and humoral immune responses and decrease in PSA levels in some patients [39–41]. Phase I dose-escalation study of PPV for CRPC with 1, 3, and 5 mg/peptide injection showed that a dose of 3 mg/peptide injection was better than those of 1 and 5 mg/peptide injections in terms of the induction of cellular immune responses to peptides, although the maximum tolerated dose (MTD) was not estimated [39]. In a phase I/II study, 58 patients with HLA-A2$^{+}$ or HLA-A24$^{+}$ with CRPC were treated with a combination of PPV and low-dose estramustine phosphate (EMP) [42]. As a result, the majority (76 %) of patients showed a decreased serum PSA level, along with a median survival time (MST) of 17 months (95 % confidence interval: 95 % CI, 12–25 months). In addition, this study showed that a small number of lymphocytes, a negative immunological response after PPV, and poor performance status were independent predictors of disease-related death. In this study, long MST with the combination therapy supports the hypothesis that this combination with a low-dose cytotoxic drug produces additional antitumor effects with minimum immunosuppression. Sequentially, we conducted a randomized, crossover, phase II trial of PPV plus low-dose EMP comparing standard-dose

**Table 11.2** Clinical trials of personalized peptide vaccination for advanced cancer

| Tumor site | Disease status | Phase | HLA restriction | Total no. of pts | Humoral response | Cellular response | Clinical response | Grade 3/4 toxicities | MST (months) | Ref. |
|---|---|---|---|---|---|---|---|---|---|---|
| Prostate | Advanced CRPC | PI | A-24 | 10 | 60 % | 40 % | SD 50 % | 0 | Not ref. | [40] |
| | Advanced CRPC | PI | A-2 | 10 | 70 % | 40 % | SD 30 % | 0 | 22 | [41] |
| | Advanced CRPC | PI/II | A-2/A-24 | 58 | 88 % | 78 % | PR 24 % | G3, 7 % | 17 | [42] |
| | Localized PC | PII | A-24 | 10 | 80 % | 80 % | PR 20 % | 0 | Not ref. | [5] |
| | Advanced CRPC | PI, extension | A-24 | 15 | 47 % | 67 % | PR 13 % | 0 | 24 | [39] |
| | Advanced CRPC | PII, randomized | A-2/A-24 | 57 | 64 % | 50 % | PFS | 0 | | [43] |
| | | | | | | | 8.5 vs 2.8 M | | 22.4 vs 16.1 | |
| | Advanced CRPC | PII | A-2/A-24/ | 42 | 44 % | 34 % | PR 12 % | 0 | 17.8 | [44] |
| | | | A-3sup/ A-26 | | | | | | | |
| Brain | Advanced malignant glioma | PI | A-2/A24 | 21 | 40–64 % | 50–82 % | PR 24 %, SD 38 % | 0 | Not reached | [45] |
| | Advanced glioblastoma multiforme | PI, extension | A-24 | 12 | 17 % | 75 % | PR 17 %, SD 42 % | 0 | 10.6 | [46] |
| Lung | Advanced lung cancer | PI | A-24 | 10 | 40 % | 40 % | SD 80 % | 0 | 15.2 | [56] |
| | Refractory SCLC | PII | A-2/A-24 | 10 | 83 % | 83 % | SD 20 % | G3, 4 % | 6.2 | [58] |
| | | | A-3sup/ A-26 | | | | | | | |
| | Refractory NSCLC | PII | A-2/A-24 | 41 | 49 % | 34 % | SD 56 % | G3, 7 % | 10.1 | [57] |
| | | | A-3sup/ A-26 | | | | | | | |

(continued)

**Table 11.2** (continued)

| Tumor site | Disease status | Phase | HLA restriction | Total no. of pts | Humoral response | Cellular response | Clinical response | Grade 3/4 toxicities | MST (months) | Ref. |
|---|---|---|---|---|---|---|---|---|---|---|
| Colorectal | Advanced colorectal cancer | PI | A-24 | 10 | 70 % | 50 % | PR 10 % | 0 | Not ref. | [53] |
| | Advanced colorectal cancer | PI/II | A-2/A-24 | 7 | 71 % | 57 % | SD 14 % | G3, 20 % | Not ref. | [54] |
| Pancreas | Advanced pancreatic cancer | PI | A-2/A-24 | 13 | 69 % | 69 % | PR 15 %, SD 54 % | 0 | 7.6 | [47] |
| | Non-resectable pancre-atic cancer | PII | A-2/A-24 | 21 | 72 % | 78 % | PR 33 %, SD 43 % | 0 | 9 | [48] |
| Stomach | Advanced gastric cancer | PI | A-2/A-24 | 13 | 80 % | 50 % | SD 45 % | 0 | Not ref. | [55] |
| Kidney | Metastatic RCC | PI | A-2/A-24 | 10 | 80 % | 5 % | SD 60 % | 0 | 23 | [60] |
| Skin | Malignant melanoma | PI | A-2/A-24 | 7 | 57 % | 86 % | SD 43 % | 0 | Not ref. | [61] |
| Uterine | Recurrent gynecologic cancer | PI | A-2/A-24 | 14 | 86 % | 85 % | SD 36 % | G3, 8 % | Not ref. | [59] |
| Bladder | Advanced urothelial cancer | PI | A-2/A-24 | 10 | 80 % | 80 % | CR 10 %, PR 10 % | 0 | 24 | [62] |

*A-3sup* A-3 supertype, *CR* complete response, *CRPC* castration-resistant prostate cancer, *G3* grade 3, *HLA* human leukocyte antigen, *MST* median survival time, *NSCLC* non-small cell lung cancer, *PI* phase I clinical trial, *PC* prostate cancer, *PD* progressive disease, *PFS* progression-free survival, *PR* partial response, *RCC* renal cell carcinoma, *SCLC* small-cell lung cancer, *SD* stable disease, *Total No. of Pts* total number of patients

EMP in HLA-A2$^+$ or HLA-A24$^+$ patients with CRPC [43]. Median progression-free survival (PFS) was 8.5 months in the PPV group and 2.8 months in the EMP group with a hazard ratio (HR) of 0.28 (95 % CI, 0.14–0.61; log-rank $p = 0.0012$), and the MST for the PPV plus low-dose EMP group was 22.4 months, while the MST for the standard-dose EMP group was 16.1 months (95 % CI, 8.0–13.4 months) ($P = 0.0328$). The HR for overall survival was 0.3 in favor of the PPV plus low-dose EMP group. These results suggest that PPV is well tolerated and active in CRPC patients. In another phase II study, we compared the MST in docetaxel-based chemotherapy (DBC)-resistant CRPC patients treated by PPV ($n = 20$) with a historical control ($n = 17$) [44]. MST from the first day of progressive disease (PD) was 17.8 and 10.5 months in DBC-resistant CRPC patients receiving PPV and those with no PPV, respectively. These encouraging preliminary study results suggested that PPV warrants further study as a novel therapy for CRPC patients with PD after DBC. Now, a phase III randomized clinical trial of PPV is under way in DBC-resistant CRPC patients.

### *11.3.2 Glioblastoma Multiforme (GBM)*

Although immunotherapy is theoretically attractive due to the discovery of TAAs and peptides capable of inducing specific immunity in patients with GBM, previously conducted immunotherapy trials failed to provide evidence of any definite clinical benefit in patients with GBM. One of the potential hurdles hindering the development of effective immunotherapy for the treatment of GBMs is the blood-brain barrier, but recent studies have shown that it does not always function in cases involving recurrent GBMs. We previously showed the feasibility of vaccination with PPV for advanced GBM patients in a phase I study [45]. Twenty-one patients received more than six vaccinations, and clinical responses were 5 cases of partial response (PR), 8 of stable disease (SD), and 8 of PD with MST of 20.7 months in this study. More importantly, significant levels of peptide-specific IgG were detected in the postvaccination tumor cavity or spinal fluid of all of the tested patients who showed favorable clinical responses. Another clinical study showed the safety and increased immune boosting with potential clinical benefits in cases of recurrent or progressive GBM, even in temozolomide-refractory settings [46]. On the basis of these promising results, double-blind randomized phase III trials are currently underway in GBM patients.

### *11.3.3 Pancreatic Cancer and Biliary Tract Cancer*

We have conducted a phase I trial of PPV in 13 HLA-A2$^+$ or HLA-A24$^+$ patients with advanced pancreatic cancer, where the patients were treated by PPV at three different doses (1, 2, or 3 mg/peptide) in combination with gemcitabine (GEM)

[47]. This combination therapy was well tolerated, and 11 of 13 patients (85 %) showed reduced tumor sizes and/or levels of tumor markers. Peptide-specific CTL responses were augmented at each dose level, and the increment of peptide-specific IgG antibodies was dependent on the peptide dose. These findings suggested that GEM did not inhibit the immune responses induced by PPV. Subsequently, we conducted a phase II trial of PPV in combination with GEM to evaluate the safety, clinical efficacy, and antigen-specific immune responses as a frontline therapy for 21 HLA-A2$^{+}$ or HLA-A24$^{+}$ nonresectable patients with advanced pancreatic cancer [48]. This combination therapy was also well tolerated, and the best clinical responses were PR in 7, SD in 9, and PD in 5 patients. The MST of all 21 patients was 9 months with a 1-year survival rate of 38 %, which was better than that reported for GEM alone (MST of 5.7 months with a 1-year survival rate of 18 %) [49]. Importantly, the MST was 15 months in patients who showed immunological responses to vaccine peptides. We also conducted a phase II clinical trial of PPV in 25 HLA-A2$^{+}$ or HLA-A24$^{+}$ chemotherapy-resistant patients with advanced biliary tract cancer [50]. When two to four vaccine peptides selected by preexisting immunity were administered to the patients in this study, humoral and/or T-cell responses specific to the vaccine antigens were substantially induced in a subset of the patients without severe adverse events. Greater numbers of selected and vaccinated peptides were significantly favorable factors for overall survival (HR = 0.258, 95 % CI = 0.098–0.682, $P$ = 0.006) in this study.

### 11.3.4 Colorectal and Gastric Cancer

We reported previously that SART3 is expressed in the majority of colorectal cancers and that two to three SART3-derived peptides are present in the majority of cancer patients with HLA-A24$^{+}$ and HLA-A2$^{+}$ [21, 51–53]. In a phase I clinical trial of PPV on ten patients with advanced colorectal cancer, we observed one PR and one SD continuing for more than 6 months [53]. These PR and SD cases were vaccinated with three kinds of SART3- and p56$^{lck}$-derived peptides, suggesting that the combination of these peptides might constitute a promising vaccine strategy for advanced colorectal carcinomas. In addition, a phase I/II clinical trial of PPV in combination with oral administration of a 5-fluorouracil derivative (TS-1) in advanced gastric or colorectal cancer patients indicated that administration of the standard dose of TS-1 in combination with PPV does not necessarily impede immunological responses in these cancer patients and actually maintains or augments them [54]. Another phase I clinical trial of PPV in 13 patients with advanced gastric cancer demonstrated prolonged survival and cellular and humoral immune responses to the vaccinated peptides in the postvaccination samples, including those of all four patients with the scirrhous type [55]. Even though only a small number of selected patients were treated, the encouraging clinical response warrants further studies of PPV in colorectal and gastric cancers.

### *11.3.5 Lung Cancer*

The prognosis of advanced lung cancer patients remains very poor with a median survival time of around 6–10 months. Phase I and II studies of PPV in a small number of patients with refractory non-small cell lung cancer (NSLC) showed longer survival (MST of 10.1–15.2 months) [56, 57] than in previous reports. A clinical study of advanced small-cell lung cancer (SCLC) showed the feasibility of PPV since there were higher rates of peptide-specific immunological boosting after PPV [58]. In order to identify potential biomarkers for predicting overall survival in advanced lung cancer patients, we retrospectively analyzed pre-vaccination clinical findings and laboratory data. In patients with refractory NSLC, a higher C-reactive protein (CRP) level before vaccination and a low frequency of $CD3^{+}CD26^{+}$ cells after vaccination were significant predictors of unfavorable overall survival [57]. In patients with refractory SCLC, the number of previous chemotherapy treatments and the frequency of $CD3^{+}CD26^{+}$ cells in PBMCs before vaccination were potential prognostic predictors in patients who received PPV [58]. These findings demonstrate that less inflammation may contribute to better responses to the PPV, suggesting that evaluation of the inflammatory factors before vaccination could be useful for selecting appropriate cancer patients for PPV.

### *11.3.6 Other Cancers*

We have also conducted phase I clinical trials for other advanced cancers including metastatic renal cell carcinoma (RCC), malignant melanoma, gynecologic cancers, and bladder cancer [59–62]. All of these studies demonstrated that PPV was safe and well tolerated with no major adverse effects and that more immune responses were observed in the majority of patients after PPV than with the predesignated peptide vaccination. Some patients treated by PPV showed objective clinical responses evaluated by the Response Evaluation Criteria in Solid Tumors with boosted immune responses: CR in one patient with chemotherapy-resistant advanced bladder tumor and PR in two patients with cervical cancer [59, 62]. These results indicate that PPV can be applied in further clinical trials aimed at the treatment of these cancers.

### *11.3.7 Biomarkers for PPV*

Recent clinical trials of cancer immunotherapies, including peptide-based cancer vaccines, have demonstrated that only a subset of patients show clinical benefits. Furthermore, unexpectedly, some large clinical trials in the past several years have demonstrated that cancer vaccines might sometimes show worse clinical outcomes

[4, 63]. It would thus be important to identify predictive biomarkers that could accurately assess antitumor immune responses and predict patient prognosis following the administration of cancer vaccines. In some clinical trials, several postvaccination biomarkers, including CTL responses, Th1 responses, delayed-type hypersensitivity (DTH), and autoimmunity, have been reported to be associated with clinical responses [64–67]. However, there are currently no validated biomarkers for cancer vaccines in widespread use.

To identify biomarkers for PPV, we statistically reviewed 500 advanced cancer patients undergoing PPV from October 2000 to October 2008 [29]. Both lymphocyte counts before vaccination ($P = 0.0095$) and increased IgG response ($P = 0.0116$) to the vaccine peptides after vaccination, along with performance status ($P < 0.0001$), were well correlated with overall survival. In CRPC patients treated with PPV ($n = 40$), a comprehensive study of soluble factors assessed by multiplexed bead array in plasma and gene expression profiles by DNA microarray in PBMC demonstrated that higher IL-6 level and granulocytic myeloid-derived suppressor cells (MDSC) in the peripheral blood before vaccination were closely related to poorer prognosis in the vaccinated patients [68]. By multivariate Cox regression analyses in patients with refractory NSCLC ($n = 41$), higher C-reactive protein (CRP) level before vaccination was a significant predictor of unfavorable overall survival (HR = 10.115, 95 % CI = 2.447–41.806, $P = 0.001$) [57]. In addition, in refractory biliary tract cancer patients ($n = 25$), multivariate Cox regression analyses showed that higher IL-6 and lower albumin levels before vaccination were significantly unfavorable factors for overall survival [HR = 1.123, 95 % CI = 1.008–1.252, $P = 0.035$; HR = 0.158, 95 % CI = 0.029–0.860, $P = 0.033$, respectively] [50].

Collectively, these findings suggested that less inflammation may contribute to better responses to PPV, indicating that the evaluation of inflammatory factors before vaccination could be useful for selecting cancer patients who are appropriate for PPV. An early-phase clinical trial is under way to reveal whether or not the blockage of IL-6-mediated inflammatory signaling with a humanized anti-IL-6 receptor monoclonal antibody, tocilizumab, would be beneficial for enhancing the immune and/or clinical responses after PPV in advanced cancer patients who show higher plasma IL-6 levels [69, 70].

## 11.4 Conclusions

The field of immunotherapy has advanced dramatically during the past 20 years, but there have remained several issues to be addressed in order to achieve successful cancer vaccine development. In view of the complexity and diversity of the immunological characteristics of tumors and the immune cell repertoires of hosts, selection of suitable peptide vaccines for individual patients based on the preexisting host immunity before vaccination could induce potent antitumor responses that provide clinical benefit to cancer patients. We have shown promising results of PPV as a new treatment modality for patients with various types of advanced cancer. Further randomized phase III clinical trials are essential to prove the clinical benefits of PPV. In addition, novel biomarkers for selecting patients who would benefit most from PPV remain to be identified.

**Disclosure Statement** The author indicated no potential conflict of interest.

# References


1. Schlom J (2012) Therapeutic cancer vaccines: current status and moving forward. J Natl Cancer Inst 104:599–613
2. Kantoff PW, Higano CS, Shore ND, Berger ER, Small EJ, Penson DF et al (2010) Sipuleucel-T immunotherapy for castration-resistant prostate cancer. N Engl J Med 363:411–422
3. Hodi FS, O'Day SJ, McDermott DF, Weber RW, Sosman JA, Haanen JB et al (2010) Improved survival with ipilimumab in patients with metastatic melanoma. N Engl J Med 363:711–723
4. Sasada T, Komatsu N, Suekane S, Yamada A, Noguchi M, Itoh K (2010) Overcoming the hurdles of randomised clinical trials of therapeutic cancer vaccines. Eur J Cancer 46:1514–1519
5. Noguchi M, Yao A, Harada M, Nakashima O, Komohara Y, Yamada S et al (2007) Immunological evaluation of neoadjuvant peptide vaccination before radical prostatectomy for patients with localized prostate cancer. Prostate 67:933–942
6. van der Bruggen P, Traversari C, Chomez P, Lurquin C, De Plaen E, Van den Eynde B et al (1991) A gene encoding an antigen recognized by cytolytic T lymphocytes on a human melanoma. Science 254:1643–1647
7. Türeci O, Sahin U, Schobert I, Koslowski M, Scmitt H, Schild HJ et al (1996) The SSX-2 gene, which is involved in the t(X; 18) translocation of synovial sarcomas, codes for the human tumor antigen HOM-MEL-40. Cancer Res 56:4766–4772
8. Hu X, Chakraborty NG, Sporn JR, Kurtzman SH, Ergin MT, Mukherji B (1996) Enhancement of cytolytic T lymphocyte precursor frequency in melanoma patients following immunization with the MAGE-1 peptide loaded antigen presenting cell-based vaccine. Cancer Res 56:2479–2483
9. Rosenberg SA, Yang JC, Restifo NP (2004) Cancer immunotherapy: moving beyond current vaccines. Nat Med 10:909–915
10. Purcell AW, McCluskey J, Rossjohn J (2007) More than one reason to rethink the use of peptides in vaccine design. Nat Rev Drug Discov 6:404–414
11. Schwartzentruber DJ, Lawson DH, Richards JM, Conry RM, Miller DM, Treisman J et al (2011) gp100 peptide vaccine and interleukin-2 in patients with advanced melanoma. N Engl J Med 364:2119–2127
12. Yamada A, Sasada T, Noguchi M, Itoh K (2013) Next-generation peptide vaccines for advanced cancer. Cancer Sci 104:15–21
13. Perez SA, von Hofe E, Kallinteris NL, Gritzapis AD, Peoples GE, Papamichail M et al (2010) A new era in anticancer peptide vaccines. Cancer 116:2071–2080
14. Schreiber RD, Old LJ, Smyth MJ (2011) Cancer immunoediting: integrating immunity's roles in cancer suppression and promotion. Science 331:1565–1570
15. Bei R, Scardino A (2010) TAA polyepitope DNA-based vaccines: a potential tool for cancer therapy. J Biomed Biotechnol 2010:102758. doi:10.1155/2010/102758
16. Yewdell JW, Bennink JR (1999) Immunodominance in major histocompatibility complex class I-restricted T lymphocyte responses. Annu Rev Immunol 17:51–88

17. Chen W, McCluskey J (2006) Immunodominance and immunodomination: critical factors in developing effective CD8+ T-cell-based cancer vaccines. Adv Cancer Res 95:203–247
18. Itoh K, Yamada A (2006) Personalized peptide vaccines: a new therapeutic modality for cancer. Cancer Sci 97:970–976
19. Mochizuki K, Sato Y, Tsuda N, Shomura H, Sakamoto M, Matsuura K et al (2004) Immunological evaluation of vaccination with pre-designated peptides frequently selected as vaccine candidates in an individualized peptide vaccination regimen. Int J Oncol 25:121–131
20. Pilla L, Rivoltini L, Patuzzo R, Marrari A, Valdagni R, Parmiani G (2009) Multipeptide vaccination in cancer patients. Expert Opin Biol Ther 9:1043–1055
21. Nakao M, Shichijo S, Imaizumi T, Inoue Y, Matsunaga K, Yamada A et al (2000) Identification of a gene coding for a new squamous cell carcinoma antigen recognized by the CTL. J Immunol 164:2565–2574
22. Shichijo S, Nakao M, Imai Y, Takasu H, Kawamoto M, Niiya F et al (1998) A gene encoding antigenic peptides of human squamous cell carcinoma recognized by cytotoxic T lymphocytes. J Exp Med 187:277–288
23. Harashima N, Tanaka K, Sasatomi T, Shimizu K, Miyagi Y, Yamada A et al (2001) Recognition of the Lck tyrosine kinase as a tumor antigen by cytotoxic T lymphocytes of cancer patients with distant metastases. Eur J Immunol 31:323–332
24. Yamada A, Kawano K, Koga M, Matsumoto T, Itoh K (2001) Multidrug resistance-associated protein 3 is a tumor rejection antigen recognized by HLA-A2402-restricted cytotoxic T lymphocytes. Cancer Res 61:6459–6466
25. Harada M, Kobayashi K, Matsueda S, Nakagawa M, Noguchi M, Itoh K (2003) Prostate-specific antigen-derived epitopes capable of inducing cellular and humoral responses in HLA-A24+ prostate cancer patients. Prostate 57:152–159
26. Inoue Y, Takaue Y, Takei M, Kato K, Kanai S, Harada Y et al (2001) Induction of tumor specific cytotoxic T lymphocytes in prostate cancer using prostatic acid phosphatase derived HLA-A2402 binding peptide. J Urol 166:1508–1513
27. Kobayashi K, Noguchi M, Itoh K, Harada M (2003) Identification of a prostate-specific membrane antigen-derived peptide capable of eliciting both cellular and humoral immune responses in HLA-A24+ prostate cancer patients. Cancer Sci 94:622–627
28. Yoshida K, Noguchi M, Mine T, Komatsu N, Yutani S, Ueno T et al (2011) Characteristics of severe adverse events after peptide vaccination for advanced cancer patients: analysis of 500 cases. Oncol Rep 25:57–62
29. Noguchi M, Mine T, Komatsu N, Suekane S, Moriya F, Matsuoka K et al (2011) Assessment of immunological biomarkers in patients with advanced cancer treated by personalized peptide vaccination. Cancer Biol Ther 10:1266–1279
30. Avogadri F, Merghoub T, Maughan MF, Hirschhorn-Cymerman D, Morris J, Ritter E et al (2010) Alphavirus replicon particles expressing TRP-2 provide potent therapeutic effect on melanoma through activation of humoral and cellular immunity. PLoS One 5:e12670
31. Hong S, Qian J, Li H, Yang J, Lu Y, Zheng Y et al (2012) CpG or IFN-α are more potent adjuvants than GM-CSF to promote anti-tumor immunity following idiotype vaccine in multiple myeloma. Cancer Immunol Immunother 61:561–571
32. Melief CJ, van der Burg SH (2008) Immunotherapy of established (pre)malignant disease by synthetic long peptide vaccines. Nat Rev Cancer 8:351–360
33. Bijker MS, van den Eeden SJ, Franken KL, Melief CJ, Offringa R, van der Burg SH (2007) CD8+ CTL priming by exact peptide epitopes in incomplete Freund's adjuvant induces a vanishing CTL response, whereas long peptides induce sustained CTL reactivity. J Immunol 179:5033–5040
34. Toes RE, Offringa R, Blom RJ, Melief CJ, Kast WM (1996) Peptide vaccination can lead to enhanced tumor growth through specific T-cell tolerance induction. Proc Natl Acad Sci U S A 93:7855–7860
35. Kenter GG, Welters MJ, Valentijn AR, Lowik MJ, Berends-van der Meer DM, Vloon AP et al (2008) Phase I immunotherapeutic trial with long peptides spanning the E6 and E7 sequences of high-risk human papillomavirus 16 in end-stage cervical cancer patients shows low toxicity and robust immunogenicity. Clin Cancer Res 14:169–177

36. Kenter GG, Welters MJ, Valentijn AR, Lowik MJ, Berends-van der Meer DM, Vloon AP et al (2009) Vaccination against HPV-16 oncoproteins for vulvar intraepithelial neoplasia. N Engl J Med 361:1838–1847
37. Leffers N, Lambeck AJ, Gooden MJ, Hoogeboom BN, Wolf R, Hamming IE et al (2009) Immunization with a P53 synthetic long peptide vaccine induces P53-specific immune responses in ovarian cancer patients, a phase II trial. Int J Cancer 125:2104–2113
38. Welters MJ, Kenter GG, Piersma SJ, Vloon AP, Löwik MJ, Berends-van der Meer DM et al (2008) Induction of tumor-specific CD4+ and CD8+ T-cell immunity in cervical cancer patients by a human papillomavirus type 16 E6 and E7 long peptides vaccine. Clin Cancer Res 14:178–187
39. Noguchi M, Uemura H, Naito S, Akaza H, Yamada A, Itoh K (2011) A phase I study of personalized peptide vaccination using 14 kinds of vaccine in combination with low-dose estramustine in HLA-A24-positive patients with castration-resistant prostate cancer. Prostate 71:470–479
40. Noguchi M, Kobayashi K, Suetsugu N, Tomiyasu K, Suekane S, Yamada A et al (2003) Induction of cellular and humoral immune responses to tumor cells and peptides in HLA-A24 positive hormone-refractory prostate cancer patients by peptide vaccination. Prostate 57:80–92
41. Noguchi M, Itoh K, Suekane S, Yao A, Suetsugu N, Katagiri K et al (2004) Phase I trial of patient-oriented vaccination in HLA-A2 positive patients with metastatic hormone refractory prostate cancer. Cancer Sci 95:77–84
42. Noguchi M, Mine T, Yamada A, Obata Y, Yoshida K, Mizoguchi J et al (2007) Combination therapy of personalized peptide vaccination and low-dose estramustine phosphate for metastatic hormone refractory prostate cancer patients: an analysis of prognostic factors in the treatment. Oncol Res 16:341–349
43. Noguchi M, Kakuma T, Uemura H, Nasu Y, Kumon H, Hirao Y et al (2009) A randomized phase II trial of personalized peptide vaccine plus low dose estramustine phosphate (EMP) versus standard dose EMP in patients with castration resistant prostate cancer. Cancer Immunol Immunother 59:1001–1009
44. Noguchi M, Moriya F, Suekane S, Matsuoka K, Arai G, Matsueda S et al (2012) Phase II study of personalized peptide vaccination for castration-resistant prostate cancer patients who failed in docetaxel-based chemotherapy. Prostate 72:834–845
45. Yajima N, Yamanaka R, Mine T, Tsuchiya N, Homma J, Sano M et al (2005) Immunologic evaluation of personalized peptide vaccination for patients with advanced malignant glioma. Clin Cancer Res 11:5900–5911
46. Terasaki M, Shibui S, Narita Y, Fujimaki T, Aoki T, Kajiwara K et al (2011) Phase I trial of a personalized peptide vaccine for patients positive for human leukocyte antigen–A24 with recurrent or progressive glioblastoma multiforme. J Clin Oncol 29:337–344
47. Yanagimoto H, Mine T, Yamamoto K, Satoi S, Terakawa N, Takahashi K et al (2007) Immunological evaluation of personalized peptide vaccination with gemcitabine for pancreatic cancer. Cancer Sci 98:605–611
48. Yanagimoto H, Shiomi H, Satoi S, Mine T, Toyokawa H, Yamamoto T et al (2010) A phase II study of personalized peptide vaccination combined with gemcitabine for non-resectable pancreatic cancer patients. Oncol Rep 24:795–801
49. Burris HA, Moore MJ, Andersen J, Green MR, Rothenberg ML, Modiano MR et al (1997) Improvements in survival and clinical benefit with gemcitabine as first-line therapy for patients with advanced pancreas cancer: a randomized trial. J Clin Oncol 15:2403–2413
50. Yoshitomi M, Yutani S, Matsueda S, Ioji T, Komatsu N, Shichijo S et al (2012) Personalized peptide vaccination for advanced biliary tract cancer: IL-6, nutritional status and pre-existing antigen-specific immunity as possible biomarkers for patient prognosis. Exp Ther Med 3:463–469
51. Ito M, Shichijo S, Miyagi Y, Kobayashi T, Tsuda N, Yamada A et al (2000) Identification of SART3-derived peptides capable of inducing HLA-A2-restricted and tumor-specific CTLs in cancer patients with different HLA-A2 subtypes. Int J Cancer 88:633–639

52. Yang D, Nakao M, Shichijo S, Sasatomi T, Takasu H, Matsumoto H et al (1999) Identification of a gene coding for a protein possessing shared tumor epitopes capable of inducing HLA-A24-restricted cytotoxic T lymphocytes in cancer patients. Cancer Res 59:4056–4063
53. Sato Y, Maeda Y, Sasatomi T, Takahashi M, Une Y, Kondo M et al (2004) A phase I trial of CTL-precursor-oriented peptide vaccine for colorectal carcinoma patients. Br J Cancer 90:13334–13342
54. Sato Y, Fujiwara T, Mine T, Shomura H, Homma S, Maeda Y et al (2007) Immunological evaluation of personalized peptide vaccination in combination with a 5-fluorouracil derivative (TS-1) for advanced gastric or colorectal carcinoma patients. Cancer Sci 98:1113–1119
55. Sato Y, Shomura H, Maeda Y, Mine T, Une Y, Akasaka Y et al (2003) Immunological evaluation of peptide vaccination for patients with gastric cancer based on pre-existing cellular response to peptide. Cancer Sci 94:802–808
56. Mine T, Gouhara R, Hida N, Imai N, Azuma K, Rikimaru T et al (2003) Immunological evaluation of CTL precursor-oriented vaccines for advanced lung cancer patients. Cancer Sci 94:548–556
57. Yoshiyama K, Terazaki Y, Matsueda S, Shichijo S, Noguchi M, Yamada A et al (2012) Personalized peptide vaccination in patients with refractory non-small cell lung cancer. Int J Oncol 40:1492–1500
58. Terazaki Y, Yoshiyama K, Matsueda S, Watanabe N, Kawahara A, Naito Y et al (2012) Immunological evaluation of personalized peptide vaccination in refractory small cell lung cancer. Cancer Sci 103:638–644
59. Tsuda N, Mochizuki K, Harada M, Sukehiro A, Kawano K, Yamada A et al (2004) Vaccination with pre-designated or evidence-based peptides for patients with recurrent gynecologic cancers. J Immunother 27:60–67
60. Suekane S, Nishitani M, Noguchi M, Komohara Y, Kokubu T, Naitoh M et al (2007) Phase I trial of personalized peptide vaccination for cytokine-refractory metastatic renal cell carcinoma patients. Cancer Sci 98:1965–1968
61. Tanaka S, Harada M, Mine T, Noguchi M, Gohara R, Azuma K et al (2003) Peptide vaccination for patients with melanoma and other types of cancer based on pre-existing peptide-specific cytotoxic T-lymphocyte precursors in the periphery. J Immunother 26:357–366
62. Matsumoto K, Noguchi M, Satoh T, Tabata K, Fujita T, Iwamura M et al (2011) A phase I study of personalized peptide vaccination for advanced urothelial carcinoma patients who failed treatment with methotrexate, vinblastine, adriamycin and cisplatin. BJU Int 108:831–838
63. Eggermont AM (2009) Therapeutic vaccines in solid tumours: can they be harmful? Eur J Cancer 45:2087–2090
64. Disis ML (2011) Immunologic biomarkers as correlates of clinical response to cancer immunotherapy. Cancer Immunol Immunother 60:433–442
65. Hoos A, Eggermont AM, Janetzki S, Hodi FS, Ibrahim R, Anderson A et al (2010) Improved endpoints for cancer immunotherapy trials. J Natl Cancer Inst 102:1388–1397
66. Amos SM, Duong CP, Westwood JA, Ritchie DS, Junghans RP, Darcy PK et al (2011) Autoimmunity associated with immunotherapy of cancer. Blood 118:499–509
67. López MN, Pereda C, Segal G, Muñoz L, Aguilera R, González FE et al (2009) Prolonged survival of dendritic cell-vaccinated melanoma patients correlates with tumor-specific delayed type IV hypersensitivity response and reduction of tumor growth factor beta-expressing T cells. J Clin Oncol 27:945–952
68. Komatsu N, Matsueda S, Tashiro K, Ioji T, Shichijo S, Noguchi M et al (2012) Gene expression profiles in peripheral blood as a biomarker in cancer patients receiving peptide vaccination. Cancer 118:3208–3221
69. Sansone P, Bromberg J (2012) Targeting the interleukin-6/jak/stat pathway in human malignancies. J Clin Oncol 30:1005–1014
70. Nishimoto N, Kishimoto T (2006) Interleukin 6: from bench to bedside. Nat Clin Pract Rheumatol 2:619–626

# Chapter 12
# WT1 Peptide Vaccine for the Treatment of Malignancies: Its Development, Recent Progress, and Future Perspectives

**Yoshihiro Oka, Akihiro Tsuboi, Hiroko Nakajima, Fumihiro Fujiki, Sumiyuki Nishida, Soyoko Morimoto, Jun Nakata, Yoshiki Nakae, Satoshi Takashima, Naoya Tatsumi, Naoki Hosen, Yusuke Oji, and Haruo Sugiyama**

**Abstract** Wilms' tumor gene (*WT1*) possesses oncogenic functions and is expressed in various hematological malignancies and solid cancers, and the gene product WT1 protein is highly immunogenic, which indicates that WT1 should be a promising target antigen for cancer immunotherapy. The identification of human WT1 cytotoxic T lymphocyte (CTL) epitopes and the demonstration using a mouse model that WT1 could serve in vivo as a target antigen for cancer immunotherapy were reported in 2000. Based on these findings, clinical trials for WT1 peptide

Y. Oka (✉)
Department of Cancer Immunology, Graduate School of Medicine, Osaka University, 1-7 Yamada-oka, Suita, Osaka 565-0871, Japan

Department of Respiratory Medicine, Allergy and Rheumatic Diseases, Graduate School of Medicine, Osaka University, Osaka, Japan

Department of Immunopathology, WPI Immunology Frontier Research Center, Osaka University, Osaka, Japan
e-mail: yoshi@imed3.med.osaka-u.ac.jp

A. Tsuboi • J. Nakata • N. Tatsumi
Department of Cancer Immunotherapy, Graduate School of Medicine, Osaka University, Osaka, Japan

H. Nakajima • F. Fujiki • S. Morimoto • H. Sugiyama (✉)
Department of Cancer Immunology, Graduate School of Medicine, Osaka University, 1-7 Yamada-oka, Suita, Osaka 565-0871, Japan
e-mail: sugiyama@sahs.med.osaka-u.ac.jp

S. Nishida • S. Takashima
Department of Respiratory Medicine, Allergy and Rheumatic Diseases, Graduate School of Medicine, Osaka University, Osaka, Japan

Y. Nakae
Department of Hematology, Kitano Hospital, Osaka, Japan

N. Hosen • Y. Oji
Department of Cancer Stem Cell Biology, Graduate School of Medicine, Osaka University, Osaka, Japan


Y. Yamaguchi (ed.), *Immunotherapy of Cancer*,
DOI 10.1007/978-4-431-55031-0_12

vaccine were started. The early clinical trials demonstrated that the WT1 peptide vaccination could induce WT1-specific immunological response such as an increase in WT1-specific CTL frequency, resulting in occurrence of clinical response such as a decrease in leukemia/solid tumor load, which strongly suggested the therapeutic potential of the WT1 peptide vaccine for the treatment of malignancies. A review article published in 2009 in a prestigious journal gave WT1 the highest ranking as a target antigen for cancer immunotherapy. Now, cases which showed immunological and/or clinical responses with treatment by WT1 peptide vaccine are being accumulated. Some of the recent clinical trials showed noteworthy results, such as the demonstration that WT1 peptide vaccination may lead acute myeloid leukemia patients with minimal residual disease to a cure and that the vaccination may prevent relapse of patients with hematological malignancies who have received allogeneic hematopoietic stem cell transplantation but are at high risk of relapse. In addition, clinical usefulness of the WT1 peptide vaccine combined with chemotherapy drugs or molecular target-based drugs was also suggested. Continuing progress of WT1-targeting immunotherapy, a translational research based on basic research, should lead to innovative development of cancer immunotherapy. Furthermore, comprehensive analysis of the samples obtained from the patients treated with the WT1-targeting immunotherapy, a reverse-translational research, should contribute to the elucidation of cancer immunity mechanisms.

**Keywords** WT1 • Immunotherapy • Cancer vaccine • Peptide vaccine • Cancer antigen

## 12.1 WT1 as a Prime Target Antigen for Cancer Immunotherapy: The Highest Ranking as the Target Antigen Has Been Given to WT1

In a review article of a prestigious journal, Clinical Cancer Research, published in 2009, Wilms' tumor gene (*WT1*) product, WT1 protein, was rated as the most promising target antigen for cancer immunotherapy among many such target antigens identified until then [1]. Its primacy was determined based on results of a series of investigations, some of which are referred to in this article. Although the ratings of the target antigens may vary depending on how the authors weigh criteria for evaluation, it has become clear that WT1 is one of the prime target antigens for cancer immunotherapy [1–3].

One of the crucial reasons for this highest ranking is that *WT1* possesses an essentially appropriate character so that the gene product WT1 could serve as a target antigen for cancer immunotherapy. The crucial character of the gene is that it plays important roles in maintaining oncogenic function of cancer cells [3–5]. In view of the gene's character, it seems unlikely that cancer cells escape from immunological attack when WT1 is used as a target antigen for immunotherapy [3]. Another advantage of WT1 is that it is expressed in various neoplasms, including hematological malignancies such as leukemia and many kinds of solid cancers, for which we can apply WT1-targeting immunotherapy [2, 6–8]. Furthermore, it was reported that acute myeloid leukemia (AML) stem cells expressed WT1, which suggested that WT1-directed immunotherapy could target leukemia/cancer stem cells [9]. In addition, it was reported that not only cancer cells themselves but also tumor vessels express WT1, indicating the possibility that tumor vessels could also become a target for WT1-directed immunotherapy [10].

Besides oncogenic function of *WT1* gene and its expression in various kinds of cancer and tumor vessels, the high immunogenicity of WT1 protein, which was demonstrated in a series of investigations and is described later in this chapter, is also an advantageous character of WT1 to become a prime target antigen for cancer immunotherapy.

## 12.2 Identification of WT1 CTL Epitopes, Which Is Really the Start for the Invention and Development of WT1-Targeting Cancer Immunotherapy

To activate WT1-specific cytotoxic T lymphocytes (CTLs) in patients, we perform intradermal or subcutaneous injection of WT1 CTL epitope peptides with immunoadjuvant. Therefore, identification of WT1 protein-derived peptides that are able to induce WT1-specific CTLs, i.e., WT1 CTL epitopes, is essential for development of WT1 peptide vaccine. And, the successful identification of the WT1 CTL epitopes indicates that WT1 is a tumor-associated antigen (TAA), a target antigen for cancer immunotherapy.

The principle of WT1 peptide vaccination is as follows [11]. We inject WT1 CTL peptides with an adjuvant into the skin. The adjuvant activates dendritic cells (DCs) present in the skin, and the injected peptides bind to HLA class I molecules on the surface of the DCs. The activated DCs with the CTL peptides then move to lymph nodes, where the DCs activate the "WT1 CTL peptide/HLA class I molecule" complex-specific T cell receptor (TCR)-bearing $CD8^+$ T cells, which become the WT1 peptide-specific CTLs with the restriction of the HLA class I type. On the other hand, since WT1 protein, a target antigen, in tumor cells is divided to small pieces of peptides, followed by presentation of the peptides with HLA class I molecules on the cell surface of the tumor cells, the WT1-specific CTLs are able to attack the tumor cells through recognition of the "WT1 peptide/HLA class I molecule" complex on the cell surface.

Identification of human WT1 CTL epitope was first reported independently by three groups, including ours, in 2000 (Table 12.1). In 2000, we, Oka et al., reported on identification of two WT1 CTL epitopes, the 9-mer WT1-126 and WT1-187 peptides, with the restriction of HLA-A*02:01, which is one of the most common HLA class I types [12]. For example, about 50 % of Caucasians and 20 % of Japanese, respectively, possess HLA-A*02:01. Soon after the publication of our

**Table 12.1** Identification of WT1 cytotoxic T lymphocyte (CTL) epitope peptides

| **Human** | | | |
|---|---|---|---|
| **HLA-A*02:01** restriction | | | |
| Publication year | Peptide name[a] | Peptide sequence | References |
| 2000 | WT1-126[b] | RMFPNAPYL | Oka et al. [12] and Gao et al. [13][c] |
| 2000 | WT1-187[d] | SLGEQQYSV | Oka et al. [12] |
| 2005[e] | WT1-37 | VLDFAPPGA | Rezvani et al. [18][e] |
| 2006 | WT1-126 modified | <u>Y</u>MFPNAPYL[f] | Pinilla-Ibarz et al. [21] |
| **HLA-A*24:02** restriction | | | |
| 2000 | WT1-235[g] | CMTWNQMNL | Ohminami et al. [15] |
| 2002 | WT1-235 modified | C<u>Y</u>TWNQMNL[h] | Tsuboi et al. [16] |
| 2002 | WT1-417 | RWPSCQKKF | Azuma et al. [17] |
| **HLA-A*01** restriction | | | |
| 2006 | WT1-317 | TSEKRPFMCAY | Asemissen et al. [20] |
| **Mouse** | | | |
| **H-2D[b]** restriction | | | |
| 2000 | WT1-126[b] | RMFPNAPYL | Oka et al. [35] |
| **H-2K[b]** restriction | | | |
| 2007 | WT1-330[i] | CNKRYFKL | Ramirez et al. [38] |

[a]Peptide names in this table are based on positions of the starting amino acids (N terminus) of each peptide and the nomenclature in the original articles (reference papers)
[b]RMFPNAPYL is a common sequence between human and mouse, while anchor residues are located at different positions between A*02:01of human and H-2D[b] of mouse
[c]Gao et al. identified WT1-126 using allogeneic experimental system (see details in the text and Ref. [13])
[d]**A*02:06** restriction was also shown by Li et al. later in 2008 [24]
[e]Rezvani et al. referred to ASH meeting in 2001 (Smithgall et al. [19])
[f]Underlined amino acid (Y: first) is the modified one
[g]**A*02:01** restriction was also shown by Bellantuono et al. later in 2002 (allogeneic experimental system) [22] and by Li et al. in 2005 [23], respectively
[h]Underlined amino acid (Y: second) is the modified one
[i]Ramirez et al. identified WT1-330 using allogeneic experimental system (see details in the text and ref. [38])
Besides WT1 peptides shown in this table, identification of immunogenic WT1 peptides based on peptide mapping was recently performed. See details in the reference papers [25–27]

study, Gao et al. also reported on identification of WT1-126 peptide as an HLA-A*02:01-restricted CTL epitope, using allo-restricted CTL approach that should be independent of immunologic tolerance, in which they showed that WT1-126 peptide-specific CTLs with HLA-A*02:01 restriction could be generated from HLA-A*02:01-negative donors [13]. It was afterward confirmed by another group that both WT1-126 and WT1-187 could serve as CTL peptides in humans [14]. As for HLA class I types other than A*02:01, Ohminami et al. reported, also in 2000, identification of a WT1 CTL epitope, 9-mer WT1-235 peptide, with the restriction of HLA-A*24:02, which is the most frequent (50–60 %) HLA class I type in Japanese, while a considerable proportion (about 20 %) of Caucasians possess this HLA class I type [15]. Subsequently, we, Tsuboi et al., found that a modified WT1-235 peptide (CYTWNQMNL) generated by a single amino acid substitution at one of the two anchor positions of the natural WT1-235 peptide (CMTWNQMNL) was able to induce a more robust WT1-specific CTL response with the restriction of HLA-A*24:02, which was reported later in 2002 [16] (Table 12.1). These WT1 CTL peptides, WT1-126, WT1-235, and modified WT1-235, became prototypes of WT1 CTL epitope peptides used for clinical trials of the WT1 peptide vaccine and analyses of WT1-specific CTL responses. Besides them, other WT1 CTL peptides have also been identified [17–21], and furthermore, some of WT1 CTL peptides were shown to cross-react to other HLA class I molecules [22–24] (Table 12.1). Recently, the results of epitope mapping-based analysis of immunogenic WT1 epitopes were also reported [25–27].

## 12.3 Evidence for High Immunogenicity of WT1 Protein/ Peptide in Humans

A series of investigations demonstrated that humoral and cellular immune response against WT1 is naturally generated in patients with malignancies, thus indicating a high immunogenicity of WT1.

We, Elisseeva et al., reported the detection of anti-WT1 antibodies of IgG as well as IgM type more frequently in peripheral blood (PB) of patients with hematological malignancies than in that of healthy donors [28]. This finding indicated that not only WT1-specific humoral immune response but also WT1-specific cellular immune response, which is needed to induce immunoglobulin class switch from IgM to IgG, was generated in these patients. Our subsequent investigation showed that the IgG type WT1-directed humoral immune response in patients with hematological malignancies was Th1 biased, which is essentially important for WT1-targeting immunotherapy [29]. More recently, we, Oji et al, demonstrated that non-small cell lung cancer (NSCLC) patients with stages I–III who showed elevation of IgG type anti-WT1 antibody had longer disease-free survival than those who did not show the elevation. This finding suggested that WT1-directed immunity was elicited in patients with NSCLC, and furthermore, that such WT1-directed immunity might perform an important role in suppression of tumor growth in this disease [30]. Another group, Gaiger et al., also reported on the detection of anti-WT1 antibody in leukemia patients [31].

A series of investigations demonstrated spontaneous induction of a WT1-directed cellular immune response, i.e., CTL response, in patients with malignancies [2, 32–34]. It is noteworthy that it was also found that WT1-specific CTLs may contribute to induction of the graft-versus-leukemia (GVL) effect after hematopoietic stem cell transplantation (HSCT) [33, 34]. This prompted us to perform

WT1 peptide vaccination after HSCT to enhance the GVL effect, as is described later in this chapter.

## 12.4 Mouse Models That Suggested In Vivo Efficacy of WT1 Peptide Vaccination

To examine whether WT1 can serve as a target antigen for cancer immunotherapy, mouse in vivo models are crucial. In 2000, we, Oka et al., demonstrated that C57/BL6 mice, which had MHC class I H-2D$^b$, vaccinated with H-2D$^b$-restricted WT1 peptide could reject the transplanted H-2D$^{b+}$ tumor cells with *WT1* expression [35] (Table 12.1). The mouse WT1 peptide identified in this study was WT1-126 [35], which happens to have the same amino acid sequence as HLA-A*02:01-restricted human WT1-126, although mouse H-2D$^b$ and human HLA-A*02:01 have different anchor positions for peptide binding. This mouse study [35], the study of identification of human WT1-126 CTL peptide reported by us [12], and the study of identification of human WT1-235 CTL peptide reported by Ohminami et al. [15], all of which were published in 2000, demonstrated the possibility that immunization of patients with "the patient-bearing HLA class I-restricted WT1 CTL peptide" could break tolerance to self-antigen WT1, thus leading to induction of WT1-specific anticancer effect (Table 12.1).

In addition, in this in vivo mouse experiment, it is noteworthy that *WT1*-expressing normal tissues, including kidney, were not damaged, even though WT1-specific CTLs were induced by immunization of mice with the WT1 peptide, leading to rejection of *WT1*-expressing tumor. This result strongly suggested that WT1 peptide vaccination would not damage normal tissues in clinical settings, either. Results of a subsequent series of in vivo mouse experiments for WT1 peptide (WT1-126) vaccine further demonstrated that WT1 peptide vaccination damaged tumors but not normal organs with *WT1* expression, including kidney and bone marrow (BM) progenitor cells [36, 37].

As a mouse CTL epitope besides WT1-126, Ramirez et al. identified H-2K$^b$-restricted WT1-330, which could induce allo-MHC-restricted CTLs, while the authors did not show the in vivo killing activity [38].

In some investigations, immunodeficient mice were used as a vehicle to examine in vivo activity of human WT1-specific CTLs [14, 39]. In such an experimental setting, human *WT1*-expressing tumor cells and human WT1-specific CTLs with restriction of the tumor's HLA class I type were transplanted into the immunodeficient mice, followed by examination of the CTL activity. For example, Doubrovina et al. demonstrated that WT1-specific CTLs with restriction of HLA-A*02:01 were accumulated in HLA-A*0201-positive tumor sites, leading to regression of the tumor [14].

## 12.5 Early and the Subsequent Clinical Trials That Demonstrated the Therapeutic Potential of the WT1 Peptide Vaccine: "Proof of Concept" for the WT1 Peptide Vaccine

### *12.5.1 The First Case Reports of Clinical Response-Positive WT1 Peptide Vaccination for Patients with Common HLA Class I Types*

In 2003, we, Oka et al., reported two HLA-A*24:02-positive myelodysplastic syndrome (MDS)-related cases which showed reduction of leukemic cells and/or *WT1* mRNA levels, a marker of leukemic cell load, with the treatment by WT1 peptide vaccine composed of HLA-A*24:02-restricted modified WT1-235 peptide and Montanide ISA51 adjuvant [40]. This report in 2003 was the first study that clearly demonstrated the vaccine's therapeutic potential in clinical setting (Table 12.2). In this report, not only the successful reduction of leukemic cell load but also leukocytopenia was observed. It was interpreted that most of the blood cells in these patients with the MDS-related disease were derived from *WT1*-expressing abnormal hematopoietic stem or progenitor cells, and therefore, hematopoiesis of the patients was mainly sustained by these abnormal blood cells, which were attacked by the vaccination-activated WT1-specific CTLs, thus resulting in the leukocytopenia. The leukocytopenia could therefore be regarded as a reflection of the vaccine's clinical effect, as well as a side effect specific to MDS.

As for HLA-A*02:01 type, Mailänder et al. reported for the first time an WT1-126 peptide-treated AML case in 2004, in which a reduction of blast cells and the subsequent long-lasting complete remission (CR) by the treatment with an HLA-A*02:01-restricted WT1 peptide (WT1-126) vaccine were shown [41]. The two abovementioned reports are the first description of the clinical courses of the patients with HLA-A*24:02 and the patient with HLA-A*02:01, respectively, in which the WT1 peptide vaccine was shown to have the therapeutic potential (Table 12.2). The vaccination-associated immunological response, such as an increase in frequencies of WT1-tetramer$^{+}$ CD8$^{+}$ T cells, was also observed.

### *12.5.2 Accumulation of Clinical Studies with Positive Results, Including Those That Show "Proof of Concept" for WT1 Peptide Vaccine*

In order to confirm that the clinical response observed after the WT1 peptide vaccination is actually induced by the vaccination, it is essential to ascertain the occurrence of the vaccination-induced immunological response and, furthermore, a correlation between the immunological and the clinical response, which would lead

**Table 12.2** Clinical trials: WT1 peptide vaccination (monotherapy)-induced immunological and/or clinical responses

| Publication year | Disease | Immunological response | Clinical response (or usefulness, significance) | HLA class I | Peptide | References |
|---|---|---|---|---|---|---|
| 2003 | MDS-related diseases[a] | Increase in WT1-specific CTLs | Reduction of blast and/or *WT1* mRNA levels | A*24:02 | WT1-235m[b] | Oka et al. [40] |
| 2004 | AML | Increase in WT1-specific CTLs, increase in WT1 specifically IFNγ-secreting CD8 T cells | Reduction of blast | A*02:01 | WT1-126 | Mailänder et al. [41] |
| 2004 | Lung cancer[c] | Increase in WT1 specifically IFNγ-secreting CD8 T cells, enhancement of WT1-specific DTH | Reduction of tumor marker, which was maintained durably | A*24:02 | WT1-235 | Tsuboi et al. [48] |
| 2004 | MDS-related diseases, AML, lung cancer, breast cancer | Increase in WT1-specific CTLs, a correlation between immuno-logical response and clinical response | Reduction of blast and/or *WT1* mRNA levels in AML, tumor reduction and/or decrease in tumor marker in solid tumor | A*24:02 | WT1-235<br>WT1-235m | Oka et al. [42][d] |
| 2006 | Various solid cancer | Not evaluated | Confirmation that the toxicity level of WT1 peptide vaccine is acceptable | A*24:02 | WT1-235m | Morita et al. [57] |
| 2007 | MDS | Increase in WT1-specific CTLs with very low dose of WT1 peptide vaccine | Reduction of abnormal cells with very low dose of WT1 peptide vaccine | A*24:02 | WT1-235m | Kawakami et al. [46] |
| 2007 | Renal cancer | Increase in WT1-specific CTLs, induction of WT1 peptide-specific DTH | Long-term SD (stable disease) | A*24:02 | WT1-235m | Iiyama et al. [49] |
| 2007 | Multiple myeloma | Increase in $CD107^+$ cells in $WT1\text{-tetramer}^+$ CD8 T cells | Reduction of myeloma cell and M protein, improvement in bone scintigraphic examination | A*24:02 | WT1-235m | Tsuboi et al. [47] |
| 2008 | AML, MDS | Increase in WT1-specific CTLs | Reduction of *WT1* mRNA levels | A*02:01 | WT1-126 | Rezvani et al. [43] |

| | | | | | | |
|---|---|---|---|---|---|---|
| 2008 | GBM | No detection of immunological response after the vaccination (high frequencies of WT1-specific CTLs before the vaccination) | PR (partial response), SD, long-term SD, suggestion that WT1 vaccine is active for the treatment of GBM | A*24:02 | WT1-235m | Izumoto et al. [55] |
| 2009 | Rhabdomyosarcoma[e] (childhood) | Increase in WT1-specific CTLs | Disappearance of bone metastasis | A*24:02 | WT1-235m | Ohta et al. [56] |
| 2009 | AML, MDS | Emergence of WT1-specific CTLs | Reduction of blast in AML, improvement of anemia in MDS | A*24:02 | WT1-235 | Yasukawa et al. [45] |
| 2009 | AML, MDS | Increase in WT1-specific CTLs | Reduction of blast, reduction of molecular disease marker such as trisomy 8, disease stabilization, neutrophil response in MDS | A*02:01 | WT1-126 | Keilholz et al. [44] |
| 2009 | Gynecological cancer | Emergence of WT1-specific DTH | Reduction of tumor size or marker | A*24:02 | WT1-235m | Ohno et al. [50] |
| 2010 | AML | Increase in WT1-specific CTLs, increase in WT1 specifically IFN-secreting T cells, induction of WT1-specific CD4 T cell response, induction of WT1-specific DTH | Difficult to be evaluated | A*02:01 and others | WT1-126m, DR-binding peptides | Maslak et al. [58] |
| 2010 | Sarcoma, ALL (childhood) | Increase in WT1-specific CTLs | CR in rhabdomyosarcoma, SD in liposarcoma | A*24:02 | WT1-235m | Hashii et al. [59] |
| 2010 | Mesothelioma, lung cancer | Induction of WT1-specific CD8 T cell response, induction of WT1-specific CD4 T cell response | Difficult to be evaluated | A*02:01 and others | WT1-126m, DR-binding peptides | Krug et al. [60] |
| 2011 | Salivary gland cancer | Difficult to be evaluated | Stabilization of tumor growth | A*24:02 | WT1-235m | Sasabe et al. [52] |

(continued)

**Table 12.2** (continued)

| Publication year | Disease | Immunological response | Clinical response (or usefulness, significance) | HLA class I | Peptide | References |
|---|---|---|---|---|---|---|
| 2011 | Ovarian cancer[f] | Not evaluated | Disappearance of pleural effusion, reduction of tumor size, long-term SD | A*24:02 | WT1-235m | Dohi et al. [61] |
| 2012 | AML, ALL (CR[g] after allogeneic HSCT[h] but at high risk of relapse) (childhood) | Increase in WT1-specific CTLs | Decrease in *WT1* or *AML/MTG8* mRNA, persistence of CR for more than 2 years in 2 of the 3 patients, which suggested a cure | A:24:02 | WT1-235m | Hashii et al. [62] |
| 2012 | Salivary gland cancer | Increase in WT1-specific CTLs, emergence of WT1-specific DTH | Stabilization of tumor growth | A*2402 | WT1-235m | Shirakata et al. [53] |
| 2012 | Melanoma | Emergence of WT1-specific DTH, infiltration of CD8 T cells in a tumor site | Stabilization of tumor growth | A*24:02 | WT1-235m | Nishioka et al. [54] |
| 2012 | AML (CR after chemo therapy but at high risk of relapse) | Increase in WT1-specific CTLs, emergence of functional WT1-specific CTLs | Reduction of *WT1* mRNA, persistence of CR for more than 8 years in 3 of the 8 patients, which suggested a cure | A*24:02 | WT1-235, WT1-235m | Tsuboi et al. [63] |
| 2012 | Various solid cancer | Not evaluated | Safety of addition of GM-CSF or CpG-ODN to WT1 peptide vaccine | A*02:01<br>A*02:06<br>A*24:02 | WT1-187, WT1-235m | Ohno et al. [64] |

| | | | | | | |
|---|---|---|---|---|---|---|
| 2013 | Gynecological malignancies | Emergence of WT1-specific DTH | Asscciation of emergence of WT1-specific DTH and overall survival | A*24:02 | WT1-235m | Miyatake et al. [51] |
| 2013 | AML, ALL (after allogeneic HSCT) | Increase in WT1-specific CTLs | Reduction of *WT1* or *MLL/AF4* mRNA levels, persistence of CR in several patients | A*2402 | WT1-235m | Maeda et al. [65] |

Abbreviations for disease names, *MDS* myelodysplastic syndromes, *AML* acute myeloid leukemia, *ALL* acute lymphoblastic leukemia, *GBM* glioblastoma multiforme

These cases with MDS-related diseases[a] and with lung cancer[c] were used in Ref [42][d] for the further analysis

[b]M modified peptide. See text for details

[e]The clinical course of this case is also shown in Ref [59]

[f]This case is one of the cases that appeared in Ref [50]

[g]Complete remission

[h]Hematopoietic stem cell transplantation

to establishment of "proof of concept" for the vaccine's therapeutic potential. In 2004, we, Oka et al., reported a positive correlation between the WT1 vaccination-induced immunological response, i.e., an increase in the frequencies of WT1-specific CTLs in PB, and the emergence of clinical response of the patients with AML, MDS, breast cancer, and lung cancer [42]. This finding clearly demonstrated the potential capability of the WT1 peptide vaccine to induce WT1-specific immunological response and the resultant clinical response.

Subsequently, the induction of WT1 peptide vaccination-induced immunological and/or clinical response for a number of patients with hematological malignancies, AML and MDS, was reported by Rezvani et al. and Keilholz et al., respectively [43, 44]. In the former, of note, an increase in WT1-specific CTL numbers in PB was shown to be associated with a decrease in a minimal residual disease (MRD) marker of the patients, which provided further evidence that WT1 peptide vaccination is able to induce WT1-specific immunological response, leading to emergence of clinical response, which, in addition to our work mentioned above, should also form a "proof of concept" for the WT1 vaccine's therapeutic potential [42, 43]. In the latter, the study reported by Keilholz et al., among the cases reported, a clinical course of an especially interesting case with secondary AML from MDS was described [44]. Treatment of this patient by the WT1 peptide vaccine resulted in the disappearance of trisomy 8, a molecular marker of the disease, which was associated with an improvement of anemia. It seems likely that the vaccination reduced the abnormal hematological clones, which subsequently led to the recovery of normal hematopoiesis, resulting in the improvement of anemia. Such disappearance of a disease-specific molecular marker, other than *WT1* mRNA level, in association with WT1 peptide vaccination should establish solid evidence for the therapeutic potential of the vaccine. In consistence with the clinical course of this case, Yasukawa et al. also reported an improvement of anemia in MDS patient treated with WT1 peptide vaccine [45].

To summarize, WT1 peptide vaccination-induced clinical response was first reported in patients with MDS-related diseases in 2003, followed by accumulation of clinical studies in which the WT1 peptide vaccination as a monotherapy, not combination therapy with other anticancer agents, could induce WT1-specific immunological and/or clinical response. The promising results of these clinical studies provided us with evidence for the WT1 peptide vaccine's therapeutic potential.

In addition to the findings of the clinical studies mentioned above, interesting clinical results obtained from monotherapy with WT1 peptide vaccine have been accumulated steadily. One of the noteworthy findings among them is the clinical course of an MDS patient treated with a reduced dose of WT1 peptide vaccine [46]. As we experienced, when MDS cases, in which hematopoiesis is mainly sustained by abnormal hematological clones, are treated by WT1 peptide vaccine, leukocytopenia, as well as reduction of leukemic blast cells, may be induced [40]. To avoid such a too rapid reduction of the WBC counts, we treated a patient with chronic myelomonocytic leukemia, a type of MDS, with a very low dose of the WT1 peptide vaccine, which produced a successful result, showing a gradual decrease in leukocyte and monocyte counts in association with an increase in frequencies of WT1 tetramer$^{+}$ CD8$^{+}$ T cells in PB [46]. This outcome indicated that low-dose WT1 peptide vaccination may be a safe and promising treatment for MDS patients. For hematological malignancies other than AML and MDS, we reported a multiple myeloma case that showed the vaccination-associated clinical response consisting of a reduction of myeloma cells in BM and that of M protein, as well as a decrease in the abnormal uptake of the myeloma lesion in a bone scintigram examination [47].

Besides the abovementioned reports, a considerable numbers of investigations showed the therapeutic potential of the WT1 vaccine for various kinds of tumors, such as lung cancer [48], renal cancer [49], gynecological malignancies including ovarian cancer [50, 51], salivary gland cancer [52, 53], malignant melanoma [54], malignant glioma [55], and rhabdomyosarcoma [56]. Importantly, WT1 peptide vaccine therapy for childhood patients was already reported in 2009 [56]. To summarize, representative clinical trial results of the WT1 peptide vaccine as a monotherapy, including those that were not yet referred to here [57–65], are listed in Table 12.2, although some of the studies focused on verification of the vaccine's safety and analyses of WT1-specific immunological response. As shown in Table 12.2, patients treated by WT1 peptide vaccine as a monotherapy are still being accumulated. Among those listed in Table 12.2, the WT1 vaccine therapies aiming at long-term survival (or a cure) [62, 63, 65], which have been performed recently as "the next stage" of the WT1 vaccine trial, are referred to later in 12.7 of this chapter.

It should be noted that emergence of WT1 peptide-specific delayed-type hypersensitivity (DTH) reaction, as well as ex vivo/in vitro immunological response such as an increase in WT1 tetramer$^{+}$ CD8$^{+}$ T cells, after the vaccination was suggested to be associated with clinical response [49, 51, 53, 54]. In addition, as an evidence for WT1 peptide vaccination-associated immune response, CD8$^{+}$ T cell infiltration in the metastatic lesion after the vaccination was detected [54].

## 12.6 Strategies to Enhance the Efficacy and Clinical Usefulness of the WT1 Peptide Vaccine

As mentioned above, since WT1 CTL epitope peptides were identified (Table 12.1), WT1 peptide-based clinical trials have been performed to treat various kinds of malignancies, which clearly demonstrated the therapeutic potential of the WT1 peptide vaccine. However, its efficacy is still limited, which prompted us to devise strategies for enhancement of the clinical effectiveness and usefulness of this vaccine (Table 12.3).

It seems obvious that the lower the tumor load is, the more effective a cancer vaccine becomes [3]. Therefore, although we treated only advanced stage cancer patients by WT1 peptide vaccine in the early clinical trials because the primary aim

**Table 12.3** Strategies that are expected to enhance clinical usefulness of WT1 peptide vaccine

| |
|---|
| WT1 peptide vaccination at MRD[a] state |
| After operation, chemotherapy, radiotherapy |
| After allogeneic HSCT[b] with or without low-dose immunosuppressive agents to prevent GVHD[c] |
| WT1 peptide vaccination in combination with other modalities other than immune-related ones |
| With chemotherapy, including gemcitabine |
| With molecular target-based drugs, including tyrosine kinase inhibitors |
| WT1 peptide vaccination in combination with other immune-related modalities |
| <cancer antigen specific> |
| WT1-specific helper peptide vaccine |
| Other tumor-associated antigen-targeting cancer vaccine |
| After allogeneic HSCT[b] |
| <cancer antigen independent> |
| Immuno-checkpoint modulators targeting CTLA-4, PD-1, PD-L1, etc. |
| Cytokines, including interferons |
| Novel immunoadjuvant, including CpG-ODN |
| After allogeneic HSCT[b] |

[a]*MRD* minimal residual disease
[b]*HSCT* hematopoietic stem cell transplantation. Patients after allogeneic HSCT are generally in MRD state, and HSCT itself is also immunotherapy targeting various antigens such as cancer antigens, including WT1, and minor histocompatibility antigens. See details in the text
[c]*GVHD* graft-versus-host disease

was to determine its safety, it is expected that WT1 peptide vaccination for patients in relatively good condition and with a relatively low tumor load after prior treatments will yield better clinical outcomes. The immune-recovering phase after HSCT should also be a candidate of favorable situations for the WT1 peptide vaccination. Patients who have received HSCT have MRD, thus not a high tumor load, so that the WT1 peptide vaccine may give clinical usefulness to such patients who have received HSCT but are still at high risk of relapse [3, 66]. Transient lymphopenia is induced after HSCT by irradiation or chemotherapeutic regimens, and this situation should allow expansion of leukemia antigen-reactive T cells without exhaustion that might be induced by the T cells' long-term exposure to abundant leukemic cells, because the T cells educated by the WT1 peptide vaccination are derived from the healthy donors without leukemia. If leukemia antigen-associated peptides are presented to the proliferating T cells during the period of lymphopenia and the subsequent T cell recovery, the host may be repopulated with T cells that contain a considerable proportion of leukemia-reactive T cells [66]. WT1-targeting vaccination after allogeneic HSCT can therefore be expected to enhance the GVL effect while minimizing graft-versus-host disease (GVHD).

For patients with a high tumor load, monotherapy with the WT1 peptide vaccine does not seem to be strong enough to durably suppress tumor growth. To solve this problem, WT1 peptide vaccine therapy combined with chemotherapy or molecular target-based drugs is thought to be more useful [11]. In fact, recent investigations showed that some chemotherapy drugs, including gemcitabine, are advantageous when combined with immunotherapy [67].

Combined therapy using two different kinds of immunotherapy is also promising. The following two strategies seem to be particularly worth mentioning here.

First is a combination therapy consisting of WT1 CTL peptides and WT1 helper peptides. After the identification of WT1 CTL epitope peptides, we and others identified WT1 protein-derived peptides that could induce WT1-specific $CD4^+$ helper T cell response, i.e., WT1 helper epitope peptides [68–74]. The representative WT1 helper peptides were listed in Table 12.4. In addition, as mentioned in 12.2, the results of epitope mapping-based analysis of immunogenic WT1 epitopes, including those with HLA class II restriction, were also reported [26, 27]. Combined administration of WT1 CTL peptides and WT1 helper peptides is expected to induce a more robust WT1-specific CTL response than can be attained with administration of WT1 CTL peptides alone, as shown in in vitro experiments [72]. It is of note that many of helper peptides are able to bind to multiple HLA class II types, i.e., promiscuous [73, 75, 76]. Furthermore, such a combined administration may induce more WT1-specific memory-type CTLs [77], which leads to a more long-term effect.

Another noteworthy combination therapy is a therapy consisting of "cancer antigen-specific" immunotherapy, which includes the WT1 peptide vaccine, and "cancer antigen-independent" immunotherapy, which includes immuno-checkpoint modulators. Recently, monoclonal antibodies that inhibit CTLA-4 or PD1/PD-L1 signals, known as immuno-checkpoint inhibitors, were developed [78–80]. Freeing T cells from their immunologically suppressive state by means of these immuno-checkpoint inhibitors, that is, a "cancer antigen-independent" immunotherapy, may enhance the efficacy of WT1 peptide vaccination, that is, a "cancer antigen-specific" immunotherapy.

Besides, cytokines, including interferons [37, 81], and novel immunoadjuvants [36, 54, 64, 82], including CpG oligodeoxynucleotides [64], may enhance the efficacy of the peptide vaccine.

## 12.7 Recent Clinical Trials, Including Noteworthy Ones That Show Us the Future Directions

The abovementioned early clinical trials, including the earliest one reported by Oka et al. in 2003 [40], of the WT1 peptide vaccination demonstrated its therapeutic potential. WT1-targeting immunotherapies other than WT1 peptide-based therapy, such as *WT1* mRNA-based DC therapy [83], also induced robust clinical as well as immunological response, further indicating the superiority of WT1 as a target antigen for cancer immunotherapy. Following a series of these investigations that demonstrated the therapeutic potential of the WT1 peptide vaccine, we proceeded

**Table 12.4** Identification of WT1 helper epitope peptides

| Publication year | Peptide name[a] | Peptide sequence | HLA class II restriction | References |
|---|---|---|---|---|
| 2002 | WT1-124 (WT1-12e)[b] | PQQMGSDVRDLNALL | HLA-DRB1*04:01 | Knights et al. [68] |
| 2003 | WT1-331 | NKRYFKLSHLQMHSR | HLA-DRB1*04:01 | Müller et al. [69] |
| 2005 | WT1-337 | LSHLQMHSRKH | HLA-DP5 | Guo et al. [70] |
| 2007 | WT1-332[c] | KRYFKLSHLQMHSRKH | HLA-DRB1*04:05 (and others[c]) | Fujiki et al. [72] |
| 2007 | WT1-423 (WT1-427 long)[d] | RSDELVRHHNMHQRNMTKL | Multiple HLA-DR types[e] | May et al. [73] |
| 2007 | WT1-328 (WT1-331 long)[f] | PGCNKRYFKLSHLQMHSRKHTG | Multiple HLA-DR types[e] | May et al. [73] |
| 2007 | WT1-122 | SGQARMFPNAPYLPSCLES | Multiple HLA-DR types[e] | May et al. [73] |
| 2007 | WT1-122 modified[g] | SGQAYMFPNAPYLPSCLES[g] | Multiple HLA-DR types[e] | May et al. [73] |
| 2008 | WT1-84 ($WT1_{333\text{-}347}$)[h] | RYFKLSHLQMHSRKH | HLA-DRB1*04:02 | Lehe et al. [74] |

[a]Peptide names in this table are based on positions of the starting amino acids (N terminus) of each peptide and the nomenclature in the original articles (reference papers)

[b]WT1-124 was called WT1-12e later in Ref [69]. The nomenclature of this peptide was explained in Cancer Immunol. Immunother. vol. 51, p.349, 2002

[c]WT1-332 was later shown to bind to multiple HLA class II types, i.e., DRB1*15:01, DRB1*15:02, DPB1*09:01, DRB1*07:01, DRB3*02:02 (ref [75, 76])

[d]WT1-423 was called "WT1-427 long" later in Ref [58, 60]

[e]See details in the ref [73] for these peptides' promiscuity of HLA binding

[f]WT1-328 was called "WT1-331 long" later in Ref [58, 60]

[g]Underlined amino acid (Y: fifth) is the modified one

[h]Lehe et al. claimed that this peptide could induce regulatory T cells

Besides WT1 peptides shown in this table, as described in text and Table 12.1, identification of immunogenic WT1 peptides based on peptide mapping was recently performed. See details in the reference papers [26, 27]

to the next stage of clinical trials to further enhance the vaccine's clinical usefulness, based on the strategies listed in Table 12.3.

To maximize the potency of the WT1 peptide vaccine in clinical settings, the effector (CTLs)/target (tumor cells) ratio, or E/T ratio, should be as high as possible. This can be best realized for patients with a low tumor load, including MRD state after surgery, chemotherapy, radiotherapy, or HSCT [3, 66, 84]. Recently, we reported on the results of WT1 peptide vaccination performed in two MRD settings, one for patients with MRD of AML after chemotherapy [63] and another for those with MRD of AML and acute lymphoblastic leukemia (ALL) after HSCT [62]. As for the former state, MRD following chemotherapy, Tsuboi et al. showed that long-term vaccination with the WT1 peptide might lead AML patients with MRD, who were at high risk of hematological relapse, to long-term CR [63]. In this paper, three among the eight AML patients maintained their hematological CR for more than 8 years due to continuous treatment with the WT1 peptide vaccine, and the *WT1* mRNA levels in PB, which reflect the leukemia load, finally decreased to normal levels, thus indicating molecular CR. This result suggested that the WT1 peptide vaccine had the potential to lead AML patients with MRD to molecular CR and, furthermore, possibly to eradication of the disease or a cure. As for the latter state, MRD following HSCT, Hashii et al. showed that favorable clinical courses could be realized for pediatric patients with hematological malignancies, who had received allogeneic HSCT but possessed the molecular MRD marker, and therefore were treated with the WT1 peptide vaccine to prevent relapse [62]. In terms of the short-term antileukemia effect, *WT1* mRNA levels, a molecular MRD marker, showed reduction after the vaccination in all the three patients, indicating the vaccine's antileukemia effect for ALL as well as AML. Besides, in an AML patient who had *AML/MTG8* transcripts as an MRD marker, the *AML/MTG8* levels also decreased after the vaccination, further indicating antileukemia effect of the WT1 peptide vaccine. In terms of the long-term effect, two of the three patients, all of whom were at high risk of relapse, sustained long-term remission, suggesting that the WT1 peptide vaccine might be able to enhance the GVL effect [62]. Very recently, in consistence with the study by Hashii et al., Maeda et al. also showed promising results of WT1 peptide vaccination for adult patients with hematological malignancies who had received HSCT but were at high risk of relapse [65]. These investigations about WT1 peptide vaccination for patients after HSCT showed the potential of the WT1 peptide vaccine to provide patients (children and adults) after HSCT with clinical usefulness, that is, prevention of relapse, leading to long-term maintenance of CR and possibly a cure.

For patients with cancer at advanced stages, combined therapy of the WT1 peptide vaccine and chemotherapy should be promising, because it was reported that some chemotherapy drugs, including gemcitabine, might affect antitumor immunity favorably [67]. Kaida et al. reported on the result of a clinical trial for pancreas cancer patients with advanced stages treated by gemcitabine and WT1 peptide vaccine, which showed the safety of the combined therapy [85]. More recently, we, Nishida et al., also reported on the result of a clinical trial using a combination therapy of the WT1 peptide vaccine and gemcitabine for patients with advanced stages of pancreatic cancer [86]. In this clinical study, a significant association was observed between longer survival and occurrence of DTH to WT1 peptide after the vaccination. Such an occurrence of the DTH after the vaccination may reflect the development and persistence of WT1-specific memory-type immunity [86, 87]. Consistent with this observation, longer-term survivors featured higher proportions of WT1-specific CTLs with memory phenotype before and after this combined therapy. Taken together, these findings suggested that memory-type cellular immunity to WT1 might contribute considerably to longer survival of the patients. In addition, of note, histopathologic examination of a tumor site could be performed in one case with a favorable clinical course, in which infiltration of a considerable numbers of WT1-specific CTLs was suggested [86].

Not only conventional chemotherapy drugs but also molecular target-based drugs should be the promising partners for the WT1 peptide vaccine in combination therapy. In fact, chronic myeloid leukemia patients treated with a combination of imatinib and WT1 peptide vaccine showed favorable clinical courses in association with induction of WT1-specific immunological responses [88, 89].

These WT1 CTL peptide-based clinical trials suggestive of future directions are also listed with other WT1 peptide vaccine trials in Table 12.2 (for monotherapy) and Table 12.5 (for combined therapy).

## 12.8 WT1 Peptide-Based DC Therapy That Shows the Primacy of WT1 as the Target Antigen

We perform intradermal or subcutaneous injection of WT1 peptide for the peptide vaccine therapy, using the resident DCs of the patients' skin as antigen-presenting cells, while injection of the WT1 peptide-pulsed DCs that were obtained through manipulation from the patients' blood is also able to induce the WT1 peptide-specific CTL response. So far, promising results of DC therapies targeting WT1, as well as the WT1 peptide vaccine therapies, have been reported. The interesting result of *WT1* mRNA-based DC therapy was already referred to in 12.7 of this chapter [83]. The results of clinical trials for WT1 peptide-based DC therapies that showed the primacy of WT1 as a target antigen for cancer immunotherapy were also reported [90–92]. Particularly, of note, in the recent clinical study of TAA peptide-based DC therapy for patients with NSCLC, multivariate analyses revealed that the use of WT1 CTL peptides favorably affected the overall survival of the patients [91]. Another study suggested the usefulness of the use of DCs co-pulsed with WT1 CTL peptide and WT1 helper peptide in combined therapy of DC and gemcitabine for patients with pancreas cancer [92]. Representative WT1 peptide-based DC therapies that showed the primacy of WT1 antigen/peptide were listed in Table 12.6.

TAA-targeting DC therapies are described in detail elsewhere in this book.

**Table 12.5** Clinical trials: WT1 peptide vaccination (combined with other therapy)-induced immunological and/or clinical response

| Publication year | Disease | Combined therapy | Immunological response | Clinical response (or usefulness, significance) | HLA class I | Peptide | References |
|---|---|---|---|---|---|---|---|
| 2010 | CML | Imatinib | Emergence of WT1-specific CTLs | Reduction of *bcr-abl* mRNA level after adding WT1 peptide vaccine on imatinib | A*24:02 | WT1-235m[a] | Narita et al. [88] |
| 2010 | CML | Imatinib | Increase in WT1-specific CTLs, emergence of WT1-specific DTH | Reduction of *bcr-abl* mRNA level after adding WT1 peptide vaccine on imatinib | A*24:02 | WT1-235m | Oji et al. [89] |
| 2011 | Pancreas cancer, biliary tract cancer | Gemcitabine | Emergence of WT1-specific CTLs | Safety of combination therapy of WT1 peptide vaccine and gemcitabine | A*02:01 A*02:06 | WT1-126 | Kaida et al. [85] |
| | | | | | A*24:02 | WT1-235m | |
| 2014 | Pancreas cancer | Gemcitabine | Emergence of WT1-specific DTH | Correlation between emergence of WT-specific specific DTH and overall survival | A*24:02 | WT1-235m | Nishida et al. [86] |

Abbreviation for disease name, *CML* chronic myeloid leukemia

[a]Modified peptide. See text and Table 12.1 for details

**Table 12.6** Representative WT1 peptide-based dendritic cell (DC) therapies that showed the primacy of WT1 as a target antigen for cancer immunotherapy[a]

| Publication year | Disease | Combined therapy | Immunological and clinical response/features/significance | HLA class I | HLA class II | WT1 peptides[b] | Reference |
|---|---|---|---|---|---|---|---|
| 2011 | AML | – | Emergence of WT1-specific CTLs, transient decrease in leukemic cells, disease stabilization | A*24:02 | No restriction for enrollment | WT1-235m[c] | Kitawaki et al. [90] |
| 2013 | NSCLC | – | Multivariate analysis-based indication that the use of WT1 peptides favorably affected the survival of the patients[d] | A*02:01<br>A*02:06<br>A*24:02 | No restriction for enrollment | WT1-126<br>WT1-235m | Takahashi et al. [91] |
| 2014 | Pancreas cancer | Gemcitabine | Possible association of the activation of WT1-specific immune response by DCs co-pulsed with WT1 CTL peptides and WT1 helper peptides with disease stabilization | A*02:01<br>A*02:06<br>A*24:02 | DRB1*04:05<br>DRB1*08:03<br>DRB1*15:01<br>DRB1*15:02<br>DPB1*05:01<br>DPB1*09:01 | WT1-126<br>WT1-235m<br>WT1-332 | Koido et al. [92] |
| 2010 | AML | – | Increase in WT1-specific CTLs in A*02:01$^+$ patients, induction to complete remission | No restriction for enrollment | No restriction for enrollment | *WT1* mRNA[a] | Van Tendeloo et al. [83][a] |

Abbreviations for disease names, *AML* acute myeloid leukemia, *NSCLC* non-small cell lung cancer

[a]Not only WT1 peptide-based DC therapies but also WT1 mRNA-based DC therapy that matched the aim of this table are listed, because the study by Van Tendeloo et al. [83] has a great impact to show the primacy of WT1 as a target antigen for cancer immunotherapy

[b]Only WT1-332 is a helper epitope, while the others are CTL epitopes. WT1-332 is promiscuous in HLA class II restriction. See details in text, Tables 12.1 and 12.4

[c]Modified peptide. See details in text and Table 12.1

[d]Tumor antigen-derived peptides other than WT1 peptides were also used in this study

## 12.9 Conclusion and Future Perspectives

After identification of WT1 CTL epitopes for humans and demonstration using a mouse experiment that WT1 protein/peptide could serve in vivo as a target antigen for cancer immunotherapy, both of which were reported in 2000 (Table 12.1), clinical trials for WT1-targeting cancer immunotherapy, a translational research based on the basic research, have been started and are now growing. Early clinical trials, which were summarized in this article, demonstrated that WT1 CTL epitope peptide-based vaccination had the therapeutic potential for patients with malignancies, because the vaccination undoubtedly induced WT1-specific CTL responses, resulting in the emergence of clinical response in some proportions of the patients [2, 3]. Recent novel findings, including WT1 expression in leukemia stem cells [9], and *WT1*'s important role in tumor angiogenesis [10, 93], also support the primacy of WT1 as a target antigen for cancer immunotherapy. Now, the next stage of clinical trials has been started aiming at enhancement of the vaccine's efficacy, resulting in more evident clinical usefulness. WT1 peptide vaccination that is scheduled to be performed for patients with MRD, such as those who have undergone chemotherapy, radiotherapy, surgery, or HSCT, is expected to prevent relapse of the diseases, leading to long-term remission or possibly a cure. On the other hand, the WT1 vaccine therapy combined with chemotherapy may provide cancer patients at advanced stages with additive efficacy, compared with chemotherapy alone. Regarding these topics, some recent clinical studies have shown promising results. Furthermore, combination therapies of the WT1 CTL peptide-based vaccine and other immunological modulators, such as WT1 helper peptide and immuno-checkpoint inhibitors, also seem to be promising. In the future, further development of the WT1 peptide vaccine in the various kinds of clinical settings may thus yield innovative change for cancer immunotherapy, while issues to be solved, including optimization of peptide dose and vaccination interval, choice of immunoadjuvant, and injection method (intradermal or subcutaneous), remain [94].

We and others have provided evidence that the WT1 peptide vaccine has therapeutic potential for the treatment of patients with malignancies and currently the patients who have shown the vaccination-associated clinical responses are further being accumulated. Intensive and comprehensive analysis of the clinical samples obtained from responders and nonresponders, which is known as a reverse-translational research, should be very useful for elucidation of cancer immunity mechanisms in humans. In fact, some interesting findings about WT1-specific CTLs were reported recently [95–97]. Of note, very recently, we observed an interesting phenomenon that WT1-specific CTLs with effector memory phenotype (WT1-EM cells) were divided into molecularly defined two different populations, a population of "quiescent" state and that of "activated" state, in the WT1 peptide-vaccinated AML patients, and that the WT1-EM cells in responders shifted to "quiescent" state and those in nonresponders shifted to "activated" state, respectively, after the vaccination [97]. Further novel findings about cancer immunity are expected to be obtained, because the clinical samples obtained from the

WT1-targeting immunotherapy are being accumulated in each institute, including ours.

Continuing progress of translational and reverse-translational research regarding WT1-targeting immunotherapy should lead to further development of cancer immunotherapy and elucidation of cancer immunity mechanisms.

**Acknowledgement and Conflict of Interest** We, the authors of this chapter, greatly appreciate the contribution by all the collaborators. We express our special thanks to Ms. Tomoe Umeda for her sincere contribution to the practice of clinical studies performed in Osaka University Hospital. We apologize to the authors whose works were not cited in this chapter due to unavoidable reasons, including lack of space.

The preparation of this review chapter was in part supported by Japan Society for the Promotion of Science (JSPS) through grants for Scientific Research from Ministry of Education, Science, Sports, Culture, and Technology. Department of Cancer Immunology is a department in collaboration with Otsuka Pharmaceutical Co., Ltd., and is supported with a grant from the company. The company had no role in the design of the preparation of this chapter.

## References

1. Cheever MA, Allison JP, Ferris AS, Finn OJ, Hastings BM, Hecht TT et al (2009) The prioritization of cancer antigens: a national cancer institute pilot project for the acceleration of translational research. Clin Cancer Res 15:5323–5337
2. Oka Y, Tsuboi A, Oji Y, Kawase I, Sugiyama H (2008) WT1 peptide vaccine for the treatment of cancer. Curr Opin Immunol 20:211–220
3. Oka Y, Sugiyama H (2010) WT1 peptide vaccine, one of the most promising cancer vaccine: its present status and the future prospects. Immunotherapy 2:591–594
4. Yamagami T, Sugiyama H, Inoue K, Ogawa H, Tatekawa T, Hirata M et al (1996) Growth inhibition of human leukemic cells by WT1 (Wilms tumor gene) antisense oligodeoxynucleotides: implications for the involvement of WT1 in leukemogenesis. Blood 87:2878–2884
5. Sugiyama H (1998) Wilms tumor gene (WT1) as a new marker for the detection of minimal residual disease in leukemia. Leuk Lymphoma 30:55–61
6. Inoue K, Sugiyama H, Ogawa H, Nakagawa M, Yamagami T, Miwa H et al (1994) WT1 as a new prognostic factor and a new marker for the detection of minimal residual disease in acute leukemia. Blood 84:3071–3079
7. Oji Y, Miyoshi S, Maeda H, Hayashi S, Tamaki H, Nakatsuka S et al (2002) Overexpression of the Wilms' tumor gene WT1 in de novo lung cancers. Int J Cancer 100:292–303
8. Nakatsuka S-I, Oji Y, Horiuchi T, Kanda T, Kitagawa M, Takeuchi T et al (2006) Immunohistochemical detection of WT1 protein in a variety of cancer cells. Mod Pathol 19:804–814
9. Saito Y, Kitamura H, Hijikata A, Tomizawa-Murasawa M, Tanaka S, Takagi S et al (2010) Identification of therapeutic targets for quiescent, chemotherapy-resistant human leukemia stem cells. Sci Transl Med 2:17ra9
10. Wagner N, Michiels JF, Schedi A, Wagner KD (2008) The Wilms' tumour suppressor WT1 is involved in endothelial cell proliferation and migration: expression in tumour vessels in vivo. Oncogene 27:3662–3672
11. Oka Y, Tsuboi A, Fujiki F, Shirakata T, Nishida S, Hosen N et al (2008) "Cancer antigen WT1 protein-derived peptide"-based treatment of cancer—toward the further development—. Curr Med Chem 15:3053–3061

12. Oka Y, Elisseeva OA, Tsuboi A, Ogawa H, Tamaki H, Li H et al (2000) Human cytotoxic T-lymphocyte responses specific for peptides of the wild-type Wilms' tumor gene (WT1) product. Immunogenetics 51:99–107
13. Gao L, Bellantuono I, Elsasser A, Marley SB, Gordon MY, Goldman JM et al (2000) Selective elimination of leukemic CD34$^+$ progenitor cells by cytotoxic T lymphocytes specific for WT1. Blood 95:2198–2203
14. Doubrovina ES, Doubrovin MM, Lee S, Shieh J-H, Heller G, Pamer E et al (2004) In vitro stimulation with WT1 peptide-loaded Epstein-Barr virus-positive B cells elicit high frequencies of WT1 peptide-specific T cells with in vitro and in vivo tumoricidal activity. Clin Cancer Res 10:7202–7219
15. Ohminami H, Yasukawa M, Fujita S (2000) HLA class I-restricted lysis of leukemia cells by a CD8$^+$ cytotoxic T-lymphocyte clone specific for WT1 peptide. Blood 95:286–293
16. Tsuboi A, Oka Y, Udaka K, Murakami M, Masuda T, Nakano A et al (2002) Enhanced induction of human WT1-specific cytotoxic T lymphocytes with a 9-mer WT1 peptide modified at HLA-A*2402-binding residues. Cancer Immunol Immunother 51:614–620
17. Azuma T, Makita M, Ninomiya K, Fujita S, Harada M, Yasukawa M (2002) Identification of a novel WT1-derived peptide which induces human leucocyte antigen-A24-restricted anti-leukaemia cytotoxic T lymphocytes. Br J Haematol 116:601–603
18. Rezvani K, Brenchley JM, Price DA, Kilical Y, Gostick A, Sewell AK et al (2005) T-cell responses directed against multiple HLA-A*0201-restricted epitopes derived from Wilms' tumor 1 protein in patients with leukemia and healthy donors: identification, quantification, and characterization. Clin Cancer Res 11:8799–8807
19. Smithgall A, Misher L, Spies G, Cheever MA, Gaiger A (2001) Identification of novel WT1 HLA-A*0201-restricted CTL epitope using whole gene in vitro priming. ASH meeting
20. Asemissen AM, Keilholz U, Tenzer S, Müller M, Walter S, Stevanovic S et al (2006) Identification of a highly immunogenic HLA-A*01-binding T cell epitope of WT1. Clin Cancer Res 12:7476–7482
21. Pinilla-Ibarz J, May RJ, Korontsvit T, Gomez M, Kappel B, Zakhaleva V et al (2006) Improved human T-cell responses against synthetic HLA-0201 analog peptides derived from the WT1 oncoprotein. Leukemia 20:2025–2030
22. Bellantuono I, Gao L, Parry S, Marley S, Dazzi F, Apperley J et al (2002) Two distinct HLA-A0201-presented epitopes of the Wilms tumor antigen 1 can function as targets for leukemia-reactive CTL. Blood 100:3835–3837
23. Li Z, Oka Y, Tsuboi A, Masuda T, Tatsumi N, Kawakami M et al (2005) $WT1_{235}$, a ninemer peptide derived from Wilms' tumor gene product, is a candidate peptide for the vaccination of HLA-A*0201-positive patients with hematopoietic malignancies. Int J Hematol 82:458–459
24. Li Z, Oka Y, Tsuboi A, Fujiki F, Harada Y, Nakajima H et al (2008) Identification of a WT1 protein-derived peptide, WT1187, as a HLA-A*0206-restricted, WT1-specific CTL epitope. Microbiol Immunol 52:551–558
25. Wolfl M, Kuball J, Ho WY, Nguyen H, Manley TJ, Bleakley M et al (2007) Activation-induced expression of CD137 permits detection, isolation, and expansion of the full repertoire of CD8$^+$ T cells responding to antigen without requiring knowledge of epitope specificities. Blood 110:201–210
26. Doubrovina E, Carpenter T, Pankov D, Selvakumar A, Hasan A, O'Reilly RJ (2012) Mapping of novel peptides of WT-1 and presenting HLA alleles that induce epitope-specific HLA-restricted T cells with cytotoxic activity against WT1$^+$ leukemias. Blood 120:1633–1646
27. Weber G, Caruana I, Rouce RH, Barrett AJ, Gerdemann U, Leen AM et al (2013) Generation of tumor antigen-specific T cell lines from pediatric patients with acute lymphoblastic leukemia—implications for immunotherapy. Clin Cancer Res 19:5079–5091
28. Elisseeva OA, Oka Y, Tsuboi A, Kim EH, Soma T, Tamaki H et al (2002) Humoral immune responses against Wilms' tumor gene WT1 product in patients with hematopoietic malignancies. Blood 99:3272–3279

29. Wu F, Oka Y, Tsuboi A, Elisseeva OA, Nakajima H, Fujiki F et al (2005) Th1-biased humoral immune responses against Wilms tumor gene WT1 product in the patients with hematopoietic malignancies. Leukemia 19:268–274
30. Oji Y, Kitamura Y, Kamino E, Kitano A, Sawabata N, Inoue M et al (2009) WT1 IgG antibody for early detection of non-small cell lung cancer and as its prognostic factor. Int J Cancer 125:381–387
31. Gaiger A, Carter L, Greinix H, Carter D, McNeill PD, Houghton RL et al (2001) WT1-specific serum antibodies in patients with leukemia. Clin Cancer Res 7:761s–765s
32. Scheibenbogen C, Letsch A, Thiel E, Schmittel A, Mailaender V, Baerwolf S et al (2002) CD8-T cell responses to Wilms tumor gene product WT1 and proteinase 3 in patients with acute myeloid leukemia. Blood 100:2132–2137
33. Rezvani K, Yong AS, Savani BL, Mielke S, Keyvanfar K, Gostic E (2007) Graft-versus-leukemia effects associated with detectable Wilms tumor-1 specific T lymphocytes after allogeneic stem-cell transplantation for acute lymphoblastic leukemia. Blood 110:1924–1937
34. Morita Y, Heike Y, Kawakami M, Miura O, Nakatsuka S, Ebisawa M et al (2006) Monitoring of WT1-specific cytotoxic T lymphocytes after allogeneic hematopoietic stem cell transplantation. Int J Cancer 119:1360–1367
35. Oka Y, Udaka K, Tsuboi A, Elisseeva OA, Ogawa H, Aozasa K et al (2000) Cancer immunotherapy targeting Wilms' tumor gene WT1 product. J Immunol 164:1873–1880
36. Nakajima H, Kawasaki K, Oka Y, Tsuboi A, Kawakami M, Ikegame K et al (2004) WT1 peptide vaccination combined with BCG-CWS is more efficient for tumor eradication than WT1 peptide vaccination alone. Cancer Immunol Immunother 53:617–624
37. Nakajima H, Oka Y, Tsuboi A, Tatsumi N, Yamamoto Y, Fujiki F et al (2012) Enhanced tumor immunity of WT1 peptide vaccination by interferon-β administration. Vaccine 30:722–729
38. Ramirez F, Ghani Y, Gao L, Stauss H (2007) Dendritic cell immunization induces non-protective WT1-specific CTL responses in mouse. J Immunother 30:140–149
39. Makita M, Hiraki A, Azuma T, Tsuboi A, Oka Y, Sugiyama H et al (2002) Antilung cancer effect of WT1-specific cytotoxic T lymphocytes. Clin Cancer Res 8:2626–2631
40. Oka Y, Tsuboi A, Murakami M, Hirai M, Tominaga N, Nakajima H et al (2003) Wilms tumor gene peptide-based immunotherapy for patients with overt leukemia from myelodysplastic syndrome (MDS) or MDS with myelofibrosis. Int J Hematol 78:56–61
41. Mailänder V, Scheibenbogen C, Thiel E, Letsch A, Blau IW, Keilholz U (2004) Complete remission in a patient with recurrent acute myeloid leukemia induced by vaccination with WT1 peptide in the absence of hematological or renal toxicity. Leukemia 18:165–166
42. Oka Y, Tsuboi A, Taguchi T, Osaki T, Kyo T, Nakajima H et al (2004) Induction of WT1 (Wilms' tumor gene)-specific cytotoxic T lymphocytes by WT1 peptide vaccine and the resultant cancer regression. Proc Natl Acad Sci U S A 101:13885–13890
43. Rezvani K, Yong ASM, Mielke S, Savini BN, Musse L, Superata J et al (2008) Leukemia-associated antigen-specific T-cell responses following combined PR1 and WT1 peptide vaccination in patients with myeloid malignancies. Blood 11:236–242
44. Keilholz U, Letsch A, Busse A, Asemissen AM, Bauer S, Brau IW et al (2009) A clinical and immunologic phase 2 trial of Wilms tumor gene product 1 (WT1) peptide vaccination in patients with AML and MDS. Blood 113:6541–6548
45. Yasukawa M, Fujiwara H, Ochi T, Suemori K, Narumi H, Azuma T et al (2009) Clinical efficacy of WT1 peptide vaccination in patients with acute myelogenous leukemia and myelodysplastic syndrome. Am J Hematol 84:314–315
46. Kawakami M, Oka Y, Tsuboi A, Harada Y, Elisseeva OA, Furukawa Y et al (2007) Clinical and immunological responses to very low dose vaccination with WT1 peptide (5μg/body) in a patient with chronic myelomonocytic leukemia. Int J Hematol 85:426–429
47. Tsuboi A, Oka Y, Nakajima H, Fukuda Y, Elisseeva OA, Yoshihara S et al (2007) Wilms' tumor gene WT1 peptide-based immunotherapy induced minimal response in a patient with advanced, therapy-resistant multiple myeloma. Int J Hematol 86:414–417

48. Tsuboi A, Oka Y, Osaki T, Kumagai T, Tachibana I, Hayashi S et al (2004) WT1 peptide-based immunotherapy with lung cancer: report of two cases. Microbiol Immunol 48:175–184
49. Iiyama T, Udaka K, Takeda S, Takeuchi T, Adachi YC, Ohtsuki Y et al (2007) WT1 (Wilms' tumor 1) peptide immunotherapy for renal cell carcinoma. Microbiol Immunol 51:519–530
50. Ohno S, Kyo S, Myojo S, Dohi S, Ishizaki J, Miyamoto K et al (2009) Wilms' tumor 1 (WT1) peptide immunotherapy for gynecological malignancy. Anticancer Res 29:4779–4784
51. Miyatake T, Ueda Y, Morimoto A, Enomoto T, Nishida S, Shirakata T et al (2013) WT1 peptide immunotherapy for gynecologic malignancies resistant to conventional therapies: a phase II trial. J Cancer Res Clin Oncol 139:457–463
52. Sasabe E, Hamada F, Iiyama T, Udaka K, Sugiyama H, Yamamoto T (2011) Wilm's tumor gene WT1 peptide immunotherapy for pulmonary metastasis from adenoid cystic carcinoma of the salivary gland. Oral Oncol 47:77–78
53. Shirakata T, Oka Y, Nishida S, Hosen N, Tsuboi A, Oji Y et al (2012) WT1 peptide therapy for a patient with chemotherapy-resistant salivary gland cancer. Anticancer Res 32:1081–1086
54. Nishioka M, Tanemura A, Nishida S, Nakano A, Tsuboi A, Oji Y et al (2012) Vaccination with the WT-1 (Wilms' tumor gene-1) peptide and the BCG-CWS in melanoma: a case report. Eur J Dermatol 22:258–259
55. Izumoto S, Tsuboi A, Oka Y, Suzuki T, Hashiba T, Kagawa N et al (2008) Phase II clinical trial of Wilms tumor 1 peptide vaccination for patients with recurrent glioblastoma. J Neurosurg 108:963–971
56. Ohta H, Hashii Y, Yoneda A, Takizawa S, Kusuki S, Tokimasa S et al (2009) WT1 (Wilms' tumor 1) peptide immunotherapy for childhood rhabdomyosarcoma: a case report. Pediatr Hematol Oncol 26:74–83
57. Morita S, Oka Y, Tsuboi A, Kawakami M, Maruno M, Izumoto S et al (2006) A phase I/II trial of a WT1 (Wilms' tumor gene) peptide vaccine in patients with solid malignancy; safety assessment based on the phase I data. Jpn J Clin Oncol 36:231–236
58. Maslak PG, Dao T, Krug LM, Chanel S, Korontsvit T, Zakhaleva V et al (2010) Vaccination with synthetic analog peptide derived from WT1 oncoprotein induces T-cell responses in patients with complete remission from acute myeloid leukemia. Blood 116:171–179
59. Hashii Y, Sato E, Ohta H, Oka Y, Sugiyama H, Ozono K (2010) WT1 peptide vaccination for cancer in children and young adults. Pediatr Blood Cancer 55:352–355
60. Krug LM, Dao T, Brown AB, Maslak P, Travis W, Bekele S et al (2010) WT1 peptide vaccinations induce CD4 and CD8 T cell immune responses in patients with mesothelioma and non-small cell lung cancer. Cancer Immunol Immunother 59:1467–1479
61. Dohi S, Ohno S, Ohno Y, Takakura M, Kyo S, Soma G-I et al (2011) WT1 peptide vaccine stabilized intractable ovarian cancer patient for one year: a case report. Anticancer Res 31: 2441–2446
62. Hashii Y, Sato-Miyashita E, Matsumura R, Kusui S, Yoshida H, Ohta H et al (2012) WT1 peptide vaccination following allogeneic stem cell transplantation in pediatric leukemic patients with high risk for relapse: successful maintenance of durable remission. Leukemia 26:530–532
63. Tsuboi A, Oka Y, Kyo T, Katayama Y, Elisseeva OA, Kawakami M et al (2012) Long-term WT1 peptide vaccination for patients with minimal residual disease. Leukemia 26:1410–1413
64. Ohno S, Okuyama R, Aruga A, Sugiyama H, Yamamoto M (2012) Phase I trial of Wilms' tumor 1 (WT1) peptide vaccine with GM-CSF or CpG in patients with solid malignancies. Anticancer Res 32:2263–2269
65. Maeda T, Hosen N, Fukushima K, Tsuboi A, Morimoto S, Matsui T et al (2013) Maintenance of complete remission after allogeneic stem cell transplantation in leukemia patients treated with Wilms tumor 1 (WT1) peptide vaccine. Blood Cancer J 3:e130
66. Rezvani K (2011) Posttransplantation vaccination: concepts today and on the horizon. Hematol Am Soc Hematol Educ Program 2011:299–304

67. Suzuki K, Kapoor V, Jassar AS, Kaiser LR, Albelda SM (2005) Gemcitabine selectively eliminates splenic Gr-1+/CD11b+ myeloid suppressor cells in tumor-bearing animals and enhances antitumor immune activity. Clin Cancer Res 11:6713–6721
68. Knights AJ, Zaniou A, Rees RC, Pawelec G, Müller L (2002) Prediction of an HLA-DR-binding peptide derived from Wilms' tumour 1 protein and demonstration of in vitro immunogenicity of WT1 (124–138)-pulsed dendritic cells generated according to an optimized protocol. Cancer Immunol Immunother 51:271–281
69. Müller L, Knights A, Pawelec G (2003) Synthetic peptides derived from the Wilms' tumor 1 protein sensitize human T lymphocytes to recognize chronic myelogenous leukemia. Hematol J 4:57–66
70. Guo Y, Niiya H, Azuma T, Uchida N, Yakushijin I, Sakai Y et al (2005) Direct recognition and lysis of leukemia cells by WT1-specific CD4+ T lymphocytes in an HLA class II-restricted manner. Blood 106:1415–1418
71. Kobayashi H, Nagato T, Aoki N, Sato K, Kimura S, Tateno M et al (2006) Defining MHC class II T helper epitopes for WT1 tumor antigen. Cancer Immunol Immunother 55:85–60
72. Fujiki F, Oka Y, Tsuboi A, Kawakami M, Kawakatsu M, Nakajima H et al (2007) Identification and characterization of a WT1(Wilms' tumor gene) protein-derived HLA-DRB1*0405-restricted 16-mer helper peptide that promotes the induction and activation of WT1-specific cytotoxic T lymphocytes. J Immunother 30:282–293
73. May RJ, Dao T, Pinilla-Ibarz J, Korontsvit T, Zakhaleva V, Zhang RH et al (2007) Peptide epitopes from the Wilms' tumor 1 oncoprotein stimulate CD4+ and CD8+ T cells that recognize and kill human malignant mesothelioma tumor cells. Clin Cancer Res 13:4547–4555
74. Lehe C, Ghebeh H, Al-Sulaiman A, Qudaihi GA, Al-Hussein K, Almohareb F et al (2008) The Wilms' tumor antigen is a novel target for human $CD4^+$ regulatory T cells: implications for immunotherapy. Cancer Res 68:6350–6359
75. Fujiki F, Oka Y, Kawakatsu M, Tsuboi A, Nakajima H, Elisseeva OA et al (2008) A WT1 protein-derived, naturally processed 16-mer peptide, $WT1_{332}$, is a promiscuous helper peptide for induction of WT1-specific Th1-type $CD4^+$ T cells. Microbiol Immunol 52:591–600
76. Anguille S, Fujiki F, Smits EL, Oji Y, Lion E, Oka Y et al (2013) Identification of a Wilms' tumor 1-derived immunogenic $CD4^+$ T-cell epitope that is recognized in the context of common Caucasian HLA-DR haplotypes. Leukemia 27:748–750
77. Janssen E, Lemmens E (2003) CD4+ T cells are required for secondary expansion and memory in CD8+ T lymphocytes. Nature 421:852–856
78. Hodi FS, O'Day SJ, McDermott DF, Weber RW, Sosman JA, Haanen JB et al (2010) Improved survival with ipilimumab in patients with metastatic melanoma. N Engl J Med 363:711–723
79. Topalian SN, Hodi FS, Bramer JR, Gettinger SN, Smith DC, McDermott DF et al (2012) Safety, activity, and immune correlates of anti-PD-1 antibody in cancer. N Engl J Med 366: 2443–2454
80. Bramer JR, Tykodi SS, Chow LQM, Hwu W-J, Topalian SL, Hwu P et al (2012) Safety and activity of anti-PD-L1 antibody in patients with advanced cancer. N Engl J Med 366: 2455–2465
81. Kaneshima H, Tsuruma T, Kutomi G, Shima H, Imamura M, Torigoe T et al (2013) Immunotherapeutic benefit of α-interferon (IFNα) in survivin2B-derived peptide vaccination for advanced pancreatic cancer patients. Cancer Sci 104:124–129
82. Yano A, Komatsu T, Ishibashi M, Udaka K (2007) Potent CTL induction by a whole cell pertussis vaccine in anti-tumor peptide immunotherapy. Microbiol Immunol 51:685–699
83. Van Tendeloo VF, Van de Velde A, Van Driessche A, Cools N, Anguille S, Price DA et al (2010) Induction of complete and molecular remissions in acute myeloid leukemia by Wilms' tumor 1 antigen-targeted dendritic cell vaccination. Proc Natl Acad Sci U S A 107: 13824–13829
84. Oka Y (2013) A vaccine for leukemia: one step closer? Cure-oriented WT1 peptide vaccination therapy is being developed. Clin Investig 3:1–4

85. Kaida M, Morita-Hoshi Y, Soeda A, Wakeda T, Yamaki Y, Kojima Y et al (2011) Phase I trial of Wilms tumor 1 (WT1) peptide vaccine and gemcitabine combination therapy in patients with advanced pancreatic or biliary tract cancer. J Immunother 34:92–99
86. Nishida S, Koido S, Takeda Y, Homma S, Komita H, Takahara A et al (2014) Wilms' tumor gene 1 (WT1)-peptide-based cancer vaccine combined with gemcitabine for patients with advanced pancreatic cancer. J Immunother 37:105–114
87. Disis ML (2011) Immunologic biomarkers as correlates of clinical response to cancer immunotherapy. Cancer Immunol Immunother 60:433–442
88. Narita M, Masuko M, Kurasaki T, Kitajima T, Takenouchi S, Saitoh A et al (2010) WT1 peptide vaccination in combination with imatinib therapy for a patient with CML in the chronic phase. Int J Med Sci 7:72–81
89. Oji Y, Oka Y, Nishida S, Tsuboi A, Kawakami M, Shirakata T et al (2010) WT1 vaccine induces reduction in minimal residual disease in an imatinib-treated CML patient. Eur J Hematol 85:358–360
90. Kitawaki T, Kadowaki N, Fukunaga K, Kasai Y, Maekawa T, Ohmori K et al (2011) A phase I/IIa clinical trial of immunotherapy for elderly patients with acute myeloid leukaemia using dendritic cells co-pulsed with WT1 peptide and zoledronate. Br J Haematol 153:786–799
91. Takahashi H, Okamoto M, Shimodaira S, Tsujitani S, Nagaya M, Ishidao T et al (2013) Impact of dendritic cell vaccines pulsed with Wilms' tumor-1 peptide antigen on the survival of patients with advanced non-small cell lung cancers. Eur J Cancer 49:852–859
92. Koido S, Homma S, Okamoto M, Takakura K, Mori M, Yoshizaki S et al (2014) Treatment with chemotherapy and dendritic cells pulsed with multiple Wilms' tumor 1 (WT1)-specific MHC class I/II-restricted epitopes for pancreatic cancer. Clin Cancer Res 20:4228–4239
93. Wagner K-D, Cherfils-Vicini J, Hosen N, Hohenstein P, Gilson E, Hastie ND et al (2014) The Wilms' tumour suppressor Wt1 is a major regulator of tumour angiogenesis and progression. Nat Commun. doi:10.1038/ncomms6852
94. Rezvani K, Yong AS, Mielke S, Jafarpour B, Savani BN, Le RQ et al (2011) Repeated PR1 and WT1 peptide vaccination in Montanide-adjuvant fails to induce sustained high-avidity, epitope-specific CD8+ T cells in myeloid malignancies. Hematologica 96:432–440
95. Ochsenreither S, Fusi A, Besse A, Bauer S, Scheibenbogen C, Stather D et al (2011) "Wilms tumor protein 1" (WT1) peptide vaccination-induced complete remission in a patient with acute myeloid leukemia is accompanied by the emergence of a predominant T-cell clone both in blood and bone marrow. J Immunother 34:85–91
96. Morimoto S, Oka Y, Tsuboi A, Tanaka Y, Fujiki F, Nakajima H et al (2012) Biased usage of T cell receptor β-chain variable region genes of WT1 (Wilms' tumor gene)-specific $CD8^+$ T cells in patients with solid tumors and healthy donors. Cancer Sci 103:408–414
97. Nakae Y, Oka Y, Fujiki F, Morimoto S, Kamiya T, Takashima S, et al (2015) Two distinct effector memory cell populations of WT1 (Wilms' tumor gene 1)-specific cytotoxic T lymphocytes in acute myeloid leukemia patients. Cancer Immunol Immunother 64:791–804

# Chapter 13
# Protein Vaccine

**Shinichi Kageyama**

**Abstract** Antigen proteins have potentials for multi-epitope vaccines, without restriction of HLA types in patients' eligibility. Since exogenous soluble protein antigens are in general hardly processed by MHC class I pathway, combination with suitable antigen delivery systems and/or adjuvants is required for efficient CD8+ and CD4+ T-cell inductions for the clinical development of protein vaccine. Several protein vaccine types have been studied for their safety and immune responses. Among them, NY-ESO-1 antigen has been the most investigated and the antigen-specific CD8+ and CD4+ T-cell responses were shown. As indicated in a single report in a NY-ESO-1 protein trial, caution should be taken about the possibility of antigen-specific regulatory T-cell induction by protein vaccines. The evidence-based clinical benefit of protein cancer vaccine as a single agent has not yet been demonstrated. Improvement of vaccination such as coadministration of a suitable immunoadjuvant should be made to break any possible anergy to antitumor immune responses. In addition, combination of an immune-checkpoint inhibitor and/or an effector T-cell therapy would be the further stage of clinical development of protein cancer vaccines.

**Keywords** Cancer vaccine • Protein vaccine • Antigen delivery system • NY-ESO-1

## 13.1 Protein-Based Cancer Vaccine

Cancer vaccines can be given in various forms and by using various administration methods. The administration will then activate the cancer antigen-specific immune responses of effector cells, mainly CD8+ T cells and CD4+ T cells, both of which are key players in adaptive immune responses, through antigen processing and presentation by host immune systems. For molecularly identified target antigens, vaccine antigens can be the forms of short peptides, long peptides, proteins, carbohydrate antigens, mRNA, or DNA. It is important for enhanced

S. Kageyama (✉)
Department of Immuno-Gene Therapy, Mie University Graduate School of Medicine, 2-174 Edobashi, Tsu, Mie 514-8507, Japan
e-mail: kageyama@clin.medic.mie-u.ac.jp



Y. Yamaguchi (ed.), *Immunotherapy of Cancer*,
DOI 10.1007/978-4-431-55031-0_13

immunogenicity of vaccines to administer vaccine antigens in combination with a delivery system for appropriate antigen transport and/or with immuno-potentiates, i.e., adjuvants, stimulating immune responses against vaccine antigens in the course of immune responses.

This chapter describes cancer vaccine using antigen proteins that are molecularly identified as tumor antigen.

## 13.2 Protein as an Immunogen for Cancer Vaccine

Antigen proteins that are molecularly identified are manufactured by recombination methodology. CD8+ T-cell epitopes that are already identified and still unidentified are included inside the proteins. For example, full-length protein of NY-ESO-1 antigen contains multiple HLA class I and class II epitope peptides between the 49th and 170th amino acid (Fig. 13.1) [1]. In this full-length protein, epitopes that can bind to Fab portion of monoclonal antibody are included [2]. Therefore, it is reasonable to use antigen protein to cover multiple epitopes for induction of not

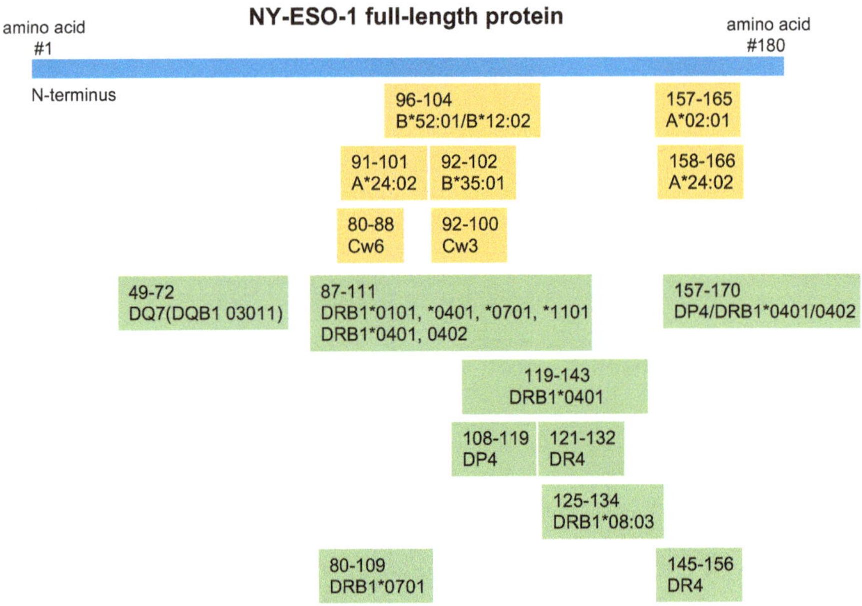


**Fig. 13.1** NY-ESO-1 full-length protein
Identified epitopes derived from NY-ESO-1 antigen that were previously published: amino acid (AA) 157-170 for HLA-DP4 [28]; AA 87-111 for HLA-DP4, including HLA-DRB1*0101, HLA-DRB1*0401, HLA-DRB1*0701, and HLA-DRB1*1101 and HLA-DPB1*0401 and HLA-DPB1*0402 [29]; AA 157-165 for HLA-A*02:01 [30]; AA 80-88 for HLA-Cw6 and AA 92-100 for HLA-Cw3 [31]; AA 125-134 for HLA-DRB1*08:03 [32]; AA 158-166 for HLA-A*24*02 [33]; AA 49-72 for HLA-DQ7 (DQB1 03011) [34]; AA 91-101 for HLA-A*24:02, AA 92-102 for HLA-B*35:01, AA 96-104 for HLA-B*52:01, and AA 96-104 for HLA-C*12:02 [35]; AA 80-109 for DRB1*0701, AA 108–119 for HLA-DP4, and AA 121–132 and 145–156 for HLA-DR4 [36]; AA 119–143 for HLA-DRB1*0401 [37, 38]

only CD8+ T cell but also CD4+ T cells and antibody, which can be called as polyvalent cancer vaccine.

In contrast to short peptide vaccines, antigen proteins can be incorporated into the antigen-presenting cells. In the process of peptide selection and its presentation to MHC class I and class II molecules, the peptides derived from the immunized protein are presented in the same way with peptides derived from tumor cells. In this sense, protein vaccines can select antigen-derived peptides through endogenous processing.

## 13.3 Protein Vaccine Comparing Other Types of Vaccine Formulations

NY-ESO-1 antigen has been most extensively investigated as cancer vaccine for protein, peptide, and DNA. As summarized in Table 13.1, in a case of NY-ESO-1 antigen, the vaccines which can induce antigen-specific immune responses are categorized as (1) epitope peptide (short peptide), (2) long peptide, (3) DNA, and (4) protein. Cytotoxic T-cell (CTL) epitope peptides are usually 8–10 mer peptides that are recognized by CD8+ T cells. In some clinical studies, they are combined with class II epitope peptides that can be recognized by CD4+ T cells. The epitope peptides are often mixed with incomplete Freund's adjuvant (IFA). The mixed emulsion is administered subcutaneously. The short peptides are easily bound to MHC class I molecules, which are abundantly distributed not only on antigen-presenting cells (APCs) but also other non-APCs like B cells and non-hematopoietic cells. It should be cautiously considered that peptides binding MHC class I without co-stimulatory signals can induce immune tolerance and anergy. In clinical trials of NY-ESO-1 short peptide, HLA-A*02:01 binding peptide, 157–165, is often used [3]. In some studies, the CTL peptide was combined with HLA class II peptide [4]. NY-ESO-1-specific T-cell responses were induced in response to the peptide administered. In a clinical trial, the melanoma patient who clinically responded to the peptide vaccine developed anti-NY-ESO-1 antibody [3]. This could be explained that the peptide vaccine induced tumor lysis by CTL, and then sequent antigen-specific humoral immune responses took place. HLA types that restrict CTL or CD4+ helper epitopes were required for the patients' selection.

Recently, peptide vaccines called long peptide that are longer than 9–11 mer peptide and compassing the minimum epitope sequences have been studied for cancer vaccine [5–7]. They are usually unable to directly bind to MHC class I molecules; thus, they should be internalized to the cytoplasm and degraded in APCs to be presented to MHC class I. In this sense, long peptide vaccines can present T-cell epitopes through selected endogenous processing. It also can avoid induction of immune tolerance and anergy. In the NY-ESO-1 long peptide vaccine study, overlapping peptides covering the full length of 180 amino acid sequences,

**Table 13.1** Vaccine formulation of NY-ESO-1 antigen

| | Epitope peptide | Long peptide | DNA | Protein |
|---|---|---|---|---|
| Vaccine formulation | HLA class I peptide | Overlapping peptides | Naked DNA | Full-length recombinant protein |
| | (A*02:01 157-165) | (79–108, 100–129, 121–150, 142–173) | Viral vector (vaccinia/fowl pox) | |
| | HLA class I peptide | 20 mer peptide | | |
| | (A*02:01 157-165 V) | (91–110) | | |
| | HLA class I peptide (A*02:01)/HLA class II peptide (DR4, DP4) | | | |
| Delivery system, adjuvant | Montanide | Montanide/poly-ICLC | None | ISCOMATRIX |
| | Montanide/CpG-DNA | Montanide/OK-432 | | Cholesteryl pullulan |
| | | | | Montanide/resiquimod |
| | | | | Montanide/CpG-DNA |
| Preconditioning | – | – | – | Low-dose cyclophosphamide |
| Immune response | Antibody, CD4+ T cell, CD8+ T cell | Antibody, CD4+ T cell, CD8+ T cell | Antibody (in case of viral vector), CD4+ T cell, CD8+ T cell | Antibody, CD4+ T cell, CD8+ T cell |
| References | [3, 4] | [5, 7] | [9–11] | [12], [13], [14, 15] |

NY-ESO-1-specific CD4+ T cells, CD8+ T cells, and antibodies were induced [5–7]. In both of the types of peptide vaccines, IFA are often used as an adjuvant, but a concern has been raised that the oil adjuvant works as a local depot so that the specific T cells are locally activated and the induced T-cell apoptosis might happen at injection sites [8].

DNA vaccines for NY-ESO-1 antigen are used in clinical trials, which included naked DNA and viral vector of vaccinia/fowl pox [9–11]. In both trials, antigen-specific CD8+ and CD4+ T cells were induced, while the antibodies were not induced in naked DNA vaccine. It has been considered that viral vector vaccines were more immunogenic than other vaccine formulations, but that the immune reactions to vector viruses limited the repeated vaccinations.

Protein vaccines of NY-ESO-1 have been studied, which included the whole naked NY-ESO-1 protein and the NY-ESO-1 protein combined with antigen delivery systems, such as ISCOMATRIX and cholesteryl pullulan (CHP) [12–16]. Valmori et al. reported that NY-ESO-1 protein was given with CpG in IFA emulsion and that CD4+ T-cell responses and antibody responses were dominantly induced first. Subsequently, NY-ESO-1-specific CD8+ T cells were induced, which means that primary immune reactions induced by protein vaccine are CD4+ T cells, and CD8+ T cells are reacted by the in vivo cross-priming mechanism [12]. Using ISCOMATRIX and CHP of protein-delivery systems, NY-ESO-1-specific CD8+ T cells were induced at the same timing as the CD4+ T cells and antibody reactions. One of the things we should consider about the protein vaccine is the possibility of regulatory T-cell (Treg) induction that is specific to tumor antigen. Ebert et al. reported that in the advanced melanoma patients vaccinated with full-length NY-ESO-1 protein/ISCOMATRIX complex, antigen-specific regulatory T cells were induced or boosted [17]. Additionally, the Tregs recognized the same peptide for the effector T cells, NY-ESO-$1_{157-170}$ for HLA-DP4 [17]. As this is only a single report, it is not fully determined the possible Treg generation with the same peptide. Still, it should be an issue to think about the inhibition of Treg in designing protein vaccine.

For manufacturing GMP-grade vaccine products for clinical trials, proteins are produced by plasmid DNA technology in microorganisms, and it takes multiple processes for extraction and purification of the protein, while peptides that have nine to ten amino acids are simpler and less costly to produce.

## 13.4 Protein Antigen Delivery System

Protein-based cancer vaccine can potentially activate both CD8+ T cells and CD4+ T cells by presenting multiple epitopes. Although exogenous soluble protein antigens incorporated by APCs are in general efficient in sensitizing CD4+ T cells, they are inefficient in sensitizing CD8+ T cells because these proteins are hardly processed by MHC class I pathway. A protein antigen delivery system consisting of cholesteryl pullulan (CHP) nanogels complexed with soluble protein molecules has been developed, in an attempt to present peptides that can bind both MHC class I and class II molecules in APCs [18]. The other antigen delivery systems, such as liposome and ISCOMATRIX, have also been reported [19, 20]. Liposome is a delivery nanoparticle consisting of bilayer phospholipid, which is broadly used as various drug delivery systems. Liposome vaccine that carries idiotype protein and adjuvant cytokines for follicular lymphoma was developed [19]. Another antigen delivery device is ISCOMATRIX with a diameter of 50 nm. It has been reported that protein/ISCOMATRIX complex induced significant CD8+ and CD4+ T-cell responses not only to viral antigens, including influenza virus, hepatitis C virus, and human papillomavirus, but also to tumor antigen, NY-ESO-1 antigen [21]. The similarity of these protein-based vaccines to CHP vaccine in terms of antigen delivery capacity is still unknown, although they are all able to present MHC class I and class II peptides, inducing antigen-specific CD8+ and CD4+ T cells.

## 13.5 Clinical Trials of Protein Vaccine

Recent publications of the clinical trials using recombinant protein are listed in Table 13.2. MAGE-A3 protein vaccine with an adjuvant AS02B for resected non-small cell lung cancer (NSCLC) patients was studied in a phase II trial. It was a randomized placebo-controlled study, and no significant difference of disease-free survival nor overall survival was seen [22]. The study was further developed as a phase III pivotal study, which unfortunately failed to detect the clinical benefit. Recombinant protein of epidermal growth factor was given to advanced NSCLC patients as a second-line therapy, which was conducted as a phase II randomized controlled trial [23]. Some trend of survival benefit was observed, and no serious adverse events were seen. NY-ESO-1 protein combined with ISCOMATRIX was studied for advanced melanoma, in which poor immunogenicity and clinical outcome were observed, and this negative effect was possibly due to Treg induction by the protein vaccination. Thus, they added low-dose cyclophosphamide to deplete Treg in the further cohort in the phase II study [13]. Although they did not detect clear Treg declines with addition of cyclophosphamide, NY-ESO-1-specific CD4+ T-cell responses were seen [13]. Another report showed that naked NY-ESO-1 protein was immunized with CpG-motif DNA and IFA, where CD4+ T-cell and antibody responses were induced and later CD8+ T-cell reactions took place [12].

CHP is an antigen delivery system, as described elsewhere. Recombinant proteins of NY-ESO-1, MAGE-A4, and HER2 were complexed with CHP, respectively, and they were immunized to therapy-resistant cancer patients [15, 16, 24–27]. The NY-ESO-1 and HER2 protein CHP complexed-vaccines induced CD8+ T-cell responses as well as CD4+ T-cell and antibody responses. This demonstrated that protein vaccine with a suitable antigen delivery system can be endogenously processed, and their CTL epitope peptides can be presented through MHC class I pathway in APCs. These CHP antigen protein vaccines have been studied as phase I trial, and further trials for estimating clinical effects are still underway.

## 13.6 Summary and Perspectives

Protein of tumor antigen as vaccine component is one of the efficient vaccines, since the protein is incorporated and processed in APCs, and multiple epitopes can be presented to MHC class II molecules, as well as class I. As soluble proteins are usually incorporated to APCs as exogenous antigens, improvements to promote cross-priming to MHC class I and II pathway are recommended, which include antigen delivery systems as described and suitable adjuvants. Several clinical trials using tumor antigen proteins demonstrated the multiple immune reactions that were induced. However, it is still underway to estimate clinical benefit and setting as a cancer treatment.

**Table 13.2** Clinical trials of recombinant protein cancer vaccine

| Recombinant protein vaccine/delivery system, adjuvant | Phase | Study population | Safety | Immune response | Clinical outcome | Reference |
|---|---|---|---|---|---|---|
| NY-ESO-1/cholesteryl pullulan (CHP) | I | Esophageal cancer, prostate cancer, melanoma | No G3/4 AE | Dose-dependent antibody response, for 200 μg<br>CD4+ T cell, CD8 T cell | Long survival in higher dose of NY-ESO-1 protein | [15, 16, 26] |
| NY-ESO-1/ISCOMATRIX, low-dose cyclophosphamide | II | Melanoma | Tolerable | CD4+ T cell | Stable disease (6/15pts) | [13] |
| NY-ESO-1/CpG, IFA | I | Melanoma, breast cancer, others | No G3/4 AE | CD4+ T cell and antibody, later CD8+ T-cell response | Not evaluated | [12] |
| MAGE-A4/cholesteryl pullulan (CHP) | I | Esophageal cancer | Tolerable | Antibody response, CD4+ T cell, CD8 T cell (antigen highly expressed tumors) | Stable disease (15/20pts) | [27] |
| MAGE-A3/AS02B | II | Non-small cell lung cancer | No difference to the control arm | Antibody response | No significance in overall survival between vaccine and control groups | [22] |
| EGF/IFA | II | Non-small cell lung cancer | No G3/4 AE | Antibody response | | [23] |
| HER2/cholesteryl pullulan (CHP) | I | Breast cancer, others | No G3/4 AE | Antibody response, CD4+ T cell, CD8 T cell | Stable disease (7/9pts) | [24] |

*AE* adverse event

It could be further developed using suitable combination with potential immunoadjuvant and/or a combined therapy with an immune-checkpoint inhibitor or an effector T-cell therapy.

## References


1. Chen YT, Scanlan MJ, Sahin U, Türeci O, Gure AO, Tsang S et al (1997) A testicular antigen aberrantly expressed in human cancers detected by autologous antibody screening. Proc Natl Acad Sci U S A 94:1914–1918
2. Komatsu N, Jackson HM, Chan KF, Oveissi S, Cebon J, Itoh K et al (2013) Fine-mapping naturally occurring NY-ESO-1 antibody epitopes in melanoma patients' sera using short overlapping peptides and full-length recombinant protein. Mol Immunol 54:465–471. doi:10.1016/j.molimm.2013.01.014
3. Jäger E, Gnjatic S, Nagata Y, Stockert E, Jäger D, Karbach J et al (2000) Induction of primary NY-ESO-1 immunity: CD8+ T lymphocyte and antibody responses in peptide-vaccinated patients with NY-ESO-1+ cancers. Proc Natl Acad Sci U S A 97:12198–12203. doi:10.1073/pnas.220413497
4. Odunsi K, Qian F, Matsuzaki J, Mhawech-Fauceglia P, Andrews C, Hoffman EW et al (2007) Vaccination with an NY-ESO-1 peptide of HLA class I/II specificities induces integrated humoral and T cell responses in ovarian cancer. Proc Natl Acad Sci U S A 104:12837–12842
5. Tsuji T, Sabbatini P, Jungbluth AA, Ritter E, Pan L, Ritter G et al (2013) Effect of Montanide and poly-ICLC adjuvant on human self/tumor antigen-specific CD4+ T cells in phase I overlapping long peptide vaccine trial. Cancer Immunol Res 1:340–350. doi:10.1158/2326-6066.CIR-13-0089
6. Wada H, Isobe M, Kakimi K, Mizote Y, Eikawa S, Sato E et al (2014) Vaccination with NY-ESO-1 overlapping peptides mixed with Picibanil OK-432 and montanide ISA-51 in patients with cancers expressing the NY-ESO-1 antigen. J Immunother 37:84–92. doi:10.1097/CJI.0000000000000017
7. Kakimi K, Isobe M, Uenaka A, Wada H, Sato E, Doki Y et al (2011) A phase I study of vaccination with NY-ESO-1f peptide mixed with Picibanil OK-432 and Montanide ISA-51 in patients with cancers expressing the NY-ESO-1 antigen. Int J Cancer 129:2836–2846. doi:10.1002/ijc.25955
8. Hailemichael Y, Dai Z, Jaffarzad N, Ye Y, Medina MA, Huang XF et al (2013) Persistent antigen at vaccination sites induces tumor-specific $CD8^+$ T cell sequestration, dysfunction and deletion. Nat Med 19:465–472. doi:10.1038/nm.3105
9. Jäger E, Karbach J, Gnjatic S, Neumann A, Bender A, Valmori D et al (2006) Recombinant vaccinia/fowlpox NY-ESO-1 vaccines induce both humoral and cellular NY-ESO-1-specific immune responses in cancer patients. Proc Natl Acad Sci U S A 103:14453–14458
10. Gnjatic S, Altorki NK, Tang DN, Tu SM, Kundra V, Ritter G et al (2009) NY-ESO-1 DNA vaccine induces T-cell responses that are suppressed by regulatory T cells. Clin Cancer Res 15:2130–2139. doi:10.1158/1078-0432.CCR-08-2632
11. Odunsi K, Matsuzaki J, Karbach J, Neumann A, Mhawech-Fauceglia P, Miller A et al (2012) Efficacy of vaccination with recombinant vaccinia and fowlpox vectors expressing NY-ESO-1 antigen in ovarian cancer and melanoma patients. Proc Natl Acad Sci U S A 109:5797–5802. doi:10.1073/pnas.1117208109
12. Valmori D, Souleimanian NE, Tosello V, Bhardwaj N, Adams S, O'Neill D et al (2007) Vaccination with NY-ESO-1 protein and CpG in Montanide induces integrated antibody/Th1 responses and CD8 T cells through cross-priming. Proc Natl Acad Sci U S A 104:8947–8952
13. Klein O, Davis ID, McArthur GA, Chen L, Haydon A, Parente P et al (2015) Low-dose cyclophosphamide enhances antigen-specific CD4(+) T cell responses to NY-ESO-1/

ISCOMATRIX™ vaccine in patients with advanced melanoma. Cancer Immunol Immunother 64:507–518. doi:10.1007/s00262-015-1656-x
14. Sabado RL, Pavlick A, Gnjatic S, Cruz CM, Vengco I, Hasan F et al (2015) Resiquimod as an immunologic adjuvant for NY-ESO-1 protein vaccination in patients with high-risk melanoma. Cancer Immunol Res 3:278–287. doi:10.1158/2326-6066.CIR-14-0202
15. Uenaka A, Wada H, Isobe M, Saika T, Tsuji K, Sato E et al (2007) T cell immunomonitoring and tumor responses in patients immunized with a complex of cholesterol-bearing hydrophobized pullulan (CHP) and NY-ESO-1 protein. Cancer Immun 7:9–19
16. Kageyama S, Wada H, Muro K, Niwa Y, Ueda S, Miyata H et al (2013) Dose-dependent effects of NY-ESO-1 protein vaccine complexed with cholesteryl pullulan (CHP-NY-ESO-1) on immune responses and survival benefits of esophageal cancer patients. J Transl Med 11: 246–255. doi:10.1186/1479-5876-11-246
17. Ebert LM, MacRaild SE, Zanker D, Davis ID, Cebon J, Chen W (2012) A cancer vaccine induces expansion of NY-ESO-1-specific regulatory T cells in patients with advanced melanoma. PLoS One 7:e48424. doi:10.1371/journal.pone.0048424
18. Ikuta Y, Katayama N, Wang L, Okugawa T, Takahashi Y, Schmitt M et al (2002) Presentation of a major histocompatibility complex class 1-binding peptide by monocyte-derived dendritic cells incorporating hydrophobized polysaccharide-truncated HER2 protein complex: implications for a polyvalent immuno-cell therapy. Blood 99:3717–3724
19. Neelapu SS, Baskar S, Gause BL, Kobrin CB, Watson TM, Frye AR et al (2004) Human autologous tumor-specific T-cell responses induced by liposomal delivery of a lymphoma antigen. Clin Cancer Res 10:8309–8317
20. Davis ID, Chen W, Jackson H, Parente P, Shackleton M, Hopkins W et al (2004) Recombinant NY-ESO-1 protein with ISCOMATRIX adjuvant induces broad integrated antibody and CD4 (+) and CD8(+) T cell responses in humans. Proc Natl Acad Sci U S A 101:10697–10702
21. Sanders MT, Brown LE, Deliyannis G, Pearse MJ (2005) ISCOM-based vaccines: the second decade. Immunol Cell Biol 83:119–128
22. Vansteenkiste J, Zielinski M, Linder A, Dahabreh J, Gonzalez EE, Malinowski W et al (2013) Adjuvant MAGE-A3 immunotherapy in resected non-small-cell lung cancer: phase II randomized study results. J Clin Oncol 31:2396–2403. doi:10.1200/JCO.2012.43.7103
23. Neninger Vinageras E, de la Torre A, Osorio Rodríguez M, Catalá Ferrer M, Bravo I, Mendoza del Pino M et al (2008) Phase II randomized controlled trial of an epidermal growth factor vaccine in advanced non-small-cell lung cancer. J Clin Oncol 26:1452–1458. doi:10.1200/JCO.2007.11.5980
24. Kitano S, Kageyama S, Nagata Y, Miyahara Y, Hiasa A, Naota H et al (2006) HER2-specific T-cell immune responses in patients vaccinated with truncated HER2 protein complexed with nanogels of cholesteryl pullulan. Clin Cancer Res 12:7397–7405
25. Kageyama S, Kitano S, Hirayama M, Nagata Y, Imai H, Shiraishi T et al (2008) Humoral immune responses in patients vaccinated with 1-146 HER2 protein complexed with cholesteryl pullulan nanogel. Cancer Sci 99:601–607
26. Aoki M, Ueda S, Nishikawa H, Kitano S, Hirayama M, Ikeda H et al (2009) Antibody responses against NY-ESO-1 and HER2 antigens in patients vaccinated with combinations of cholesteryl pullulan (CHP)-NY-ESO-1 and CHP-HER2 with OK-432. Vaccine 27: 6854–6861. doi:10.1016/j.vaccine.2009.09.018
27. Saito T, Wada H, Yamasaki M, Miyata H, Nishikawa H et al (2014) High expression of MAGE-A4 and MHC class I antigens in tumor cells and induction of MAGE-A4 immune responses are prognostic markers of CHP-MAGE-A4 cancer vaccine. Vaccine 32(45): 5901–5907. doi:10.1016/j.vaccine.2014.09.002
28. Jäger E, Jäger D, Karbach J, Chen YT, Ritter G, Nagata Y et al (2000) Identification of NY-ESO-1 epitopes presented by human histocompatibility antigen (HLA)-DRB4*0101-0103 and recognized by CD4(+) T lymphocytes of patients with NY-ESO-1-expressing melanoma. J Exp Med 191:625–630

29. Mandic M1, Castelli F, Janjic B, Almunia C, Andrade P, Gillet D, et al (2005) One NY-ESO-1-derived epitope that promiscuously binds to multiple HLA-DR and HLA-DP4 molecules and stimulates autologous CD4+ T cells from patients with NY-ESO-1-expressing melanoma. J Immunol 174:1751–1759.
30. Jäger E, Chen YT, Drijfhout JW, Karbach J, Ringhoffer M, Jäger D et al (1998) Simultaneous humoral and cellular immune response against cancer-testis antigen NY-ESO-1: definition of human histocompatibility leukocyte antigen (HLA)-A2-binding peptide epitopes. J Exp Med 187:265–270
31. Gnjatic S, Nagata Y, Jager E, Stockert E, Shankara S, Roberts BL et al (2000) Strategy for monitoring T cell responses to NY-ESO-1 in patients with any HLA class I allele. Proc Natl Acad Sci U S A 97:10917–10922
32. Mizote Y, Uenaka A, Isobe M, Wada H, Kakimi K, Saika T et al (2014) Production of NY-ESO-1 peptide/DRB1*08:03 tetramers and ex vivo detection of CD4 T-cell responses in vaccinated cancer patients. Vaccine 32:957–964
33. Yamaguchi H, Tanaka F, Ohta M, Inoue H, Mori M (2004) Identification of HLA-A24-restricted CTL epitope from cancer-testis antigen, NY-ESO-1, and induction of a specific antitumor immune response. Clin Cancer Res 10:890–896
34. Karbach J, Pauligk C, Bender A, Gnjatic S, Franzmann K, Wahle C et al (2006) Identification of new NY-ESO-1 epitopes recognized by CD4+ T cells and presented by HLA-DQ B1 03011. Int J Cancer 118:668–674
35. Eikawa S, Kakimi K, Isobe M, Kuzushima K, Luescher I, Ohue Y et al (2013) Induction of CD8 T-cell responses restricted to multiple HLA class I alleles in a cancer patient by immunization with a 20-mer NY-ESO-1f (NY-ESO-1 91-110) peptide. Int J Cancer 132: 345–354
36. Gnjatic S, Atanackovic D, Jäger E, Matsuo M, Selvakumar A, Altorki NK et al (2003) Survey of naturally occurring CD4+ T cell responses against NY-ESO-1 in cancer patients: correlation with antibody responses. Proc Natl Acad Sci U S A 100:8862–8867
37. Zeng G, Touloukian CE, Wang X, Restifo NP, Rosenberg SA, Wang RF (2000) Identification of CD4+ T cell epitopes from NY-ESO-1 presented by HLA-DR molecules. J Immunol 165: 1153–1159
38. Zarour HM, Storkus WJ, Brusic V, Williams E, Kirkwood JM (2000) NY-ESO-1 encodes DRB1*0401-restricted epitopes recognized by melanoma-reactive CD4+ T cells. Cancer Res 60:4946–4952

# Chapter 14
# Dendritic Cell-Based Vaccine for Cancer

**Masato Okamoto**

**Abstract** Although cancer vaccines could not show the evidence of their therapeutic effects in phase III clinical trials, two dendritic cell (DC)-based vaccines, sipuleucel-T (Provenge®) and DCVax®-Brain, are approved in the USA and Switzerland, respectively. Furthermore, pivotal randomized phase III trials of several DC vaccines are ongoing in the USA and Europe. The promising data are also shown in retrospective as well as prospective clinical studies by using Japanese DC vaccine Vaccell® that we are engaged in development; therefore, its large-scale prospective clinical trial is now preparing. In this chapter, I introduce the results of representative clinical trials including sipuleucel-T and DCVax® and the process of Vaccell® development, consider the advantages of the DC vaccine for conventional vaccine, and discuss the problems and future prospects of the DC vaccine.

**Keywords** Specific immunotherapy • Cancer vaccine • Dendritic cells • OK-432 • Clinical trial

## 14.1 Introduction

Although cancer vaccine that is one of the antigen specific immunotherapics has been expected for the patients with malignancies resistant to standard treatment, the therapeutic effect has not been evidenced. Even the certain cancer vaccines which showed clinical effects in early phase clinical studies [1–4] have not demonstrated clear clinical benefits in pivotal phase III trials. On July 16, 2007, the Swiss Institute of Public Health has approved the world's first therapeutic vaccine for brain cancer DCVax®-Brain (Northwest Biotherapeutics, Inc.), and on April 29, 2010, the US Food and Drug Administration (FDA) has approved sipuleucel-T (Dendreon Corp.) which is a cancer vaccine for the treatment of hormone-refractory prostate cancer. Sipuleucel-T is the only vaccine approved so far by the US FDA to treat cancer. Interestingly, both vaccines are antigen-presenting cell (APC) (mainly dendritic cell (DC))-based cancer vaccine. "Why is it DC vaccine?"

M. Okamoto (✉)
Department of Advanced Immunotherapeutics, Oncology Center, Kitasato Institute Hospital, Kitasato University School of Pharmacy, 5-9-1 Shirokane, Minato-ku, Tokyo 108-8641, Japan
e-mail: okamotom@pharm.kitasato-u.ac.jp



Y. Yamaguchi (ed.), *Immunotherapy of Cancer*,
DOI 10.1007/978-4-431-55031-0_14

## 14.2 DCs and DC Vaccine

### *14.2.1 DCs, T-Cell Response, and Clinical Outcome*

DCs are potent APCs which play a central role in initiating adaptive and innate immune responses. In most tissues, DCs are present in an immature state. The immature DCs (iDCs) are unable to stimulate T cells but are extremely well equipped to capture antigens. The iDCs are matured by the stimulation associated with capturing antigens such as bacteria, viruses, and apoptotic cancer cells and by other stimulating agents including inflammatory cytokines such as tumor necrosis factor (TNF)-α, interleukin (IL)-1β, CD40 ligand, and several conserved microbial molecules such as lipopolysaccharide (LPS), lipoprotein, CpG DNA, and double-stranded RNA [5–8]. In the primary tumor sites, iDCs phagocytize antigens from apoptotic tumor cells and the appropriately matured antigen-bearing DCs that result strongly expressing CD80, CD83, CD86, CD40, and MHC class I and MHC class II; migrate to the paracortical T-cell-rich area of the draining lymph nodes; present antigens to CD8+T cells via MHC class I and to CD4+T cells via MHC class II; and induce tumor-specific cytotoxic T lymphocytes (CTLs) as well as helper T cells to exhibit antitumor effects. The details about the cytology of DCs entrust it to other basic articles.

To generate cancer antigen-specific CTLs and to elicit anticancer effects, iDCs should be matured appropriately to derive helper T-cell type I (Th1) because it is much significant for inducing CTLs that the antigens are presented to T cells under Th1-dominant condition in cytokine balance (Fig. 14.1) [9–15]. Immunologically suppressive conditions such as Th2, Th17, and regulatory T cells (Tregs), but not Th1, may be induced in many cancer-bearing hosts. Although controversial findings have been reported in the role of Th17 in antitumor immunity, such an inhibitory condition causes the dysfunction of DCs as well as the induction of tolerogenic DCs; therefore, CTLs may not be induced, and it is also possible that the immunological tolerance even may cause the tumor progression and poor prognosis.

Actually, it has been reported that the survival of the advanced melanoma patients who received an allogeneic cancer vaccine (Canvaxin™) developed from three melanoma cell lines was shorter than that of the patients who received placebo [16, 17]. In stage III melanoma patients, the 5-year survival was 59 % for those receiving Canvaxin™ and 68 % for the untreated patients. In the stage IV melanoma patients, the median survival was 32 months for the patients treated with Canvaxin™ and was 39 months for control patients. In addition, phase III trial using a cell-based gene-transduced multi-antigen vaccine GVAX® (Cell Genesys, Inc.) showed that overall survival (OS) was shorter in the GVAX arm with median survival of 12.2 versus 14.1 months in the placebo arm ($P = 0.0076$) [18]. Cancer progression by peptide vaccine has been reported also in mouse model via induction of apoptosis of CD8+T cells [19]. These reports strongly suggest the possibility that the cancer vaccines become harmful when they do not work appropriately.

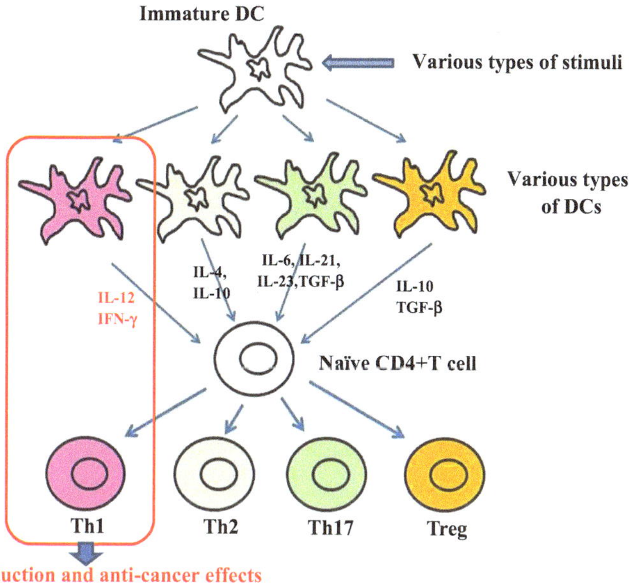


**Fig. 14.1** Effects of various DCs in CD4+ T-cell differentiation. Immature DCs which received various stimuli including bacterial components and inflammatory or anti-inflammatory cytokines, differentiate into several types of DCs which induce Th1, Th2, Th17, or Treg. It is important for making a therapeutic DC vaccine to prepare the DCs which can induce a Th1 immune response

## *14.2.2 Advantages of DC Vaccine*

In the conventional cancer vaccines in which only antigens such as peptides, proteins, nucleic acids, etc. or antigens plus immunoadjuvants are administered, we cannot reject the following possibilities that (1) the number of APCs (mainly DCs) in the patients' bodies is too small to induce antigen-specific CTLs for eliminating cancer cells, (2) the administered antigens are not presented on HLA molecules on DCs, (3) DCs do not mature appropriately, and (4) DCs differentiate into tolerogenic type. These may be the reasons why cancer vaccines could not show anticancer effect and why several vaccine protocols induced cancer progression and poor prognosis as described above.

DC vaccines were developed to clear these problems. DCs are cultured in large scale, are certainly pulsed with antigens, and are matured appropriately into Th1-inducing type ex vivo. DC vaccine is the only method at present to be able to control artificially the Th1-type host immune response that can be promising for eliciting antitumor effects (Fig. 14.1). Actually, advanced melanoma patients who received Melapuldencel-T, which is an autologous tumor-pulsed DC vaccine, showed a much prolonged survival time as compared with those who received only autologous tumor vaccine (see Sect. 14.3).

## 14.2.3 Several Types of DC Vaccines

### 14.2.3.1 Source of DCs

Although a number of basic examinations for DC induction from CD34+ hematopoietic stem cells, for expansion of peripheral blood DCs such as myeloid DCs and plasmacytoid DCs, for use of allogeneic DCs, etc. [20–24] have been done, these strategies could not be standard methods so far for clinical applications of DC vaccine. Most of DCs whose safety is established and which are used for large-scale clinical trials are autologous peripheral blood monocyte-derived DCs as described in Sects. 14.3 and 14.4.

### 14.2.3.2 Antigens Which Are Loaded Ex Vivo into DCs for Human Use

Here, I briefly describe about cancer antigens for the vaccines. Please make other chapters reference about the details.

Although several types of antigens such as apoptotic bodies, tumor lysates, or mRNAs derived from autologous or allogeneic tumors and peptides, proteins, or mRNAs for purified tumor-associated antigens (TAAs) to be pulsed into DCs for therapeutic vaccine have been reported [25–30], each type of antigens has some problems as well as advantages as shown in Table 14.1. For example, although patient-derived whole tumors include all of their TAAs, the key TAAs which are required for inducing CTLs and for eliminating cancer cells are limited. Possibly, the amounts of the key TAAs included in whole tumor cells in each patient may be too small to work for eliciting anticancer effects. If we would find key TAAs for

**Table 14.1** Antigen types which are ex vivo loaded into DCs for therapeutic vaccines

| Antigen type | | Advantage | Problem |
|---|---|---|---|
| 1. Autologous tumor | Apoptotic body | They may adapt to variety and the change of the antigens | Quantities of the key antigen may be too small |
| | Tumor lysate | | They may include suppressive components |
| | mRNA | | |
| 2. Allogeneic tumor | Apoptotic body | They may adapt to variety and the change of the antigens | Quantities of the key antigen may be too small |
| | Tumor lysate | High CTL-inducing activity by allogeneic antigens | They may include suppressive components |
| | mRNA | | Adverse allogeneic reaction |
| 3. Purified TAA | Peptide | High amounts of key antigens can be used | They may not adapt to variety and the change of the antigens profile |
| | Protein | | |
| | mRNA | | |

*CTL* cytotoxic T lymphocyte, *TAA* tumor-associated antigen key antigens: antigens required for inducing CTLs and for eliminating cancer cells

each patient, the synthetic peptides, proteins, or nucleic acids for the key TAAs are able to be effectively used.

In 2009, Cheever et al. have reported the prioritization of cancer antigens as vaccines for cancer patients [31]. In my opinion, the significant points as an antigen for therapeutic vaccine are that the antigen(s) (1) are overexpressed in cancer cells but not in normal cells, (2) have high activity for inducing CTLs, (3) are expressed on cancer stem cells (cancer stemlike cells, cancer-initiating cells), and (4) have a function to be critical for cancer cells to survive. Especially, (3) and (4) are important in vaccine therapy to prevent cancer cells from escaping out of immunosurveillance. Recently, lots of investigators including our group are trying to find the cancer antigen(s) that satisfied the above requirements (most equally to "key TAAs") to develop more effective cancer vaccine; therefore, in the near future, multi-peptides (or proteins or nucleic acids) for TAAs may become the main antigens for the therapeutic DC vaccine (also see Sect. 14.4.3), although autologous tumors have been mainly used for large-volume clinical trials so far (see Sect. 14.3 and Table 14.2).

In addition, we have reported most recently that the vaccination with vascular progenitor cells derived from induced pluripotent stem (iPS) cells elicits antitumor immunity targeting vascular and tumor cells in basic examination [32]. Such a strategy also will be carried out with the progress of the science for regenerative medicine.

## 14.3 Development of Therapeutic DC Vaccines

It was much difficult for the investigators to conduct a large-scale clinical trial of the DC vaccine because the cell processing process should be required to make the therapeutic DC vaccine. Therefore, the evidence for the anticancer effect of the DC vaccine has not been provided even if there are a lot of reports from relatively small-size clinical trials. However, recent progress of cell processing system under the GCP management has made DC vaccine to be provided to lots of patients and the investigators to be able to conduct a large-scale, pivotal phase III clinical trial.

Here, I introduce the DC vaccines which have already been approved in the USA or Europe or the DC vaccines whose phase III study is ongoing in the USA (Table 14.2).

### *14.3.1 DCVax® (Northwest Biotherapeutics, Inc.)*

DCVax®-Brain which is an autologous peripheral blood monocyte-derived DC vaccine loaded with the patients' own glioblastoma cell lysate has been approved by the Swiss Institute of Public Health as the world's first commercially available therapeutic vaccine for brain cancer in 2007. DCVax®-Brain delayed disease

**Table 14.2** DC vaccine products which are already approved or whose phase III trial is ongoing

| Products | Company | APCs | Antigens | Cancer type | Phase III trials authorized by the US FDA | Approval |
|---|---|---|---|---|---|---|
| DCVax®-Brain | Northwest Biotherapeutics, Inc. | Autologous monocyte DCs | Autologous GBM tumor lysate | GBM | | Approved by the Swiss Institute of Public Health on 2007 |
| DCVax®-L (same as DCVax®-Brain) | Northwest Biotherapeutics, Inc. | Autologous monocyte DCs | Autologous GBM tumor lysate | GBM | A phase III trial is ongoing [NCT00045968] | |
| Sipuleucel-T (Provenge®) | Dendreon Corp. | Autologous APCs (mainly DCs) | Recombinant PAP protein | Hormone-refractory prostate cancer | A phase III IMPACT trial is completed [NCT00065442] | Approved by the US FDA on 2010 |
| Melapuldencel-T (also called DC-TC) | NeoStem, Inc. | Autologous monocyte DCs | Irradiated, autologous tumor cells | Advanced melanoma | A phase III trial is ongoing [NCT01875653] | |
| AGS-003 | Argos Therapeutics, Inc. | Autologous monocyte DCs | Autologous tumor-derived RNA | Metastatic RCC | A phase III ADAPT trial [NCT01582672] | |
| ICT-107 | Immunocellular therapeutics, Ltd. | Autologous monocyte DCs | Six peptides: AIM-2, MAGE1, TRP-2, gp100, HER2, IL-13Ra2 | Newly diagnosed GBM | A phase III study is now being prepared | |

*APC* antigen-presenting cells, *GBM* glioblastoma multiform, *PAP* prostatic acid phosphatase, protein, *RCC* renal cell carcinoma

recurrence from 6.9 to 18.1 months for newly diagnosed glioblastoma patients and extends OS from 14.6 months to more than 33 months [33–35].

In the USA, a phase III clinical trial evaluating DCVax®-L (other names: DCVax®-Brain, DCVax®) for the treatment of glioblastoma multiforme (GBM) is now ongoing, authorized by the US FDA. The primary endpoint is progression-free survival (PFS), and the secondary endpoints are OS, immune response, and also safety.

### *14.3.2 Sipuleucel-T (Provenge®, Dendreon Corp.)*

Sipuleucel-T is the only vaccine approved so far by the US FDA to treat cancer. Administration of sipuleucel-T which is autologous APCs (mainly DCs) pulsed with the fusion protein (prostatic acid phosphatase (PAP)-granulocyte-macrophage colony-stimulating factor (GM-CSF)) extended 4.1 months in median OS compared to the placebo control group (25.8 months vs 21.7 months) and reduced the risk of death by 22.5 % compared to the control in phase III IMPACT trial, a 512-patient, multicenter, randomized, double-blind, placebo-controlled study [36]. Antigen-specific immune responses were detected in patients who received sipuleucel-T. Further study also showed that sipuleucel-T administration elicits a recruitment of activated effector T cells into a tumor microenvironment as well as a systemic antigen-specific T-cell response [37].

### *14.3.3 Melapuldencel-T (NeoStem, Inc.)*

Melapuldencel-T (also called DC-TC) is a monocyte-derived therapeutic DC vaccine which is loaded with irradiated, ex vivo proliferated, autologous tumor cells for patients with malignant melanoma.

Results of phase II clinical trial that were presented at the 2014 ASCO Annual Meeting are based on further analysis of previously published data from 170 melanoma patients enrolled in three studies including (1) a single-arm phase II trial of only irradiated, autologous tumor cells [38], (2) a single-arm phase II trial of Melapuldencel-T [39], (3) and a randomized phase II trial comparing Melapuldencel-T and only irradiated, autologous tumor vaccine [40]. Patients were classified as no evidence of disease (NED) or non-NED. In all patients, 5-year OS rate was 50 % for the Melapuldencel-T group vs. 32 % for control patients who received autologous tumor vaccine alone ($p = 0.004$). In the subset of NED patients, 5-year OS was 73 % for the Melapuldencel-T group vs. 43 % for control patients ($p = 0.015$) [41, 42]. In non-NED patients, 5-year OS rate was higher in the Melapuldencel-T group (33 %) than in control group (20 %) ($p = 0.025$).

NeoStem, Inc. is initiating a phase III, randomized, double-blind, multicenter trial of Melapuldencel-T for patients with previously treated, advanced melanoma under a Special Protocol Assessment (SPA) agreement with the US FDA [NCT01875653], and this DC vaccine has been granted fast-track designation by the agency as well.

### 14.3.4 AGS-003 (Argos Therapeutics, Inc.)

AGS-003 is an autologous monocyte-derived DC vaccine loaded with autologous tumor RNA and CD40 ligand RNA. On July 3, 2012, the US FDA has approved the SPA for pivotal phase III clinical trial of AGS-003 for the treatment of metastatic renal cell carcinoma (mRCC) [NCT01582672] based on the highly encouraging long-term survival observed in the phase II trial. In the 21 metastatic clear-cell RCC patients (11 intermediate risk and 10 poor risk) enrolled in this study, the median OS was 30.2 months and the median PFS was 11.2 months. The median OS for the intermediate risk population was 57.1 month, and 52 % of all 21 patients achieved OS $\geq$30 months and 33.3 % of the patients were still alive at 48 months after registration. Five of 21 patients have exceeded or are currently nearing the 5-year plus survival mark [43, 44].

This phase III trial (ADAPT study) is now ongoing. The protocol focused on a primary endpoint of improving OS for patients with mRCC randomized to receive AGS-003 combined with sunitinib vs. sunitinib alone [NCT01582672] [45].

### 14.3.5 ICT-107 (ImmunoCellular Therapeutics, Ltd.)

ICT-107 is an autologous monocyte-derived DC vaccine pulsed with six synthetic class I peptides from AIM-2, MAGE1, TRP-2, gp100, HER2/neu, and IL-13Ra2 for patients with newly diagnosed GBM [46]. Results of a randomized, double-blind, placebo-controlled phase II study were presented on the 2014 ASCO Annual Meeting [47]. HLA-A1+ and/or HLA-A2+ resected GBM patients with residual tumor $<1$ cm$^3$ who received 6 weeks of concurrent temozolomide (TMZ) and radiation. One hundred twenty-four patients were randomized 2:1 to ICT-107 group or control group who received unpulsed DCs in combination with TMZ. In HLA-A2 patients with unmethylated MGMT, median OS was 15.8 months for ICT-107 group and 11.8 months for control group, and median PFS was 10.5 months for ICT-107 group and 6.0 months for control group. Much interestingly, in HLA-A2 patients with methylated MGMT, median PFS was 24.1 months for ICT-107 group and 8.5 months for control group. In the ICT-107 group, IL-12 production and HLA-DR expression were predictive of OS ($p$-values $<0.05$).

Both the US FDA and European National Regulatory Authorities provided encouraging suggestions for advancing ICT-107 into phase III trial.

## 14.4 Development of Japanese DC Vaccine, Vaccell®

Our group (the DC Vaccine Study Group at the Japan Society of Innovative Cell Therapy (J-SICT)) is also developing the DC vaccine "Vaccell®" for cancer in Japan. The original methodology using peripheral blood monocytes for making this vaccine has been developed by Yamashita and Takahashi based on the method reported by Banchereau, Steinman, Akagawa, Zhou, and Tedder et al. [6, 48, 49]. Then, in this vaccine, the condition for DC maturation was optimized by Okamoto et al., the antigens pulsed into the DCs were examined and selected also by Okamoto et al., and then, finally, the vaccine was adjusted as the product by Yonemitsu et al. The Vaccell® whose standard operating procedure (SOP) has been established as described above has been served to patients with various malignancies, and not only large-scale retrospective but also prospective studies have been done or are ongoing.

### *14.4.1 Phase I Clinical Trial Using the DC Vaccine Made by Original Method*

Yamashita et al. has carried out phase I clinical trial of monocyte-derived DC vaccine pulsed with autologous tumor lysates made by their original methodology in ten patients with stage IV advanced melanoma and six patients with advanced thyroid cancer including five papillary and one follicular types [50–52].

The DC vaccine could be safely harvested, cryopreserved, and administrated to patients without obvious complications. These patients were vaccinated weekly with $10^7$ DCs for 10 weeks and given 350–700 kIU of IL-2 three times per week. Of the ten melanoma patients, one showed stable disease (SD), seven showed progressive disease (PD), and two showed mixed response including partial tumor regression. Of the six thyroid cancer patients, disease was assessed as SD in two and as PD in four. Tumor growth rate appeared to be reduced during DC vaccination in four PD patients as well as two SD patients.

Although these studies showed limited clinical benefits for cancer patients, the improvement of clinical efficacy will require further research.

### *14.4.2 Induction of Mature DCs by Using OK-432*

In the 1990s and early 2000s, the investigators used cytokine cocktail including tumor necrosis factor (TNF)-α to mature DCs; however, much more effective mature DCs (mDCs) were required for therapeutic cancer vaccines. We expected it in OK-432 (Chugai Pharmaceutical Co., Ltd, Tokyo, Japan) which is a

*Streptococcus*-derived immunoadjuvant in Japan. Here, I focused on our experimental findings of OK-432.

#### 14.4.2.1 Streptococcal Adjuvant OK-432 Induces Th1 via TLRs

OK-432, a penicillin-killed and lyophilized preparation of a low-virulence strain of *Streptococcus pyogenes* (group A) [53], has been successfully used as an immunotherapeutic agent in many types of malignancies [54–58]. We have also reported that OK-432-based immunotherapy has a marked therapeutic effect in patients with head and neck cancer [59–62]. OK-432 elicits antitumor effects by stimulating immunocompetent cells such as macrophages, T cells, and natural killer (NK) cells and by inducing multiple cytokines [63–65]. In addition, the most important function of OK-432 is to induce IL-12 strongly and to polarize the T-cell response to a Th1-dominant state [66].

OK-432 consists of whole bacterial bodies and contains many components. We have reported that the agonists of Toll-like receptor (TLR) 4/MD-2 complex and TLR9 derived from the OK-432 induce Th1-type immune response and enhance antitumor immunity both in human and in mice [61, 67–69] (Fig. 14.2).

#### 14.4.2.2 DC Maturation, CTL Induction, and Antitumor Effect by OK-432

Next, we have shown that the expression of TLR4 on DCs is significant for anticancer effect of DC-based immunotherapy in combination with OK-432

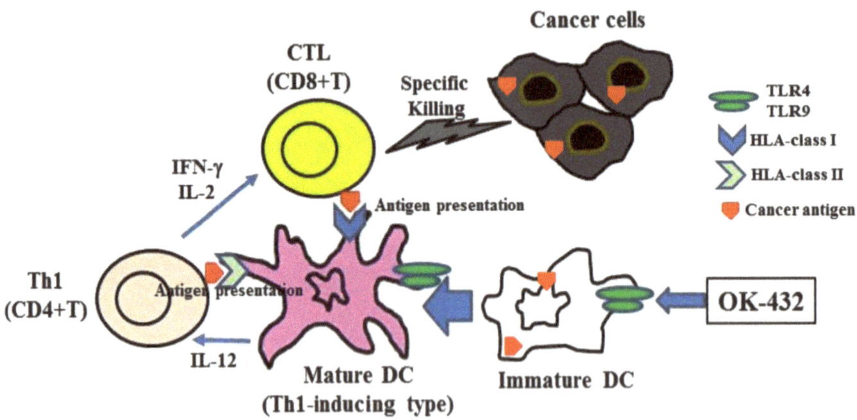


**Fig. 14.2** Generation of Th1-inducing DCs by OK-432 via TLRs and antitumor effect. DCs which were matured and differentiated into the IL-12-producing and Th1-inducing type by OK-432 stimulation present a cancer antigen to CD8+ T cells via HLA class I and to CD4+T cells via HLA class II. CD4+T cells which recognized an antigen under IL-12 stimulation, differentiate to Th1, and produce IFN-γ and IL-2. Antigen-recognizing CD8+T cells (CTLs) are activated by these Th1 cytokines, then kill cancer cells specifically to the cancer antigen

[70, 71]. OK-432 as well as OK-PSA which is an agonist for TLR4 isolated from OK-432, augmented IL-12 production as well as expression of the surface molecules (HLA class I, HLA class II, CD80, CD83, CD86, CD40, etc.) on DCs, and then DCs stimulated with OK-432 or OK-PSA markedly augmented antigen-specific CTL activities far stronger than LPS or TNF-$\alpha$. In tumor-bearing mouse model, although OK-PSA accelerated the antitumor effect of DC therapy in wild-type mice bearing syngeneic tumor, the OK-PSA effect on the DC therapy was not significant in TLR4-/- mice. Interestingly, an administration of wild-type-mouse-derived DCs plus OK-PSA exhibited a marked antitumor effect even in the TLR4-/- mice. Similar results were obtained from another experimental model by using original OK-432 but not isolated OK-PSA [70, 71]. OK-432/OK-PSA may be a potent immunoadjuvant for the DC vaccine (Fig. 14.2).

### *14.4.3 Antigens Pulsed into DCs*

So far, we mainly use WT1 and MUC1 peptides as antigen pulsed into DCs. It appears in the article by Cheever et al. [31] about their being superior to other antigens; however, we never stop searching for much better antigens for therapeutic DC vaccine (see Sect. 14.2.3.2). Most recently, we have been going to use WT1-specific MHC class II-restricted epitope combined with MHC class I-restricted epitope for our DC vaccine (see 14.5.1).

### *14.4.4 Methodology for Making a Monocyte-Derived, OK-432-Stimulated, Cancer Antigen-Pulsed DC Vaccine, Vaccell®*

According to the data described above, Vaccell® is made as follows. Peripheral blood mononuclear cells (PBMCs) were isolated from the leukapheresis products by Ficoll-Hypaque gradient density centrifugation. These PBMCs were placed on tissue culture plates, and the adherent cells were cultured in a medium containing GM-CSF and IL-4 to generate iDCs. Five days later, the DCs were stimulated with OK-432 and PGE2 for 24 h. The DCs were then pulsed with peptide antigens according to the HLA-A pattern. The DCs were cryopreserved and kept until the day of administration. The phenotype $CD14^{-/low}/HLA\text{-}DR^{+}/HLA\text{-}ABC^{+}/CD80^{+}/CD83^{+}/CD86^{+}/CD40^{+}/CCR7^{+}$ was taken to define mDCs. The DCs were prepared by well-trained technical staff in each institutional cell processing center under the SOP. Regarding release criteria, testing for sterility, mycoplasma (PCR method), and endotoxin (Endospecy™, Seikagaku Corp., Tokyo) was done using the supernatant or cell suspension just before the tube filling.

## 14.5 Reports of Clinical Observation for Vaccell®

At the point of writing, we have published 11 articles (10 original and 1 review papers) related to the clinical application of Vaccell®. Five articles described the effects of Vaccell® for pancreatic cancer [72–76], two for biliary tract cancer [77, 78], one for lung cancer [79], one for ovarian cancer [80], one for pediatric patient with relapsed leukemia [81], and one for several types of advanced cancers treated with radiation therapy in combination with DC vaccine [82].

### *14.5.1 Pancreatic Cancer*

The first paper related to the clinical application of Vaccell® has reported the results of retrospective study of the clinical and immunological evaluation of DC-based immunotherapy in combination with standard chemotherapy in 49 patients with advanced pancreatic carcinoma [72]. Prolongation of survival in this cohort was highly likely (median OS: 360 days from the first vaccination). An increased number of cancer antigen-specific CTLs and decreased Tregs were observed in several patients during vaccination, and an increased OS tended to be associated only with the latter.

We have conducted the next retrospective observation by expanding sample size to 354 patients as a multicenter analysis [73]. Of 354 patients who met the inclusion criteria, 255 patients who received standard chemotherapy combined with peptide-pulsed DC vaccines were analyzed. The mean OS from diagnosis was 16.5 months and that from the 1st vaccination was 9.9 months. Importantly, we found that delayed-type hypersensitivity (DTH) reaction after vaccination was an independent prognostic factor for better survival (Fig. 14.3a) and that OK-432 might be a good adjuvant enhancing the antitumor immunity during DC vaccination. This is the first report of a multicenter clinical study suggesting the feasibility and possible clinical benefit of an add-on DC vaccine in patients with advanced pancreatic combined with standard chemotherapy.

Next, a small-scale prospective clinical study in The Jikei University Hospital (principal investigator: Dr. Shigeo Koido) was conducted. In this trial, we loaded the WT1-specific HLA class II-restricted epitope in combination with HLA class I-restricted epitope into the DCs [74–76]. Ten stage IV patients with pancreatic ductal adenocarcinoma who showed HLA-positive for A*02:01, A*02:06, A*24:02, DRB1*04:05, DRB1*08:03, DRB1*15:01, DRB1*15:02, DPB1*05:01, or DPB1*09:01 were enrolled. The patients received one course of gemcitabine followed by biweekly intradermal vaccinations and gemcitabine. WT1-specific IFN-γ-producing CD4+T cells were significantly increased after treatment with the DCs pulsed with both WT1 class I- and II-restricted peptides (WT1-I/II). WT1 peptide-specific DTH was detected in 4 of the 7 patients who received WT1-I/II-DC and in 0 of the 3 patients who received DCs pulsed with WT1-I or WT1-II alone.

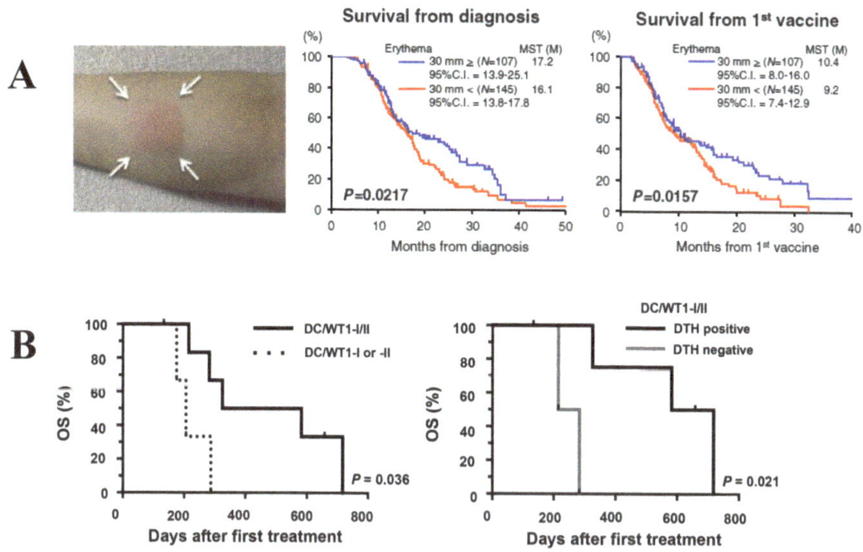


**Fig. 14.3** Japanese DC vaccine Vaccell® for pancreatic cancer patients. (**a**) Two-hundred fifty-five patients who received standard chemotherapy combined with peptide-pulsed DC vaccines were analyzed. DTH skin reaction after vaccination was an independent prognostic factor for better survival. (**b**) Seven patients who received WT1-I/II-pulsed DCs showed a markedly longer survival than three patients who received DCs pulsed with WT1-I or WT1-II alone. The WT1-specific DTH-positive patients showed significantly improved OS and PFS compared with the DTH-negative patients (These graphs and a photograph were cited from Refs. [73, 74])

The WT1-specific DTH-positive patients showed significantly improved OS and PFS compared with the DTH-negative patients (Fig. 14.3b). In particular, all three patients with strong DTH reactions had a median OS of 717 days. The decreased neutrophil/lymphocyte ratio (NLR) and the increased expression of HLA-DR and CD83 may be prognostic markers of longer survival. The activation of WT1-specific immune responses by DC vaccine pulsed with WT1-I/II in combination with chemotherapy may be associated with disease stability in advanced pancreatic cancer.

Previously, there have been some reports describing the advantage of the use of HLA class II-restricted antigen epitope(s) [83], while it is also suggested the possibility that HLA class II-restricted epitope may induce suppressive immune responses such as Th2, Th17, and Tregs. Immunoadjuvant(s), such as OK-432, should be used for inducing certain Th1. We are now planning large-scale prospective phase II/III clinical trials of the Vaccell® for pancreatic cancer patients.

### 14.5.2 Lung Cancer

Takahashi et al. reported the impact of DC vaccine pulsed with WT1 peptide antigen but not other antigens used in the current retrospective observation on the survival of patients with advanced non-small cell lung carcinomas (NSCLC) [79]. Sixty-two patients with previously treated inoperable or relapsed NSCLCs were enrolled in this study. One or more antigens (peptides for WT1, MUC1, CEA, and/or autologous tumor lysate) were pulsed into DCs according to our criteria [79]. The median survival time was 27 months (82 % in 1 year and 54 % in 2 years) from initial diagnosis and that was 12 months (48 % in 1 year and 22 % in 2 years) from the first DC vaccination. Interestingly, multivariate analyses revealed that the use of WT1 but not other antigens significantly affected the OS of the patients. DC vaccines pulsed with WT1 may hold a significant impact to prolong the overall survival of patients with advanced NSCLCs.

### 14.5.3 DC Vaccine in Combination with Radiation Therapy

Shibamoto et al. demonstrated the efficacy of DC vaccine in combination with IMRT or other conformal radiotherapy (RT), assuming minimal immunosuppression by such RT modalities [82]. Forty patients who had recurrent, metastatic, or locally advanced tumors were enrolled in the study. Although an additional effect of DC vaccine in target tumors of RT remained unclear, interestingly, 55 % of tumor control rate (22 % PR, 33 % SD) outside the RT target volume has been shown.

Abscopal effect caused after RT is often reported, and the possibility that this effect depends on antigen spreading induced by cancer-cell death by RT is being discussed. Immunotherapy combined with RT such as IMRT assuming minimal immunosuppression may be a promising strategy for the control of malignancies resistant to standard treatment.

### 14.5.4 Allogeneic DC Vaccine

Saito and Shimodaira et al. reported an important case of pediatric patients with relapsed leukemia who received allogeneic DC vaccine [81]. A 15-year-old girl with acute lymphoblastic leukemia received allogeneic WT1 peptide-pulsed DC vaccine after her third hematopoietic stem cell transplantation (HSCT). DC vaccines were generated from the third HSCT donor who was her younger sister aged 12. The patient received 14 vaccines. No vaccination-related GVHD, pancytopenia, or other systematic adverse effects developed during the 14 sessions of vaccination. WT1-specific CTL responses were detected after DC vaccination by both

WT1-tetramer and ELISPOT assays. DTH reaction on injection sites also showed good response.

After the 14th vaccination, the patient maintained complete hematological remission with complete donor chimerism. Then, vaccination was discontinued at the request of the patient and her parents. Unfortunately, a 4th relapse occurred 44 months after the 3rd HSCT, which was 14 months after the final DC vaccination.

This strategy is promising and may be safe, tolerable, and even feasible for patients with a relapse after HSCT. If DC vaccine was continued, did the relapse occur or not? We must make use of this experience in the next step.

## 14.6 Future Strategy for Improving Clinical Effects of DC Vaccine

To let cancer vaccine work effectively, three critical points will be required: (1) development of more effective and easily prepared DC vaccine, (2) canceling an immunosuppressive condition in patients, and (3) development of predictive biomarkers for selecting patients who are expected to obtain clinical benefit by DC vaccine and for developing novel immunological therapeutic strategy for cancer patients.

### *14.6.1 Development of More Effective and Easily Prepared DC Vaccine*

#### 14.6.1.1 Source of DCs

Although several investigators are now trying the induction of functional DCs from pluripotent stem cells such as iPS cells [84, 85], they are not yet the DC sources superior to autologous peripheral blood monocytes because of the problems such as a culture condition, a culture period, a reliability, and harmful effects including carcinogenesis. In addition, we should also consider which source of autologous or allogeneic cells is better for therapeutic vaccine. Healthy volunteer-derived DC vaccines can be made as ready-to-use vaccines beforehand; however, allogeneic reaction may be a harmful risk. The possibility of clinical application of autologous or allogeneic PS cell-derived DCs is now being examined.

#### 14.6.1.2 DC Expansion

Peripheral blood monocyte-derived DCs are mainly used for human study because the number of DCs in blood is too small for therapeutic DC vaccine as well as cannot be expanded basically. In this case, a leukapheresis should be performed for obtaining the monocytes of the required amount. If the leukapheresis process might be skipped, the burdens of the patients in this therapy may be much decreased. At the present, lots of investigators are trying to develop the methodology for expanding the number of DCs [86, 87]. I expect it for progress of this future technology development.

### *14.6.2 Combination Immunotherapy (Canceling Immunosuppressive Condition)*

As shown in a delayed separation in survival curve, it takes time (3–6 months or more) so that vaccines elicit therapeutic effects; therefore, monotherapy of vaccine can be recommended as postoperative adjuvant therapy. In patients with advanced cancer, a combination immunotherapy such as an immunochemotherapy and an immunoradiotherapy may be recommended.

On the other hand, some populations of cancer patients are difficult to respond to cancer vaccine because an immunosuppressive state may be induced in tumor microenvironment and in systemic environment. In such cases, the therapies for canceling the immunosuppression for improving patients' immune condition may have to be combined to cancer vaccine such as DC vaccine. The methodology for canceling immunosuppression which can be combined to DC vaccine is very important to improve therapeutic effects of the vaccine, although I avoid describing the details in this chapter. A summary is shown in Table 14.3.

### *14.6.3 Predictive Biomarker*

Biomarkers which can predict the clinical outcome of the patients who received DC vaccine before treatment or at early stage during DC vaccination are required for the selection of patients who are expected to obtain clinical benefit by DC vaccine and for development of novel immunological therapeutic strategy for cancer patients.

For example, it has been reported that high serum IL-6 level was significantly correlated with poor clinical outcomes in castration-resistant prostate cancer patients, advanced biliary tract cancer patients, and advanced colorectal cancer patients who received the personalized peptide vaccine [96–98]. IL-6 blockade may cancel the immunosuppression of the patients and may improve vaccine effects. They have already started the trial of IL-6 blockade and the peptide vaccine. This is an excellent strategy.

In our Vaccell® study, strong DTH skin reaction, decreased Tregs, low NLR, low CRP, and high Alb may be predictive markers for good clinical outcome of patients with advanced pancreatic cancer. In addition, OK-432 is useful to increase

**Table 14.3** Methodology for canceling the immunosuppressive condition in cancer patients for improving the effects of cancer vaccines

| Therapies/drugs | Effects | Ref. |
|---|---|---|
| 1. Checkpoint inhibitors | T-cell activation by blocking checkpoint molecules | See other chapters |
| Anti-CTLA4, anti-TIM3 | | |
| Anti-PD-1, anti-LAG3 | | |
| Anti-PD-L1 | | |
| 2. Chemotherapeutic agents | Treg number ↓ | [88, 89] |
| Cyclophosphamide | Treg number ↓ MDSC number ↓ | [72, 89, 90] |
| Gemcitabine | DC number ↑ WT1 expression ↑ | [91, 92] |
| 5-FU/S-1 | PD-L1 expression ↓ DC function ↑ | [71, 93] |
| 3. Radiation therapy | Treg number ↓ | [94, 95] |
| | Immunogenic cell death | |
| | Antigen spreading | |

*Treg* regulatory T cell, *MDSC* myeloid-derived suppressor cell

DTH reaction [72–76]. In GBM patients who received ICT-107 vaccine, vaccine activation markers IL-12 production and HLA-DR expression were predictive of OS ($p$-values <0.05) (see Sect. 14.3.5).

In the near future, we have to identify the evidenced biomarker from large-scale, well-controlled prospective trials of DC vaccine.

## 14.7 Conclusion

I believe that there are some populations (relatively large populations) of cancer patients who can obtain clinical benefit by DC vaccine. DC vaccine has a potential to elicit antitumor effect, and we therefore have to make DC vaccine a standard treatment for cancer patients.

We will be able to make the DC vaccine much more effective by expanding DC number, by identifying more effective antigens, by developing predictive biomarkers, and by combining with the therapies for canceling an immunosuppressive condition as well as for tumor mass reduction.

**Acknowledgment** I thank Dr. Yoshiyuki Yamaguchi, an editor of this book, for giving me the opportunity to write. I also acknowledge all members of the DC Vaccine Study Group at the J-SICT for carrying out clinical studies and for giving me critical comments for the DC vaccines.

# References

1. Vansteenkiste J, Zielinski M, Linder A, Dahabreh J, Gonzalez EE, Malinowski W, Lopez-Brea M, Vanakesa T, Jassem J, Kalofonos H, Perdeus J, Bonnet R, Basko J, Janilionis R, Passlick B, Treasure T, Gillet M, Lehmann FF, Brichard VG (2013) Adjuvant MAGE-A3 immunotherapy in resected non-small-cell lung cancer: phase II randomized study results. J Clin Oncol 31:2396–2403
2. Kruit WH, Suciu S, Dreno B, Mortier L, Robert C, Chiarion-Sileni V, Maio M, Testori A, Dorval T, Grob JJ, Becker JC, Spatz A, Eggermont AM, Louahed J, Lehmann FF, Brichard VG, Keilholz U (2013) Selection of immunostimulant AS15 for active immunization with MAGE-A3protein: results of a randomized phase II study of the European Organisation for Research and Treatment of Cancer Melanoma Group in Metastatic Melanoma. J Clin Oncol 31:2413–2420
3. Butts C, Maksymiuk A, Goss G, Soulières D, Marshall E, Cormier Y, Ellis PM, Price A, Sawhney R, Beier F, Falk M, Murray N (2011) Updated survival analysis in patients with stage IIIB or IV non-small-cell lung cancer receiving BLP25 liposome vaccine (L-BLP25): phase IIB randomized, multicenter, open-label trial. J Cancer Res Clin Oncol 137:1337–1342
4. Butts C, Socinski MA, Mitchell PL, Thatcher N, Havel L, Krzakowski M, Nawrocki S, Ciuleanu TE, Bosquée L, Trigo JM, Spira A, Tremblay L, Nyman J, Ramlau R, Wickart-Johansson G, Ellis P, Gladkov O, Pereira JR, Eberhardt WE, Helwig C, Schröder A, Shepherd FA, START trial team (2014) Tecemotide (L-BLP25) versus placebo after chemoradiotherapy for stage III non-small-cell lung cancer (START): a randomised, double-blind, phase 3 trial. Lancet Oncol 15:59–68
5. Steinman RM (1991) The dendritic cell system and its role in immunogenicity. Annu Rev Immunol 9:271–296
6. Banchereau J, Steinman RM (1998) Dendritic cells and the control of immunity. Nature 392:245–252
7. Fong L, Engleman EG (2000) Dendritic cells in cancer immunotherapy. Annu Rev Immunol 18:245–273
8. Banchereau J, Briere F, Caux C (2000) Immunobiology of dendritic cells. Annu Rev Immunol 18:767–811
9. Asselin-Paturel C, Echchakir H, Carayol G, Gay F, Opolon P, Grunenwald D, Chouaib S, Mami-Chouaib F (1998) Quantitative analysis of Th1, Th2, and TGF-β1 cytokine expression in tumor, TIL and PBL of non-small cell lung cancer patients. Int J Cancer 77:7–12
10. Gorelik L, Prokhorova A, Mokyr MB (1994) Low-dose melphalan-induced shift in the production of a Th2-type cytokine to a Th1-type cytokine in mice bearing a large MOPC-315 tumor. Cancer Immunol Immunother 39:117–126
11. Mosmann TR, Cherwinski H, Bond MW, Giedlin MA, Coffman RL (1986) Two types of murine helper T cell clone. Definition according to profiles of lymphokine activities and secreted proteins. J Immunol 136:2348–2357
12. Takeuchi T, Ueki T, Sasaki Y, Kajiwara T, Li B, Moriyama L, Kawabe K (1997) Th2-like response and antitumor effect of anti-interleukin-4 mAb in mice bearing renal cell carcinoma. Cancer Immunol Immunother 43:375–381
13. Kennedy R, Celis E (2008) Multiple roles for CD4+ T cells in anti-tumor immune responses. Immunol Rev 222:129–144
14. Bailey SR, Nelson MH, Himes RA, Li Z, Mehrotra S, Paulos CM (2014) Th17 cells in cancer: the ultimate identity crisis. Front Immunol 5:276
15. Alizadeh D, Katsanis E, Larmonier N (2013) The multifaceted role of Th17 lymphocytes and their associated cytokines in cancer. Clin Dev Immunol 2013:957878
16. Morton DL, Mozzillo N, Thompson JF, Kelley MC, Faries M, Wagner J, Schneebaum S, Schuchter L, Gammon G, Elashoff R, MMAIT Clinical Trial Group (2007) An international, randomized, phase III trial of bacillus Calmette-Guerin (BCG) plus allogeneic melanoma

vaccine (MCV) or placebo after complete resection of melanoma metastatic to regional or distant sites. J Clin Oncol 25[abstract 8508]
17. Eggermont AMM (2009) Therapeutic vaccines in solid tumors: can they be harmful? Eur J Cancer 45:2087–2090
18. Small E, Demkow T, Gerritsen WR, Rolland F, Hoskin P, Smith DC, Parker C, Chondros D, Ma J, Hege K (2009) A phase III study of GVAX immunotherapy for prostate cancer in combination with docetaxel versus docetaxel plus prednisone in symptomatic, castration-resistant prostate cancer (CRPC). Genitourinary Cancers Symposium [Abstract 7]
19. Muraoka D, Kato T, Wang L, Maeda Y, Noguchi T, Harada N, Takeda K, Yagita H, Guillaume P, Luescher I, Old LJ, Shiku H, Nishikawa H (2010) Peptide vaccine induces enhanced tumor growth associated with apoptosis induction in CD8+ T cells. J Immunol 1185:3768–3776
20. Aspord C, Charles J, Leccia MT, Laurin D, Richard MJ, Chaperot L, Plumas J (2010) A novel cancer vaccine strategy based on HLA-A*0201 matched allogeneic plasmacytoid dendritic cells. PLoS ONE 5, e10458
21. Hutten T, Thordardottir S, Hobo W, Hübel J, van der Waart AB, Cany J, Dolstra H, Hangalapura BN (2014) Ex vivo generation of interstitial and Langerhans cell-like dendritic cell subset-based vaccines for hematological malignancies. J Immunother 37(5):267–277
22. Balan S, Kale VP, Limaye LS (2010) A large number of mature and functional dendritic cells can be efficiently generated from umbilical cord blood-derived mononuclear cells by a simple two-step culture method. Transfusion 50(11):2413–2423
23. Han S, Wang Y, Wang B, Patel E, Okada S, Yang LJ, Moreb JS, Chang LJ (2010) Ex vivo development, expansion and in vivo analysis of a novel lineage of dendritic cells from hematopoietic stem cells. J Immune Based Ther Vaccines 8:8
24. Palucka K, Banchereau J (2012) Cancer immunotherapy via dendritic cells. Nat Rev Cancer 12:265–277
25. Finn OJ (2008) Cancer immunology. N Engl J Med 358:2704–2715
26. Galluzzi L, Senovilla L, Vacchelli E, Eggermont A, Fridman WH, Galon J, Sautès-Fridman C, Tartour E, Zitvogel L, Kroemer G (2012) Trial watch: dendritic cell-based interventions for cancer therapy. Oncoimmunology 1:1111–1134
27. Parajuli P, Sloan AE (2004) Dendritic cell-based immunotherapy of malignant gliomas. Cancer Invest 22:405–416
28. Hadzantonis M, O'Neill H (1999) Dendritic cell immunotherapy for melanoma. Cancer Biother Radiopharm 14:11–22
29. Banchereau J, Palucka AK (2005) Dendritic cells as therapeutic vaccines against cancer. Nat Rev Immunol 5:296–306
30. Lee J, Boczkowski D, Nair S (2013) Programming human dendritic cells with mRNA. Methods Mol Biol 969:111–125
31. Cheever MA, Allison JP, Ferris AS, Finn OJ, Hastings BM, Hecht TT, Mellman I, Prindiville SA, Viner JL, Weiner LM, Matrisian LM (2009) The prioritization of cancer antigens: a national cancer institute pilot project for the acceleration of translational research. Clin Cancer Res 15:5323–5337
32. Koido S, Ito M, Sagawa Y, Okamoto M, Hayashi K, Nagasaki E, Kan S, Komita H, Kamata Y, Homma S (2014) Vaccination with vascular progenitor cells derived from induced pluripotent stem cells elicits antitumor immunity targeting vascular and tumor cells. Cancer Immunol Immunother 63:459–468
33. Knutson KL (2002) Technology evaluation: DCVax, Northwest biotherapeutics. Curr Opin Mol Ther 4:403–407
34. Wheeler CJ, Black KL (2009) DCVax-brain and DC vaccines in the treatment of GBM. Expert Opin Investig Drugs 18:509–519
35. Polyzoidis S, Keyoumars A (2014) DCVax®-L developed by Northwest Biotherapeutics. Hum Vaccin Immunother, 10:3139–3145

36. Kantoff PW, Higano CS, Shore ND, Berger ER, Small EJ, Penson DF, Redfern CH, Ferrari AC, Dreicer R, Sims RB, Xu Y, Frohlich MW, Schellhammer PF, IMPACT Study Investigators (2010) Sipuleucel-T immunotherapy for castration-resistant prostate cancer. N Engl J Med 363:411–422
37. Fong L, Carroll P, Weinberg V, Chan S, Lewis J, Corman J, Amling CL, Stephenson RA, Simko J, Sheikh NA, Sims RB, Frohlich MW, Small EJ (2014) Activated lymphocyte recruitment into the tumor microenvironment following preoperative sipuleucel-T for localized prostate cancer. J Natl Cancer Inst 106: in press
38. Dillman RO, DePriest C, DeLeon C, Barth NM, Schwartzberg LS, Beutel LD, Schiltz PM, Nayak SK (2007) Patient-specific vaccines derived from autologous tumor cell lines as active specific immunotherapy: results of exploratory phase I/II trials in patients with metastatic melanoma. Cancer Biother Radiopharm 22:309–321
39. Dillman RO, Selvan SR, Schiltz PM, McClay EF, Barth NM, DePriest C, de Leon C, Mayorga C, Cornforth AN, Allen K (2009) Phase II trial of dendritic cells loaded with antigens from self-renewing, proliferating autologous tumor cells as patient-specific antitumor vaccines in patients with metastatic melanoma: final report. Cancer Biother Radiopharm 24:311–319
40. Dillman RO, Cornforth AN, Depriest C, McClay EF, Amatruda TT, de Leon C, Ellis RE, Mayorga C, Carbonell D, Cubellis JM (2012) Tumor stem cell antigens as consolidative active specific immunotherapy: a randomized phase II trial of dendritic cells versus tumor cells in patients with metastatic melanoma. J Immunother 35:641–649
41. Dillman RO, Depriest C, Ellis RA, Cornforth AN, DeLeon C (2014) Five-year survival for patients with metastatic melanoma who had no evidence of disease at time of treatment with patient specific tumor stem cell vaccines. AACR Annual meeting [Abstract #197]
42. Dillman RO, Depriest C, Ellis RA (2014) Long-term survival for patients with detectable metastatic melanoma at time of treatment with patient-specific tumor stem cell vaccines. ASCO annual meeting [Abstract #3090]
43. Amin A, Dudek AZ, Logan TF, Lance RS, Holzbeierlein JM, Master VA, Pal SK, Knox JJ, Karsh LI, Plessinger D, Nicolette CA, Figlin RA, AGS-003-006 Study Group (2014) Long-term survival in unfavorable-risk mRCC patients treated with a combination of autologous immunotherapy (AGS-003) plus sunitinib. ASCO Annual Meeting [Abstract #4524]
44. Amin A, Dudek AZ, Logan TF, Lance RS, Holzbeierlein JM, Master VA, Pal SK, Knox JJ, Karsh LI, Plessinger D, Nicolette CA, Figlin RA (2013) Prolonged survival with personalized immunotherapy (AGS-003) in combination with sunitinib in unfavorable risk metastatic RCC (mRCC). Genitourinary Cancers Symposium [Abstract #357]
45. Figlin RA, Wood CG, ADAPT Study Group (2014) ADAPT: an ongoing international phase III randomized trial of autologous dendritic cell immunotherapy (AGS-003) plus standard treatment in advanced renal cell carcinoma (RCC). Genitourinary Cancers Symposium [Abstract #449]
46. Phuphanich S, Wheeler CJ, Rudnick JD, Mazer M, Wang H, Nuño MA, Richardson JE, Fan X, Ji J, Chu RM, Bender JG, Hawkins ES, Patil CG, Black KL, Yu JS (2013) Phase I trial of a multi-epitope-pulsed dendritic cell vaccine for patients with newly diagnosed glioblastoma. Cancer Immunol Immunother 62:125–135
47. Wen PY, Reardon DA, Phuphanich S, Aiken R, Landolfi JC, Curry WT, Zhu JJ, Glantz MJ, Peereboom DM, Markert J, LaRocca RV, O'Rourke D, Fink KL, Kim LJ, Gruber ML, Lesser GJ, Pan E, Kesari S, Hawkins ES, Yu J (2014) A randomized, double-blind, placebo-controlled phase 2 trial of dendritic cell (DC) vaccination with ICT-107 in newly diagnosed glioblastoma (GBM) patients. ASCO Annual Meeting [Abstract #2005]
48. Zhou LJ, Tedder TF (1996) CD14+ blood monocyte can differentiate into functionally mature CD83+ dendritic cells. Proc Natl Acad Sci U S A 93:2588–2592
49. Akagawa KS, Takasuka N, Nozaki Y, Komuro I, Azuma M, Ueda M, Naito M, Takahashi K (1996) Generation of CD1+RelB+ dendritic cells and tartrate-resistant acid phosphatase-positive osteoclast-like multinucleated giant cells from human monocytes. Blood 88:4029–4039

50. Nagayama H, Sato K, Morishita M, Uchimaru K, Oyaizu N, Inazawa T, Yamasaki T, Enomoto M, Nakaoka T, Nakamura T, Maekawa T, Yamamoto A, Shimada S, Saida T, Kawakami Y, Asano S, Tani K, Takahashi TA, Yamashita N (2003) Results of a phase I clinical study using autologous tumour lysate-pulsed monocyte-derived mature dendritic cell vaccinations for stage IV malignant melanoma patients combined with low dose interleukin-2. Melanoma Res 13:521–530
51. Yoshiura K, Nakaoka T, Nishishita T, Sato K, Yamamoto A, Shimada S, Saida T, Kawakami Y, Takahashi TA, Fukuda H, Imajoh-Ohmi S, Oyaizu N, Yamashita N (2005) Carbonic anhydrase II is a tumor vessel endothelium-associated antigen targeted by dendritic cell therapy. Clin Cancer Res 11:8201–8207
52. Kuwabara K, Nishishita T, Morishita M, Oyaizu N, Yamashita S, Kanematsu T, Obara T, Mimura Y, Inoue Y, Kaminishi M, Kaga K, Amino N, Kitaoka M, Ito K, Miyauchi A, Noguchi S, Uchimaru K, Akagawa E, Watanabe N, Takahashi TA, Sato K, Inazawa T, Nakaoka T, Yamashita N (2007) Results of a phase I clinical study using dendritic cell vaccinations for thyroid cancer. Thyroid 17:53–58
53. Okamoto H, Shoin S, Koshimura S, Shimizu R (1967) Studies on the anticancer and streptolysin S-forming abilities of hemolytic streptococci. Jpn J Microbiol 11:323–336
54. Torisu M, Katano M, Kimura Y, Itoh H, Takesue M (1983) New approach to management of malignant ascites with a streptococcus preparation, OK-432. I. Improvement of host immunity and prolongation of survival. Surgery 93:357–364
55. Watanabe Y, Iwa T (1987) Clinical value of immunotherapy with the streptococcal preparation OK-432 in non-small cell lung cancer. J Biol Response Mod 6:169–180
56. Kikkawa F, Kawai M, Oguchi H, Kojima M, Ishikawa H, Iwata M et al (1993) Randomised study of immunotherapy with OK-432 in uterine cervical carcinoma. Eur J Cancer 29:1542–1546
57. Maehara Y, Okuyama T, Kakeji Y, Baba H, Furusawa M, Sigimachi K (1994) Postoperative immunochemotherapy including streptococcal lysate OK-432 is effective for patients with gastric cancer and serosal invasion. Am J Surg 168:36–40
58. Kitahara S, Ikeda M, Inoue T, Matsunaga T, Yamaguchi K, Takayama E et al (1996) Inhibition of head and neck metastatic and/or recurrent cancer by local administration of multi-cytokine inducer OK-432. J Laryngol Otol 110:449–453
59. Sato M, Yoshida H, Yanagawa T, Yura Y, Urata M, Atsumi M et al (1984) Effect of intradermal administration of streptococcal preparation OK-432 on interferon and natural killer cell activities in patients with oral cancer. Int J Oral Surg 13:7–15
60. Sato M, Harada K, Yoshida H, Yura Y, Azuma M, Iga H et al (1997) Therapy for oral squamous cell carcinoma by tegafur and streptococcal agent OK-432 in combination with radiotherapy: association of the therapeutic effect with differentiation and apoptosis in the cancer cells. Apoptosis 2:227–238
61. Okamoto M, Oshikawa T, Tano T, Ohe G, Furuichi S, Nishikawa H, Ahmed SU, Akashi S, Miyake K, Takeuchi O, Akira S, Moriya Y, Matsubara S, Ryoma Y, Saito M, Sato M (2003) Involvement of Toll-like receptor 4 signaling in interferon-γ production and anti-tumor effect by a streptococcal agent OK-432. J Natl Cancer Inst 95:316–326
62. Tano T, Okamoto M, Kan S, Bando T, Goda H, Nakashiro K, Shimodaira S, Koido S, Homma S, Sato M, Fujita T, Sato M, Yamashita N, Hamakawa H, Kawakami Y (2013) Immunochemoradiotherapy for patients with oral squamous cell carcinoma: augmentation of OK-432-induced helper T-cell 1 response by 5-FU and X-ray irradiation. Neoplasia 15:805–814
63. Oshimi K, Kano S, Takaku F, Okumura K (1980) Augmentation of mouse natural killer cell activity by a streptococcal preparation, OK-432. J Natl Cancer Inst 65:1265–1269
64. Saito M, Ebina T, Koi M, Yamaguchi T, Kamade Y, Ishida N (1982) Induction of interferon-gamma in mouse spleen cells by OK-432, a preparation of *Streptococcus pyogenes*. Cell Immunol 68:187–192

65. Misaki T, Watanabe Y, Iida Y, Hidaka A, Kasagi K, Fukushima H et al (1992) Recruitment of T lymphocytes and induction of tumor necrosis factor in thyroid cancer by a local immunotherapy. Cancer Immunol Immunother 35:92–96
66. Fujimoto T, Duda RB, Azilvasi A, Chen X, Mai M, O'Donnell MA (1997) Streptococcal preparation OK-432 is a potent inducer of IL-12 and a T helper cell 1 dominant state. J Immunol 158:5619–5626
67. Okamoto M, Oshikawa T, Ohe G, Nishikawa H, Furuichi S, Tano T, Moriya Y, Saito M, Sato M (2001) Severe impairment of anti-cancer effect of lipoteichoic acid-related molecule isolated from a penicillin-killed Streptococcus pyogenes in toll-like receptor 4-deficient mice. Int Immunopharmacol 1:1789–1795
68. Okamoto M, Oshikawa T, Tano T, Ahmed SU, Kan S, Sasai A, Akashi S, Miyake K, Moriya Y, Ryoma Y, Saito M, Sato M (2006) Mechanism of anti-cancer host response induced by OK-432, a streptococcal preparation, mediated by phagocytosis and toll-like receptor 4 signaling. J Immunother 29:78–86
69. Oshikawa T, Okamoto M, Tano T, Sasai A, Kan S, Moriya Y, Ryoma Y, Saito M, Akira S, Sato M (2006) Anti-tumor effect of OK-432-derived DNA: one of the active constituents of OK-432, a streptococcal immunotherapeutic agent. J Immunother 29:143–150
70. Okamoto M, Furuichi S, Nishioka Y, Oshikawa T, Tano T, Ahmed SU, Takeda K, Akira S, Ryoma Y, Moriya Y, Saito M, Sone S, Sato M (2004) Expression of Toll-like receptor 4 on dendritic cells is significant for anti-cancer effect of dendritic cell-based immunotherapy in combination with an active component of OK-432, a streptococcal preparation. Cancer Res 64:5461–5470
71. Ahmed SU, Okamoto M, Oshikawa T, Tano T, Sasai A, Kan S, Hiroshima T, Ohue H, Moriya Y, Ryoma Y, Saito M, Sato M (2004) Anti-tumor effect of an intratumoral administration of dendritic cells in combination with TS-1, an oral fluoropyrimidine anti-cancer drug, and OK-432, a streptococcal immunopotentiator: involvement of Toll-like receptor 4. J Immunother 27:432–441
72. Kimura Y, Tsukada J, Tomoda T, Takahashi H, Imai K, Shimamura K, Sunamura M, Yonemitsu Y, Shimodaira S, Koido S, Homma S, Okamoto M (2012) Clinical and immunologic evaluation of dendritic cell-based immunotherapy in combination with gemcitabine and/or S-1 in the patients with advanced pancreatic carcinoma. Pancreas 41:195–205
73. Kobayashi M, Shimodaira S, Nagai K, Ogasawara M, Takahashi H, Abe H, Tanii M, Okamoto M, Tsujitani S, Yusa S, Ishidao T, Kishimoto J, Shibamoto Y, Nagaya M, Yonemitsu Y (2014) Prognostic factors related to add-on dendritic cell vaccines on patients with inoperable pancreatic cancer receiving chemotherapy: a multicenter analysis. Cancer Immunol Immunother 63:797–806
74. Koido S, Homma S, Okamoto M, Takakura K, Tsukinaga S, Odahara S, Koyama S, Imazu H, Mori M, Yoshizaki S, Kan S, Hayashi K, Komita H, Kamata Y, Ito M, Ishidao T, Yusa S, Shimodaira S, Matsushima M, Uchiyama K, Kajihara M, Arakawa H, Misawa T, Toyama Y, Yanagisawa S, Ikegami M, Gong J, Ohkusa T, Tajiri H (2014) Treatment with chemotherapy and dendritic cells pulsed with multiple Wilms' tumor gene 1 (WT1)-specific MHC class I/II-restricted epitopes for pancreatic cancer. Clin Cancer Res 20:4228–4239
75. Takakura K, Koido S, Kan S, Yoshida K, Mori M, Hirano Y, Ito Z, Kobayashi H, Takami S, Matsumoto Y, Kajihara M, Misawa T, Okamoto M, Homma S, Ohkusa T, Tajiri H (2015) Prognostic markers for patient outcome following vaccination with multiple MHC class I/II-restricted WT1 peptide-pulsed dendritic cells plus chemotherapy for pancreatic cancer. Anticancer Res 35(1):555–562
76. Koido S, Homma S, Okamoto M, Takakura K, Gong J, Sugiyama H, Ohkusa T, Tajiri H (2014) Chemoimmunotherapy targeting Wilms' tumor 1 (WT1)-specific cytotoxic T lymphocyte and helper T cell responses for patients with pancreatic cancer. OncoImmunology 3(10):e958950
77. Kobayashi M, Sakabe T, Abe H, Tanii M, Takahashi H, Chiba A, Yanagida E, Shibamoto Y, Ogasawara M, Tsujitani S, Koido S, Nagai K, Shimodaira S, Okamoto M, Yonemitsu Y,

Suzuki N, Nagaya M (2013) Dendritic cell-based immunotherapy targeting synthesized peptides for advanced biliary tract cancer. J Gastrointest Surg 17:1609–1617
78. Koido S, Kan S, Yoshida K, Yoshizaki S, Takakura K, Tsukinaga S, Odahara S, Kajihara M, Okamoto M, Ito M, Yusa S, Ohkusa T, Gong J, Homma S, Tajiri H (2014) Immunogenic modulation of cholangiocarcinoma cells by chemoimmunotherapy. Anticancer Res 34:6353–6361
79. Takahashi H, Okamoto M, Shimodaira S, Tsujitani S, Nagaya M, Ishidao T, Kishimoto J, Sugiyama H, Yonemitsu Y (2013) Impact of dendritic cell vaccines pulsed with Wilms' tumor-1 peptide antigen on the survival of patients with advanced non-small cell lung cancers. Eur J Cancer 49:852–859
80. Kobayashi M, Chiba A, Izawa H, Yanagida E, Okamoto M, Shimodaira S, Yonemitsu Y, Shibamoto Y, Suzuki N, Nagaya M (2014) The feasibility and clinical effects of dendritic cell-based immunotherapy targeting synthesized peptides for recurrent ovarian cancer. J Ovarian Res 7:48
81. Saito S, Yanagisawa R, Yoshikawa k, Higuchi Y, Koya T, Yoshizawa K, Tanaka M, Sakashita K, Kobayashi T, Kurata T, Hirabayashi K, Nakazawa Y, Shiohara M, Yonemitsu Y, Okamoto M, Sugiyama H, Koike K, Shimodaira S (2015) Safety and tolerability of allogeneic dendritic cell vaccination with induction of WT1-specific T cells in a pediatric donor and pediatric patient with relapsed leukemia: a case report and review of the literature. Cytotherapy 17(3):330–335
82. Shibamoto Y, Okamoto M, Kobayashi M, Ayakawa S, Iwata H, Sugie C, Mitsuishi Y, Takahashi H (2013) Immune-maximizing (IMAX) therapy for cancer: combination of dendritic-cell vaccine and intensity-modulated radiation. Mol Clin Oncol 1:649–654
83. Rosa DS, Ribeiro SP, Cunha-Neto E (2010) CD4+ T cell epitope discovery and rational vaccine design. Arch Immunol Ther Exp (Warsz) 58:121–130
84. Senju S, Hirata S, Motomura Y, Fukuma D, Matsunaga Y, Fukushima S, Matsuyoshi H, Nishimura Y (2010) Pluripotent stem cells as source of dendritic cells for immune therapy. Int J Hematol 91:392–400
85. Senju S, Haruta M, Matsumura K, Matsunaga Y, Fukushima S, Ikeda T, Takamatsu K, Irie A, Nishimura Y (2011) Generation of dendritic cells and macrophages from human induced pluripotent stem cells aiming at cell therapy. Gene Ther 18:874–883
86. Haruta M, Tomita Y, Imamura Y, Matsumura K, Ikeda T, Takamatsu K, Nishimura Y, Senju S (2013) Generation of a large number of functional dendritic cells from human monocytes expanded by forced expression of cMYC plus BMI1. Hum Immunol 74:1400–1408
87. Harada Y, Okada-Nakanishi Y, Ueda Y, Tsujitani S, Saito S, Fuji-Ogawa T, Iida A, Hasegawa M, Ichikawa T, Yonemitsu Y (2011) Cytokine-based high log-scale expansion of functional human dendritic cells from cord-blood CD34-positive cells. Sci Rep 1:174
88. Walter S, Weinschenk T, Stenzl A, Zdrojowy R, Pluzanska A, Szczylik C, Staehler M, Brugger W, Dietrich PY, Mendrzyk R, Hilf N, Schoor O, Fritsche J, Mahr A, Maurer D, Vass V, Trautwein C, Lewandrowski P, Flohr C, Pohla H, Stanczak JJ, Bronte V, Mandruzzato S, Biedermann T, Pawelec G, Derhovanessian E, Yamagishi H, Miki T, Hongo F, Takaha N, Hirakawa K, Tanaka H, Stevanovic S, Frisch J, Mayer-Mokler A, Kirner A, Rammensee HG, Reinhardt C, Singh-Jasuja H (2012) Multipeptide immune response to cancer vaccine IMA901 after single-dose cyclophosphamide associates with longer patient survival. Nat Med 18:1254–1261
89. Kan S, Hazama S, Maeda K, Inoue Y, Homma S, Koido S, Okamoto M, Oka M (2012) Suppressive effects of cyclophosphamide and gemcitabine on regulatory T cell induction in vitro. Anticancer Res 32:5363–5370
90. Ghansah T, Vohra N, Kinney K, Weber A, Kodumudi K, Springett G, Sarnaik AA, Pilon-Thomas S (2013) Dendritic cell immunotherapy combined with gemcitabine chemotherapy enhances survival in a murine model of pancreatic carcinoma. Cancer Immunol Immunother 62(6):1083–1091

91. Soeda A, Morita-Hoshi Y, Makiyama H, Morizane C, Ueno H, Ikeda M, Okusaka T, Yamagata S, Takahashi N, Hyodo I, Takaue Y, Heike Y (2009) Regular dose of gemcitabine induces an increase in CD14+ monocytes and CD11c+ dendritic cells in patients with advanced pancreatic cancer. Jpn J Clin Oncol 39:797–806
92. Takahara A, Koido S, Ito M, Nagasaki E, Sagawa Y, Iwamoto T, Komita H, Ochi T, Fujiwara H, Yasukawa M, Mineno J, Shiku H, Nishida S, Sugiyama H, Tajiri H, Homma S (2011) Gemcitabine enhances Wilms' tumor gene WT1 expression and sensitizes human pancreatic cancer cells with WI1-specific T-cell-mediated antitumor immune response. Cancer Immunol Immunother 60:1289–1297
93. Okamoto M, Tano T, Goda H, Fujita Y, Nakashiro K, Hamakawa H. Down-regulation of PD-1 ligands by chemotherapeutic agents via inhibition of STAT3 activity enhances T cell-stimulating ability of dendritic cells. AACR 102th Annual Meeting [Abstract #5033]
94. Zhou Y, Ni H, Balint K, Sanzari JK, Dentchev T, Diffenderfer ES, Wilson JM, Cengel KA, Weissman D (2014) Ionizing radiation selectively reduces skin regulatory T cells and alters immune function. PLoS ONE 9, e100800
95. Sebastian M, Papachristofilou A, Weiss C, Früh M, Cathomas R, Hilbe W, Wehler T, Rippin G, Koch SD, Scheel B, Fotin-Mleczek M, Heidenreich R, Kallen KJ, Gnad-Vogt U, Zippelius A (2014) Phase Ib study evaluating a self-adjuvanted mRNA cancer vaccine (RNActive®) combined with local radiation as consolidation and maintenance treatment for patients with stage IV non-small cell lung cancer. BMC Cancer 14:748
96. Kibe S, Yutani S, Motoyama S, Nomura T, Tanaka N, Kawahara A, Yamaguchi T, Matsueda S, Komatsu N, Miura M, Hinai Y, Hattori S, Yamada A, Kage M, Itoh K, Akagi Y, Sasada T (2014) Phase II study of personalized peptide vaccination for previously treated advanced colorectal cancer. Cancer Immunol Res 2(12):1154–1162
97. Yoshitomi M, Yutani S, Matsueda S, Ioji T, Komatsu N, Shichijo S, Yamada A, Itoh K, Sasada T, Kinoshita H (2012) Personalized peptide vaccination for advanced biliary tract cancer: IL-6, nutritional status and pre-existing antigen-specific immunity as possible biomarkers for patient prognosis. Exp Ther Med 3:463–469
98. Noguchi M, Moriya F, Suekane S, Matsuoka K, Arai G, Matsueda S, Sasada T, Yamada A, Itoh K (2012) Phase II study of personalized peptide vaccination for castration-resistant prostate cancer patients who failed in docetaxel-based chemotherapy. Prostate 72:834–845

# Part V
# Immunoadjuvants

# Chapter 15
# CpG Motif

**Masahiro Katsuda and Hiroki Yamaue**

**Abstract** The key feature of innate immune cells that enables them to detect and categorize infection seems to be their repertoire of pattern recognition receptors (PRRs). The best understood PRR family comprises the toll-likc rcccptors (TLRs), ten of which are known in humans. PRRs have recently been attributed with a critical role in eliciting anticancer immune responses, raising interest in the development of immunotherapeutic regimens based on natural or synthetic TLR agonists. In contrast to viruses and other pathogens, vaccines containing recombinant proteins or synthetic antigenic peptides usually fail to induce significant immune responses unless they include an adjuvant. Bacterial unmethylated CpG-rich oligodeoxynucleotides (ODNs), which bind to TLR9, are some of the most promising candidates for a cancer vaccine adjuvant and are currently being tested in many human clinical trials. In this context, recent clinical trials using CpG-ODN for cancer patients are summarized for consideration of the near future use and the next generation of CpG-ODNs in creating more potent cancer vaccine adjuvants.

**Keywords** TLR • CpG-ODN • Vaccine adjuvant

## 15.1 Toll-Like Receptors

The innate immune system is activated via exposure to pathogen-associated molecular patterns that are expressed by a diverse group of infectious microorganisms. The host subsequently mounts an adaptive immune response directed against determinants that are uniquely expressed by the pathogen. The resultant antigen-specific immunity is characterized by the production of high-affinity antibodies and the generation of cytotoxic T cells that provide long-lasting protection [1]. The key feature of innate immune cells that enables them to detect and categorize infection seems to be their repertoire of pattern recognition receptors (PRRs). The best understood PRR family is the toll-like receptors (TLRs), ten of which are known in humans.

---

M. Katsuda • H. Yamaue (✉)
Second Department of Surgery, Wakayama Medical University, School of Medicine, 811-1 Kimiidera, Wakayama 641-8510, Japan
e-mail: yamaue-h@wakayama-med.ac.jp



Y. Yamaguchi (ed.), *Immunotherapy of Cancer*,
DOI 10.1007/978-4-431-55031-0_15

**Table 15.1** Ligands and synthetic or purified adjuvants of TLRs

| TLRs (PRRs) | Ligands (PAMPs) | Synthetic or purified adjuvants |
|---|---|---|
| TLR2/1 or TLR2/6 | Lipoproteins, lipopeptide, peptide glycans | *Escherichia coli* heat-labile enterotoxins, MDP, MALP2 |
| TLR3 | dsRNA | Poly I:C |
| TLR4 | LPS | MDP, MPL |
| TLR5 | Flagellin | Flagellin |
| TLR7,8 | ssRNA | Imiquimod, R848, ssRNA |
| TLR9 | CpG DNA | CpG-ODNs |

*dsRNA* double-stranded RNA, *LPS* lipopolysaccharide, *MALP* macrophage-activating lipopeptide, *MDP* muramyl dipeptide, *MPL* monophosphoryl lipid A, *ODN* oligodeoxynucleotide, *PAMPs* pathogen-associated molecular patterns, *PRR* pattern recognition receptor, *ssRNA* single-stranded RNA, *TLR* toll-like receptor

TLRs are single membrane-spanning proteins known for their ability to detect microbe-associated molecular patterns; conserved microbial products, including bacterial lipopolysaccharide (mixed TLR2/TLR4 agonists) [2–4]; components of the bacterial cell wall, such as lipoteichoic acid (a specific activator of TLR2) [5]; bacterial flagellin (a pure TLR5 agonist) [6–9]; microbial DNA (a TLR9 agonist) [10]; microbial single-stranded RNA (ssRNA, which can be detected by both TLR7 and TLR8) [11–13]; and viral double-stranded RNA (dsRNA, which specifically activates TLR3) [14–16] (Table 15.1). TLRs that detect nucleic acids (i.e., TLR3, TLR7, TLR8, and TLR9) are localized to the endosomal compartment, while TLRs that mainly detect proteo-lipidic structures (i.e., TLR1, TLR2, TLR4, TLR5, TLR6, and TLR10) are exposed on the cell surface [17, 18]. As exceptions to this general pattern, TLR2 and TLR10 have been shown to co-localize at phagosomes.

## 15.2 TLR Ligands as Cancer Vaccine Adjuvants

PRRs have recently been attributed with a critical role in eliciting anticancer immune responses, raising interest in the development of immunotherapeutic regimens based on natural or synthetic TLR agonists. In contrast to viruses and other pathogens, vaccines containing recombinant proteins or synthetic antigenic peptides usually fail to induce significant immune responses unless they include an adjuvant [19, 20]. Several recently identified TLR ligands are promising vaccine adjuvants because of their high efficacy in increasing an immune response. Despite the intense wave of preclinical and clinical investigation, only three TLR agonists are currently licensed by the US Food and Drug Administration (FDA) for use in cancer patients: bacillus Calmette-Guérin (BCG), an attenuated strain of *Mycobacterium bovis* that operates as a mixed TLR2/TLR4 agonist; monophosphoryl lipid A (MPL), a derivative of *Salmonella minnesota* that functions as a potent agonist of TLR4; and imiquimod, a synthetic imidazoquinoline that activates TLR7 (Table 15.1).

## 15.3 CpG-ODN; TLR9 Agonist

Bacterial unmethylated CpG-rich oligodeoxynucleotides (ODNs), which bind to TLR9, are some of the most promising candidates for a cancer vaccine adjuvant and are currently being tested in many human clinical trials. The discovery of the CpG motif in 1995 led to a shift in the perception of the immune-stimulatory effects of oligodeoxynucleotides (ODN). Instead of an unwanted nonspecific effect, they came to be viewed as a highly evolved immune defense that can be selectively triggered for a wide range of therapeutic applications. During the last decade, dozens of human clinical trials have been conducted with different CpG-ODNs in thousands of humans for applications ranging from vaccine adjuvant to immunotherapies for allergies, cancer, and infectious diseases. Along with many positive results have come some failures, showing the limitations of several therapeutic approaches.

## 15.4 Latest Clinical Trials Using CpG-ODN for Cancer Patients

Recently completed trials have evaluated the safety and immunostimulatory profile of the TLR9 agonist IMO-2055 (also known as EMD1201081) [21, 22], which is given in combination with 5-fluorouracil, cisplatin, and cetuximab as a first-line palliative treatment to patients with recurrent/metastatic head and neck squamous cell carcinoma [23]. Agatolimod (also known as CpG 7909, PF-3512676, and Promune®), an unmethylated CpG-ODN that activates TLR9 [24], is also given in combination with tremelimumab (an experimental monoclonal antibody targeting the immune checkpoint regulator cytotoxic T lymphocyte [CTL]-associated protein 4) [25, 26] to patients affected by advanced solid tumors [27]. Most recently, the safety and therapeutic profile of GNKG168 (a CpG-ODN) [28, 29], given intravenously as a stand-alone agent, was being assessed in a cohort of relapsed acute lymphoblastic leukemia (ALL) or AML patients (NCT01743807). This study was already terminated in 2014. As a cancer vaccine adjuvant, the experimental formulation AS15, which is composed of the immune-stimulatory components CpG 7909, monophosphoryl lipid, and QS-21, a plant derivative, is being tested for its ability to boost immune responses elicited by full-length recombinant preferentially expressed antigen in melanoma in patients with non-small cell lung cancer (NSCLC) upon tumor resection (NCT01853878). AS15 has also been used to boost the immunogenicity of a *v-erb-b2* erythroblastic leukemia viral oncogene homolog 2, neuro/glioblastoma-derived oncogene homolog (avian) (ERBB2)-targeting vaccine in patients with trastuzumab-resistant ERBB2-overexpressing metastatic breast carcinoma [30]. In this phase I clinical trial, the coadministration of ERBB2-derived peptides with lapatinib was well tolerated, triggered detectable ERBB2-specific immune responses in a majority of the patients, and was associated with promising clinical benefits, which warranted the initiation of phase II/III studies.

In the adjuvant setting, no improvement in progression-free survival was observed in the phase III MAGRIT study [31]. This clinical trial summary provided the background and rationale for a randomized trial to investigate the efficacy of melanoma-associated antigen (MAGE)-A3 antigen-specific cancer immunotherapeutic agents with the adjuvant AS15 in preventing cancer relapse, when administered after tumor resection, in patients with MAGE-A3-positive stages IB, II, and IIIA NSCLC. Results for MAGRIT, which randomized 2,272 patients with NSCLC to a vaccine or placebo group after they had lung resections, showed no statistical difference between the two cohorts. We need a better understanding of mechanisms, but this result might suggest that the following factors are important in determining the efficacy of a cancer vaccine with adjuvant: (1) antigen-specific cancer immunotherapeutic agents, (2) combination agents, (3) patient status, (4) cancer type, and (5) study design. The investigator of MARGIT is planning to combine his vaccine with a checkpoint inhibitor, which may be the key to a sustained therapeutic response.

We conducted a phase I/II trial for patients with advanced esophageal squamous cell carcinoma using epitope peptides derived from novel testis cancer antigens, LY6K and TTK, in combination with CpG 7909 [32]. This study investigated the feasibility and toxicity of the combination as well as its induction of tumor antigen-specific immune responses. Patients were vaccinated on days 1, 8, 15, and 22 in each 28-day treatment cycle with peptide LY6K, peptide TTK, and CpG 7909 (level 1, 0 mg/kg; level 2, 0.02 mg/kg; level 3, 0.1 mg/kg), and all patients tolerated the treatment. Potent LY6K- and TTK-specific T-cell responses in peripheral blood mononuclear cells (PBMCs) were detected in levels 2 and 3. The frequency of LY6K-177-specific or TTK-567-specific $CD8^+$ T cells increased in patients at levels 2 and 3 (with CpG). The vaccination with peptides and CpG 7909 increased and activated both plasmacytoid dendritic cells (PDCs) and natural killer (NK) cells and increased the serum level of interferon (IFN)-$\alpha$. There were no complete or partial responses; however, one of three patients at level 1 and four of six patients at levels 2 and 3 showed stable disease. In conclusion, vaccination with LY6K-177 and TTK-567 in combination with CpG 7909 successfully elicited antigen-specific $CD8^+$ T-cell responses and enhanced the innate and acquired immunity of patients with advanced esophageal squamous cell carcinoma [32].

## 15.5 Next Generation of CpG-ODN to Enhance Adjuvant Effects

### *15.5.1 Selection of CpG-ODN Type*

In numerous murine models, TLR9 activation enhances antigen-specific cellular responses to a wide variety of antigens. The mechanism that contributes to the potent adjuvant activity of CpG-ODNs is maturation and differentiation of dendritic cells, which results in a strong induction of CTLs, even in the absence of CD4 T-cell help [33]. However, the cellular patterns of TLR expression vary between different species [28, 34]. B cells, monocytes, and all DC subsets express TLR9 in mice; however, only PDCs and B cells express TLR9 in humans [35–38]. Consequently, the murine immune system responds differently in comparison with human systems when exposed to CpG-ODN, and extrapolating the experimental results to humans is impossible. Furthermore, little is known about the mechanism by which CpG-ODNs augment acquired cellular immunity in humans, although substantial evidence shows that systemically administered CpG-ODNs augment the activity of antitumor immunity in human clinical cancer vaccine trials.

Three distinct classes of CpG-ODNs have been identified on the basis of differences in their structures and immune-stimulating effects [33, 39–41]. CpG-A (also known as D-type) induces the production of high levels of IFN-α from PDCs, with relatively little B-cell stimulation. In contrast, CpG-B (also known as K-type) induces low-level production of IFN-α but profound B-cell activation. CpG-C has intermediate immune effects with excellent in vivo stability and ease of formation (Table 15.2). To date, mostly CpG B has been applied for clinical treatments of cancer patients; however, the class of CpG-ODNs that would be the most useful as adjuvants for a human cancer vaccine remains unknown.

We examined the activity of these three types of CpG-ODNs in enhancing the induction of human peptide-specific CTLs [42]. We also used tumor antigen epitope peptide-specific CTL clones to elucidate the effect of CpG-ODNs and investigate their adjuvant mechanism in peptide vaccine therapy. Our data showed that PDCs activated by CpG-ODNs augmented the induction of peptide-specific CTLs, and CpG-A was superior to CpG-B and CpG-C in terms of the augmenting effect. CpG-A induced a much larger amount of type-1 IFNs than CpG-B and CpG-C. Moreover, we showed that type-1 IFNs produced by PBMCs stimulated by CpG-ODNs directly augmented the proliferation and cytotoxicity of peptide-specific CTL clones. Augmentation of cytotoxicity was induced through the upregulation of granzyme B. IFN-α is proposed as one of the key molecules enabling CpG-ODNs to induce adjuvant effects in peptide vaccine therapy. In addition, type-1 IFNs induced the maturation of antigen presenting cells (APCs) and activation of NK cells (Fig. 15.1). Finally, we concluded that CpG-A might be a more effective cancer vaccine adjuvant than CpG-B or CpG-C because of its production of a large amount of type-1 IFNs [42]. However, it is difficult to make a GMP-compliant material of CpG-A, because CpG-A is not soluble in phosphate-

**Table 15.2** Features of each type of CpG-ODNs

| | CpG-A (D-type) | CpG-B (K-type) | CpG-C |
|---|---|---|---|
| ODN backbone | Typically consisted of one palindromic CpG motif with PO backbone and PS poly-G tail | Consisted of PS backbone and non-palindromic multiple CpG motifs | Consisted of PS backbone and one palindromic sequence |
| High-order structure | G-tetrads | Linear | Duplex |
| Examples | D35, ODN 2216 | K3, CpG 7909 | CpG 10101, ODN 2395 |
| Main target cells | PDCs | B cells | B cells and PDCs |
| Actions | IFN-α | IL-6, PDC maturation | IFN-α, IL-6 (intermediate between the A and B type) |
| Solubility (in PBS) | Aggregation | Soluble | Soluble |

*IFN* interferon, *IL* interleukin, *ODN* oligodeoxynucleotide, *PBS* phosphate-buffered saline, *PDC* plasmacytoid dendritic cell, *PO* phosphodiester, *PS* phosphorothioate

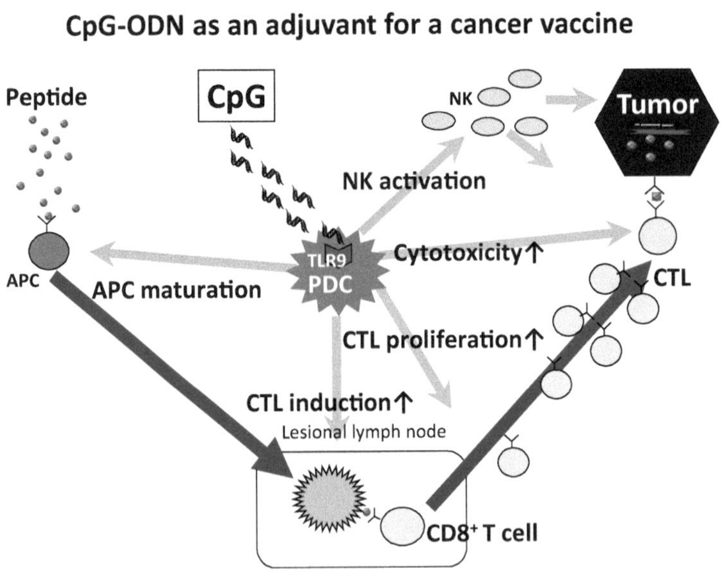


**Fig. 15.1** CpG-ODN as an adjuvant for a cancer vaccine. Type-1 IFNs produced by the stimulation of CpG-ODNs directly augmented the proliferation and cytotoxicity of peptide-specific CTL to induce adjuvant effects in peptide vaccine therapy. In addition, type-1 IFNs induced the maturation of APCs and activation of NK cells

buffered saline and agglutinates (Table 15.2). We need to overcome this problem to apply CpG-A for clinical use.

## *15.5.2 Delivery of CpG-ODN Toward Peritumoral Site*

The analysis of the tumor microenvironment indicates that the lytic activity of CTL and NK cells is suppressed by regulatory T lymphocytes (Treg), myeloid-derived suppressor cells (MDSCs), and/or M2 macrophages surrounding the tumor [43, 44]. Thus, it appears that successful immunotherapy will require both the amplification of tumor-specific immunity and reversal of tumor-associated immune suppression.

The antitumor activity of TLR agonists has generally been explored by delivering them systemically. For example, CpG-ODN administered in combination with vaccines promotes the induction of tumor-specific cellular and humoral immune responses [45–47]. However, a growing body of evidence suggests that the efficacy of TLR agonists might be improved by injecting them directly into the cancerous tissue [48, 49]. Local delivery of TLR agonists appears to interfere with the function of suppressive cells in the tumor microenvironment (Fig. 15.2). In a

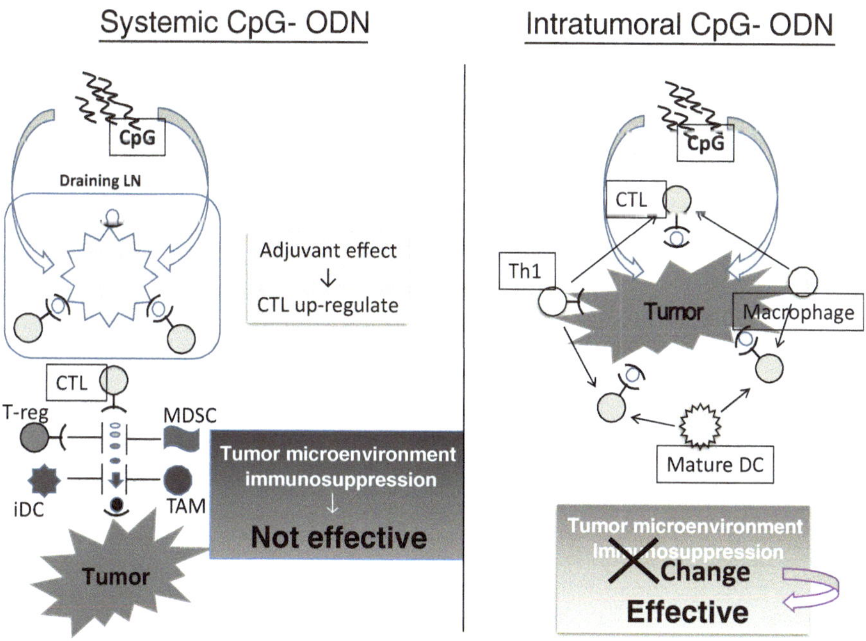


**Fig. 15.2** Systemic CpG-ODN, intratumoral CpG-ODN. Intratumoral CpG-ODN changes peritumoral immunological microenvironment and induces increased levels of tumor-specific T cells, which can subsequently exert systemic antitumor control

mouse model, intratumoral injection of CpG-ODN reduced the number of tumor-infiltrating MDSCs and their suppressive activity [49].

In clinical trials, addition of systemic administration with CpG-ODN to chemotherapy has not improved clinical outcomes versus chemotherapy alone so far, even though some papers showed increasing toxicity [50]. However, intratumoral or peritumoral injection with CpG-ODN alone for patients with basal cell carcinoma [51], metastatic melanoma [51], and recurrent glioblastoma [52] showed clinical benefits including tumor regression. Moreover, local administration of CpG-ODN increased systemic tumor-specific $CD8^+$ T-cell frequencies as well as effector NK cell rate in melanoma patients [53]. In addition, intratumoral injection of CpG-ODN combined with local radiation against mycosis fungoides [54] and B-cell lymphoma [55] induced systemic tumor regression. In these studies, the systemic tumor-reactive memory $CD8^+$ T cells were induced [54] and Tregs were reduced at the immunized sites [55]. Recently, the intratumoral administration of SD-101 (a phosphorothioate CpG-ODN) [28] is being evaluated as a means to enhance the antineoplastic effects of local irradiation in subjects bearing Hodgkin and non-Hodgkin lymphoma (NCT01745354).

These results indicate that intratumoral injection of CpG-ODN changes peritumoral immunological microenvironment and induces increased levels of tumor-specific T cells, which can subsequently exert systemic antitumor control. Therefore, local administration of CpG-ODN might be a novel systemic cancer treatment strategy. Moreover, the development of a drug delivery system toward peritumoral site with CpG-ODN could not only be a new generation anticancer drug but also a potent vaccine adjuvant.

## References

1. Klinman DM (2004) Immunotherapeutic uses of CpG oligodeoxynucleotides. Nat Rev Immunol 4(4):249–258. doi:10.1038/nri1329
2. Jiang Q, Akashi S, Miyake K, Petty HR (2000) Lipopolysaccharide induces physical proximity between CD14 and toll-like receptor 4 (TLR4) prior to nuclear translocation of NF-kappa B. J Immunol 165(7):3541–3544
3. Schroder NW, Opitz B, Lamping N, Michelsen KS, Zahringer U, Gobel UB et al (2000) Involvement of lipopolysaccharide binding protein, CD14, and toll-like receptors in the initiation of innate immune responses by Treponema glycolipids. J Immunol 165 (5):2683–2693
4. Mata-Haro V, Cekic C, Martin M, Chilton PM, Casella CR, Mitchell TC (2007) The vaccine adjuvant monophosphoryl lipid A as a TRIF-biased agonist of TLR4. Science 316 (5831):1628–1632. doi:10.1126/science.1138963
5. Hoebe K, Georgel P, Rutschmann S, Du X, Mudd S, Crozat K et al (2005) CD36 is a sensor of diacylglycerides. Nature 433(7025):523–527. doi:10.1038/nature03253
6. Hayashi F, Smith KD, Ozinsky A, Hawn TR, Yi EC, Goodlett DR et al (2001) The innate immune response to bacterial flagellin is mediated by toll-like receptor 5. Nature 410 (6832):1099–1103. doi:10.1038/35074106

7. Smith KD, Andersen-Nissen E, Hayashi F, Strobe K, Bergman MA, Barrett SL et al (2003) Toll-like receptor 5 recognizes a conserved site on flagellin required for protofilament formation and bacterial motility. Nat Immunol 4(12):1247–1253. doi:10.1038/ni1011
8. Lu J, Sun PD (2012) The structure of the TLR5-flagellin complex: a new mode of pathogen detection, conserved receptor dimerization for signaling. Sci Signal 5(223):pe11
9. Yoon SI, Kurnasov O, Natarajan V, Hong M, Gudkov AV, Osterman AL et al (2012) Structural basis of TLR5-flagellin recognition and signaling. Science 335(6070):859–864. doi:10.1126/science.1215584
10. Hemmi H, Takeuchi O, Kawai T, Kaisho T, Sato S, Sanjo H et al (2000) A toll-like receptor recognizes bacterial DNA. Nature 408(6813):740–745. doi:10.1038/35047123
11. Diebold SS, Kaisho T, Hemmi H, Akira S, Reis e Sousa C (2004) Innate antiviral responses by means of TLR7-mediated recognition of single-stranded RNA. Science 303(5663):1529–1531. doi:10.1126/science.1093616
12. Heil F, Hemmi H, Hochrein H, Ampenberger F, Kirschning C, Akira S et al (2004) Species-specific recognition of single-stranded RNA via toll-like receptor 7 and 8. Science 303 (5663):1526–1529. doi:10.1126/science.1093620
13. Hotz C, Bourquin C (2012) Systemic cancer immunotherapy with toll-like receptor 7 agonists: timing is everything. Oncoimmunology 1(2):227–228. doi:10.4161/onci.1.2.18169
14. Alexopoulou L, Holt AC, Medzhitov R, Flavell RA (2001) Recognition of double-stranded RNA and activation of NF-kappaB by toll-like receptor 3. Nature 413(6857):732–738. doi:10.1038/35099560
15. Choe J, Kelker MS, Wilson IA (2005) Crystal structure of human toll-like receptor 3 (TLR3) ectodomain. Science 309(5734):581–585. doi:10.1126/science.1115253
16. Liu L, Botos I, Wang Y, Leonard JN, Shiloach J, Segal DM et al (2008) Structural basis of toll-like receptor 3 signaling with double-stranded RNA. Science 320(5874):379–381. doi:10.1126/science.1155406
17. Hennessy EJ, Parker AE, O'Neill LA (2010) Targeting toll-like receptors: emerging therapeutics? Nat Rev Drug Discov 9(4):293–307. doi:10.1038/nrd3203
18. Jinushi M (2012) The role of innate immune signals in antitumor immunity. Oncoimmunology 1(2):189–194. doi:10.4161/onci.1.2.18495
19. Janeway CA Jr (1989) Approaching the asymptote? Evolution and revolution in immunology. Cold Spring Harb Symp Quant Biol 54(Pt 1):1–13
20. Marrack P, Kappler J (1994) Subversion of the immune system by pathogens. Cell 76 (2):323–332
21. Agrawal S, Kandimalla ER (2007) Synthetic agonists of toll-like receptors 7, 8 and 9. Biochem Soc Trans 35(Pt 6):1461–1467. doi:10.1042/BST0351461
22. Kandimalla ER, Bhagat L, Li Y, Yu D, Wang D, Cong YP et al (2005) Immunomodulatory oligonucleotides containing a cytosine-phosphate-2′-deoxy-7-deazaguanosine motif as potent toll-like receptor 9 agonists. Proc Natl Acad Sci U S A 102(19):6925–6930. doi:10.1073/pnas.0501729102
23. Machiels JP, Kaminsky MC, Keller U, Brummendorf TH, Goddemeier T, Forssmann U et al (2013) Phase Ib trial of the toll-like receptor 9 agonist IMO-2055 in combination with 5-fluorouracil, cisplatin, and cetuximab as first-line palliative treatment in patients with recurrent/metastatic squamous cell carcinoma of the head and neck. Invest New Drugs 31 (5):1207–1216. doi:10.1007/s10637-013-9933-z
24. Murad YM, Clay TM, Lyerly HK, Morse MA (2007) CPG-7909 (PF-3512676, ProMune): toll-like receptor-9 agonist in cancer therapy. Expert Opin Biol Ther 7(8):1257–1266. doi:10.1517/14712598.7.8.1257
25. Ribas A (2010) Clinical development of the anti-CTLA-4 antibody tremelimumab. Semin Oncol 37(5):450–454. doi:10.1053/j.seminoncol.2010.09.010
26. Waitz R, Fasso M, Allison JP (2012) CTLA-4 blockade synergizes with cryoablation to mediate tumor rejection. Oncoimmunology 1(4):544–546

27. Millward M, Underhill C, Lobb S, McBurnie J, Meech SJ, Gomez-Navarro J et al (2013) Phase I study of tremelimumab (CP-675 206) plus PF-3512676 (CPG 7909) in patients with melanoma or advanced solid tumours. Br J Cancer 108(10):1998–2004. doi:10.1038/bjc.2013.227
28. Krieg AM (2006) Therapeutic potential of toll-like receptor 9 activation. Nat Rev Drug Discov 5(6):471–484. doi:10.1038/nrd2059
29. Shirota H, Klinman DM (2012) Effect of CpG ODN on monocytic myeloid derived suppressor cells. Oncoimmunology 1(5):780–782. doi:10.4161/onci.19731
30. Hamilton E, Blackwell K, Hobeika AC, Clay TM, Broadwater G, Ren XR et al (2012) Phase 1 clinical trial of HER2-specific immunotherapy with concomitant HER2 kinase inhibition [corrected]. J Transl Med 10:28. doi:10.1186/1479-5876-10-28
31. Tyagi P, Mirakhur B (2009) MAGRIT: the largest-ever phase III lung cancer trial aims to establish a novel tumor-specific approach to therapy. Clin Lung Cancer 10(5):371–374. doi:10.3816/CLC.2009.n.052
32. Iwahashi M, Katsuda M, Nakamori M, Nakamura M, Naka T, Ojima T et al (2010) Vaccination with peptides derived from cancer-testis antigens in combination with CpG-7909 elicits strong specific CD8+ T cell response in patients with metastatic esophageal squamous cell carcinoma. Cancer Sci 101(12):2510–2517. doi:10.1111/j.1349-7006.2010.01732.x
33. Krieg AM (2007) Antiinfective applications of toll-like receptor 9 agonists. Proc Am Thorac Soc 4(3):289–294. doi:10.1513/pats.200701-021AW
34. Liu YJ (2005) IPC: professional type 1 interferon-producing cells and plasmacytoid dendritic cell precursors. Annu Rev Immunol 23:275–306. doi:10.1146/annurev.immunol.23.021704.115633
35. Bauer S, Kirschning CJ, Hacker H, Redecke V, Hausmann S, Akira S et al (2001) Human TLR9 confers responsiveness to bacterial DNA via species-specific CpG motif recognition. Proc Natl Acad Sci U S A 98(16):9237–9242. doi:10.1073/pnas.161293498
36. Hornung V, Rothenfusser S, Britsch S, Krug A, Jahrsdorfer B, Giese T et al (2002) Quantitative expression of toll-like receptor 1-10 mRNA in cellular subsets of human peripheral blood mononuclear cells and sensitivity to CpG oligodeoxynucleotides. J Immunol 168 (9):4531–4537
37. Kadowaki N, Ho S, Antonenko S, Malefyt RW, Kastelein RA, Bazan F et al (2001) Subsets of human dendritic cell precursors express different toll-like receptors and respond to different microbial antigens. J Exp Med 194(6):863–869
38. Vollmer J, Jurk M, Samulowitz U, Lipford G, Forsbach A, Wullner M et al (2004) CpG oligodeoxynucleotides stimulate IFN-gamma-inducible protein-10 production in human B cells. J Endotoxin Res 10(6):431–438. doi:10.1179/096805104225006534
39. Krieg AM (2004) Antitumor applications of stimulating toll-like receptor 9 with CpG oligodeoxynucleotides. Curr Oncol Rep 6(2):88–95
40. Martinson JA, Tenorio AR, Montoya CJ, Al-Harthi L, Gichinga CN, Krieg AM et al (2007) Impact of class A, B and C CpG-oligodeoxynucleotides on in vitro activation of innate immune cells in human immunodeficiency virus-1 infected individuals. Immunology 120 (4):526–535. doi:10.1111/j.1365-2567.2007.02530.x
41. Marshall JD, Fearon K, Abbate C, Subramanian S, Yee P, Gregorio J et al (2003) Identification of a novel CpG DNA class and motif that optimally stimulate B cell and plasmacytoid dendritic cell functions. J Leukoc Biol 73(6):781–792
42. Katsuda M, Iwahashi M, Matsuda K, Miyazawa M, Nakamori M, Nakamura M et al (2011) Comparison of different classes of CpG-ODN in augmenting the generation of human epitope peptide-specific CTLs. Int J Oncol 39(5):1295–1302. doi:10.3892/ijo.2011.1146
43. Muller AJ, Scherle PA (2006) Targeting the mechanisms of tumoral immune tolerance with small-molecule inhibitors. Nat Rev Cancer 6(8):613–625. doi:10.1038/nrc1929
44. Zitvogel L, Tesniere A, Kroemer G (2006) Cancer despite immunosurveillance: immunoselection and immunosubversion. Nat Rev Immunol 6(10):715–727. doi:10.1038/nri1936

45. Murad YM, Clay TM (2009) CpG oligodeoxynucleotides as TLR9 agonists: therapeutic applications in cancer. BioDrugs 23(6):361–375. doi:10.2165/11316930-000000000-00000
46. Shirota H, Klinman DM (2011) CpG-conjugated apoptotic tumor cells elicit potent tumor-specific immunity. Cancer Immunol Immunother 60(5):659–669. doi:10.1007/s00262-011-0973-y
47. Vollmer J, Krieg AM (2009) Immunotherapeutic applications of CpG oligodeoxynucleotide TLR9 agonists. Adv Drug Deliv Rev 61(3):195–204. doi:10.1016/j.addr.2008.12.008
48. Baines J, Celis E (2003) Immune-mediated tumor regression induced by CpG-containing oligodeoxynucleotides. Clin Cancer Res 9(7):2693–2700
49. Murdoch C, Muthana M, Coffelt SB, Lewis CE (2008) The role of myeloid cells in the promotion of tumour angiogenesis. Nat Rev Cancer 8(8):618–631. doi:10.1038/nrc2444
50. Hirsh V, Paz-Ares L, Boyer M, Rosell R, Middleton G, Eberhardt WE et al (2011) Randomized phase III trial of paclitaxel/carboplatin with or without PF-3512676 (toll-like receptor 9 agonist) as first-line treatment for advanced non-small-cell lung cancer. J Clin Oncol 29 (19):2667–2674. doi:10.1200/JCO.2010.32.8971
51. Hofmann MA, Kors C, Audring H, Walden P, Sterry W, Trefzer U (2008) Phase 1 evaluation of intralesionally injected TLR9-agonist PF-3512676 in patients with basal cell carcinoma or metastatic melanoma. J Immunother 31(5):520–527. doi:10.1097/CJI.0b013e318174a4df
52. Carpentier A, Metellus P, Ursu R, Zohar S, Lafitte F, Barrie M et al (2010) Intracerebral administration of CpG oligonucleotide for patients with recurrent glioblastoma: a phase II study. Neuro Oncol 12(4):401–408. doi:10.1093/neuonc/nop047
53. Molenkamp BG, Sluijter BJ, van Leeuwen PA, Santegoets SJ, Meijer S, Wijnands PG et al (2008) Local administration of PF-3512676 CpG-B instigates tumor-specific CD8+ T-cell reactivity in melanoma patients. Clin Cancer Res 14(14):4532–4542. doi:10.1158/1078-0432.CCR-07-4711
54. Kim YH, Gratzinger D, Harrison C, Brody JD, Czerwinski DK, Ai WZ et al (2012) In situ vaccination against mycosis fungoides by intratumoral injection of a TLR9 agonist combined with radiation: a phase 1/2 study. Blood 119(2):355–363. doi:10.1182/blood-2011-05-355222
55. Brody JD, Ai WZ, Czerwinski DK, Torchia JA, Levy M, Advani RH et al (2010) In situ vaccination with a TLR9 agonist induces systemic lymphoma regression: a phase I/II study. J Clin Oncol 28(28):4324–4332. doi:10.1200/JCO.2010.28.9793

# Chapter 16
# Pattern Recognition by Dendritic Cells and Its Application to Vaccine Adjuvant for Antitumor Immunotherapy

**Tsukasa Seya, Masahiro Azuma, and Misako Matsumoto**

**Abstract** Dendritic cells (DCs) initiate the maturation to a specific stage in response to stimuli with microbial pattern molecules (PAMP) and trigger activation of host immune response together with antigens (Ags). Recently, subsets of dendritic cells have been subdivided with surface markers into DCs with high Ag-presenting capacity and those with less capacity. These DC subsets have been found to induce various effectors in response to their different compositions of pattern recognition receptors (PRRs). In human, the best Ag-presenting cell is CD141+ DC, while in the mouse the best one is CD8a+ DC. In this paper, we describe the properties of PRRs in host DC subsets and outline the induction mechanism of effector cells. PAMP is usually called "adjuvant" in the field of tumor immunology. I will explain the recent launch of the obvious mechanisms by which the DC-dependent NK activation and antitumor CTL induction are promoted by adjuvants.

**Keywords** Antigen-presenting dendritic cell (CD8$\alpha^+$ DC, CD141$^+$ DC) • Pam2 lipopeptide • Poly(I:C) • NK cell activation • Toll-like receptor • INAM • Antitumor immunotherapy

## Abbreviations

| | |
|---|---|
| APC | antigen-presenting cell |
| BCGCWS | Bacillus Calmette-Guerin cell-wall skeleton |
| BDCA | Blood Dendritic Cell Antigens |
| DAMP | damage-associated molecular patterns |
| FACS | flow cytometry |
| GM-CSF | granulocyte-macrophage-coloney stimulating factor |
| INAM | IRF3-dependent NK cell activating molecule |
| IRAK | IL-1 Receptor–associated Kinase |

T. Seya (✉) • M. Azuma • M. Matsumoto
Department of Microbiology and Immunology, Graduate School of Medicine, Hokkaido University, Kita 15, Nishi 7, Kita-ku, Sapporo, Hokkaido 060-8638, Japan
e-mail: seya-tu@pop.med.hokudai.ac.jp



Y. Yamaguchi (ed.), *Immunotherapy of Cancer*,
DOI 10.1007/978-4-431-55031-0_16

| | |
|---|---|
| IRF | interferon-regulatory factor |
| Mal/TIRAP | TIRAP toll-interleukin 1 receptor (TIR) domain containing adaptor |
| MALP | macrophage-activating lipopeptide |
| MAVS | mitochondrial antiviral signaling protein |
| qPCR | quantitative PCR |
| TICAM | Toll-IL-1R homology domain-containing adaptor molecule |
| TRAM | TRIF-associated adaptor molecule |

## 16.1 Introduction

Adjuvant has been used for a long time in immunization. Oil adjuvants (Freund's complete adjuvant (FCA), Freund's incomplete adjuvant (FIA)) and aluminum hydroxide (alum) have been frequently used for an antigen conjugate that was expected to enhance antigenicity. The mechanism of potential action of adjuvant has not been clearly demonstrated in alum and oil until recently, considering the antigen "dirty" that enhance the immune function in those cases. Microbial constituents (pattern molecules) with immune-potentiating abilities have been isolated as the adjuvant components based on the functional studies and agonist search for innate immune receptors, which we called pattern recognition receptors (PRRs), and it was found that these components were agonists for PRRs such as toll-like receptors (TLRs). The impact of this finding is that the pattern molecules rather than Ags in microbes endow directionality to the immune system, which we call innate immunity (pattern sensing in dendritic cells) [1]. Reexamination to the basic concept of the immune system is carried out with this concept, and the current concept for the antitumor immunity also is in the transconversion. Crystals of alum and urea stimulate the Nod-like receptor (NLR) inflammasome system in the cytoplasm, and NLR activation induces IL-1β and IL-18 in myeloid cells. These cytokines have been found to trigger the activation of MyD88 in DC via the receptor NLR [2]. FCA includes dead mycobacteria; thus, CpG DNA, peptidoglycan (PGN), and lipoproteins are known to function as ligands for TLR9, TLR2/TLR4, and TLR2, respectively [3]. Analogs of double-stranded RNA (polyI:C) and single-stranded RNA (ssRNA) that are produced during the replication of viruses act as agonists for TLR3 and TLR7/TLR8, respectively. A flagella protein flagellin of Gram-negative bacteria and lipopolysaccharide (LPS) are ligands for TLR5 and TLR4, respectively. These led to identification of the characteristics of DC maturation inducers. Here, we summarize the properties of these adjuvants and their derivatives as DC maturation inducers (Table 16.1).

The cytokine-inducing profiles of these adjuvants and their derivatives have been clarified over a decade. However, their roles in antitumor immunity are just starting, including the mechanism of immune enhancing, effector inducibility, and dendritic cell maturation. Toxicity problem has not been always deeply considered in practical use, and the criteria for therapeutic application of adjuvant to patients have not been determined for clinical trials. Current alum and oil (Montanide)

**Table 16.1** Adjuvants for activation of MyD88 or TICAM-1

| Human TLR | Ligands | Adjuvants |
|---|---|---|
| TLR1 | Pam3 | TAN33 |
| TLR2 | Pam2, Pam3, PGN | M161Ag (MALP-2, MALP-2s) TAN33, SMP105, OM-174, K12PGN, 0111:B4PGN |
| TLR3 | dsRNA | poly(I:C), poly(I:C12U), poly(I:C)LC, (poly(A:U)) |
| TLR4 | LPS, RSV F | Lipid A, MPLA |
| TLR5 | Flagellin | sTLR5 |
| TLR6 | Pam2 | M161Ag (MALP-2, MALP2s), SMP105, PM-174 |
| TLR7 | ssRNA | imiquimod, poly-U |
| TLR8 | ssRNA | imiquimod, poly-U |
| TLR9 | CpG DNA | CpG-ODN, hemozoin |
| TLR10 | ? | ? |

therapy do not have high immune-enhancing ability, but they are activators for a standard NLR system. BCG-CWS (TLR2/TLR4), polyI:C/poly-L-lysine (TLR3), and monophospholipid A (MPLA) (TLR4) are agonists of the TLR and appear superior to alum but harbor toxicity such as inflammation symptoms and skin erosion, which would be significant side effects. Furthermore, there are some cases that cause lethal shock, disseminated coagulation, and interstitial pneumonia. Development of adjuvants to overcome these problems is being expected. In this paper, we will review the molecular mechanisms of DC maturation and effector activation by TLR agonistic adjuvants.

## 16.2 DC Maturation by TLR Agonists

The fact that the TLR agonists possess a maturation effect on DC has been shown early since TLR was discovered [4, 5]. There appear two major pathways, MyD88 pathway and TICAM-1 (TRIF) pathway, in enhancing Ag-presenting ability to mature myeloid dendritic cells (mDC) (Fig. 16.1). MyD88 constitutes a different signaling pathway from TICAM-1 as an adapter to assemble an activation platform [6]. MyD88 binds the Mal/TIRAP as a bridge in mDC TLR2/TLR4 and directly activates signal to the transcription factor NF-κB in TLR5 [6]. IL-1 receptor also recruits MyD88 to signal for the activation of NF-κB. In plasmacytoid (p)DC, TLR7 and TLR9 recruit MyD88 to activate the transcription factor IRF7 [7]. On the other hand, TICAM-1 is an adapter that only TLR3 and TLR4 can take [6]. TLR3 directly and TLR4 indirectly bind TICAM-1 via TICAM-2 (TRAM) [6]. Only TLR4 can take both MyD88 and TICAM-1 as adapters (Fig. 16.1). A typical example that both pathways are activated is endotoxin shock by LPS [8]. In this case, Gram-negative bacteria activate the TLR4/TICAM-1 pathway to induce type I IFN, which in turn activates IFNAR. IFNAR signal promotes production of caspase

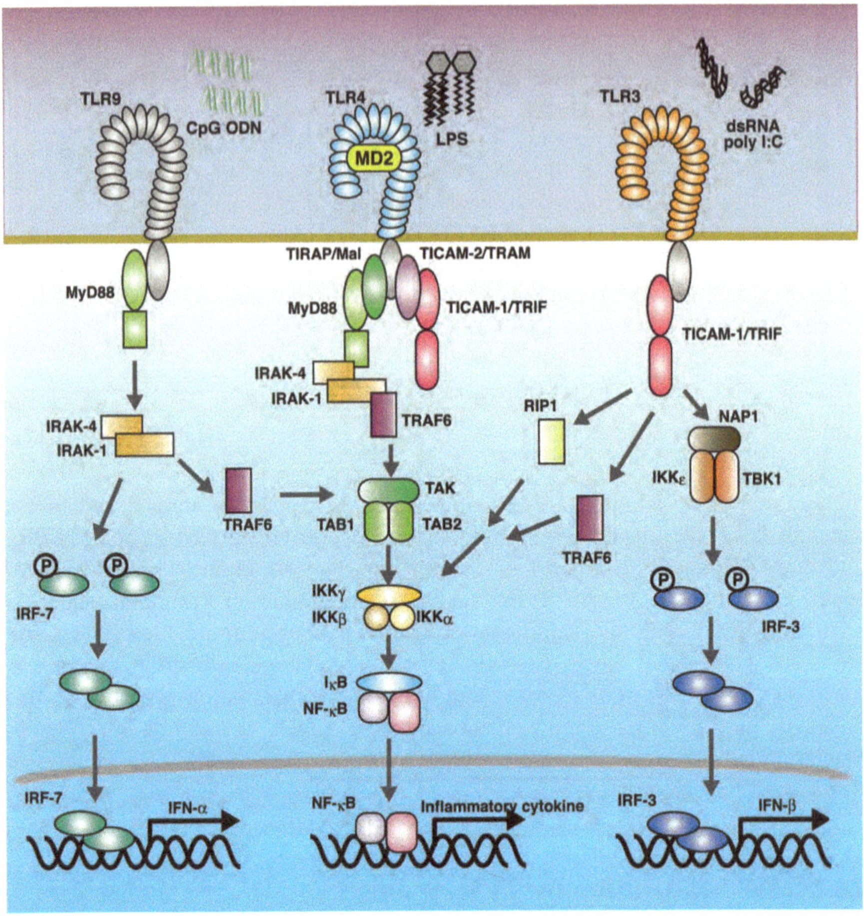


**Fig. 16.1** MyD88 pathway and TICAM-1 pathway. TICAM-1 is the adapter that only TLR3 and TLR4 participate in. In contrast, MyD88 is an adapter that all of TLRs except TLR3 use for signal. TICAM-1 activates the transcription factor IRF3/IRF7 and NF-κB, to a little late compared with MyD88. This figure refers to as an example of TLR3 and TLR4. On the other hand, MyD88 in pDC activates the pathway that primarily activates the IRF7 or NF-kB. The examples are TLR9 as for IRF7 activation and TLR4 as for MyD88 activation. TLR2 possesses only the MyD88 pathway in the examples of TLR4. Also, TLR5 binds directly to MyD88 without TIRAP. TLR7 adopts a similar MyD88 pathway to TLR9. Each TLR responses to different ligands (Table 16.1)

11. The NALP3/ASC/procaspase 1 complex, named NALP3 inflammasome, turns active by caspase 11, where procaspase 1 is converted to the active form. On the other hand, production of NALP3 and preform of IL-1β/IL-18 are upregulated by MyD88 signaling of TLR4. The caspase 1 initiates active IL-1β/IL-18 production. Thus, the mechanism of LPS endotoxin shock has been known to be complex as has been expected in humans. It is necessary to select a safe adjuvant for activating either pathway.

The MyD88 and TICAM-1 pathways both induce maturation of mDC, but their modes are different from each other. IL-12 and type I interferon (IFN) are induced depending on the TICAM-1 pathway [9]. NK activation of mDC is also activated by TICAM-1 (described below). Type I interferon (IFN) induction of MyD88 is seen only in pDC [7]. MyD88 of mDC is a strong inducer of inflammatory cytokines such as IL-1β, IL-6, and TNF-α [9]. Both MyD88 and TICAM-1 confer the cross-presentation ability on mDCs, but the molecular mechanism of this DC maturation remains to be determined.

## 16.3 TLR Expression in DC Subsets

For mice, bone marrow-derived DC (BMDC, representatives of mDC) and plasmacytoid DC (pDC) are prepared from bone marrow cells using GM-CSF or Flt3 ligand, respectively. Langerhans cells are prepared by treatment of bone marrow cells with GM-CSF, IL-4, and TGF-β. Additional DC subsets are separated from the spleen and intestine using FACS sorter. For humans, monocyte-derived DC (Mo-DC) is used as mDC, and they show significantly different properties from the CD141+ (PDCA3) DC subset, a representative APC, in peripheral blood. On the other hand, peripheral blood pDC can be separated using the PDCA4 [1, 9, 10].

Distribution of TLRs in each human DC subset is shown in Table 16.2, where the TLR proteins were determined using antihuman TLR antibody. Mouse TLRs in terms of protein expression have not been addressed with mouse BMDC or pDC, since no good mAbs are available for their assessment. However, PCR analyses suggest that mouse BMDC express TLR7 and TLR9 as in pDC, which properties entirely differ from those of human Mo-DC or CD141+ DC. Human CD141+ DC of APC do not express TLR7 or TLR9. Although mouse CD8α+ DC express minimal TLR4 and TLR5, human CD141+ DC do not express them. Human and mouse APC commonly express high levels of TLR2 family [1, 2, 6] and TLR3.

**Table 16.2** TLR expression profile in human DCs

| | Freshly isolated | | | In vitro-differentiated cells | |
|---|---|---|---|---|---|
| | Monocyte | mDC (CD141+) | pDC (BDCA4+) | Monocyte-derived DC macrophages | |
| TLR1 | ++ | + | − | + | ++ |
| TLR2 | ++ | ++ | − | ++ | ++ |
| TLR3 | − | ++ | − | ++ | + |
| TLR4 | ++ | − | − | + | + |
| TLR6 | ++ | + | − | + | + |
| TLR7 | − | − | + | − | − |
| TLR8 | + | + | − | + | + |
| TLR9 | − | − | + | − | − |

+, −: TLR7 and TLR9 are results of qPCR; others are the results of FACS

pDC generally express TLR7 and TLR9. Human but not mouse mDC express TLR8 [11]. CpG has low immune-enhancing function due to this reason that human APC DCs exert limited TLR9 compared to the mouse. The in vivo immune-enhancing function of CpG may be supported by pDC with TLR9.

## 16.4 DC Subsets and Effector Induction

Effector cells can be evaluated by the antigen-dependent activation of T cells, CTL, Th1, Th2, Th17, and Treg, and antigen-independent NK activation (Fig. 16.2). NK cells are activated by (1) NK activating ligand (a mDC side factor) and the combination of NK receptors and (2) cytokines such as IL-2, IL-15, IFN-α/β, and IL-12 (mDC side factors) [11]. CTL is the result of activation of CD8α+ T cells which process is promoted via class I presentation by mDC. Other effector is a result of the activation of CD4+ T cells by class II presentation by mDC. CD4 T cells are classified into subsets, Th1, Th2, Th17, Treg, etc. The master transcription factors to each Th1, Th2, Th17, and Treg are T-bet, GATA-3, RORgt, and FOXP3, respectively [12].

The mechanism by which DC selectively induces various effectors remains unclear. Certain DC subsets seem to associate with preferential induction of a

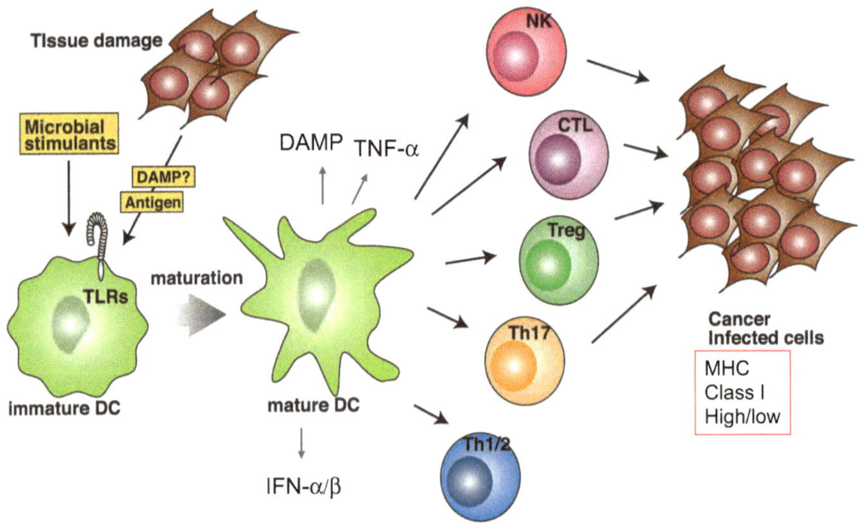


**Fig. 16.2** Induction of various effectors by TLR agonists. A variety of TLR agonists (PAMP) induces unique staged dendritic cell maturation to drive different effector cells. The adapter molecule downstream of TLRs activates the transcription factors in dendritic cells. The NK activation and CTL induction are specified in the signal in DC. Adjuvant is believed to express molecules that execute effector induction. When dendritic cells stimulated with PAMP are adoptively transferred to mice around the tumor, you can assess effector functions against the tumor

particular effector. If the root which imparts directionality to the immune system is a dendritic cell, antigen per se does not decide the strategy but determines the object for the activated immune cells. The strategy is reflected in the induced effector, such as antibody, NK, CTL, Th17, and Treg. In fact, murine splenic CD8α+ DC likely to induce Treg [13] and NK cells [14]. Lamina propria pDC in the mouse intestinal tract promote IgA production [15]. CD70+/CD11c+ DC induce Th17 cells by ATP of intestinal bacteria [16]. BMDC can activate NK cells through the TICAM-1 pathway in DC [17].

## 16.5 DC-Mediated NK Cell Activation in Tumor Immunity by Adjuvant

BMDC drive antitumor NK cell activation depending on the TICAM-1 pathway [17]. This NK activation is attributable to cell-cell contact by BMDC and NK cells rather than humoral factors such as cytokines, induced by DC [18]. Therefore, the key for the mechanisms of induction of antitumor NK cells would be a membrane molecule on DC that promotes the surface expression by the TICAM-1 pathway (Fig. 16.3). NK activation is not due to IRF3 but due to IRF7, since NK activation is not affected in IRF7 KO BMDC but is severely hampered in IRF3 BMDC [18]. Thus, NK induction pathway in mDC uses the transcription factor IRF3 in TICAM-1 downstream. With screening methods of the candidate cDNA to express lentiviral vectors in IRF3-deficient BMDC, it is possible to identify NK activation molecule [18]. We have identified the INAM as an NK activation molecule of dendritic cells. INAM was a specific NK activation molecule that connects BMDC with NK cells (Fig. 16.3). This molecule strongly promoted NK activation in DC but did not induce NK activation in a BaF3 strain which overexpresses INAM. INAM is a membrane protein similar to tetraspanin of molecular weight 45,000 and had a sugar chain with posttranslational modification. INAM is mainly distributed to the spleen and lymph tissue. INAM is expected to make a loop-like structure in two locations on the cell surface from the predicted sequence [18].

INAM is presumed to be involved in the configuration of the immune synapse of the BMDC-NK inter-surface. When the BMDC overexpressing INAM are adoptively transferred to tumor-bearing mice, regression of NK-sensitive tumor occurs rapidly [19]. If NK cells are removed from the mice by NK1.1 Ab, tumor regression no longer occurs [18]. This suggests that INAM is a direct factor that drives the induction of antitumor NK cells.

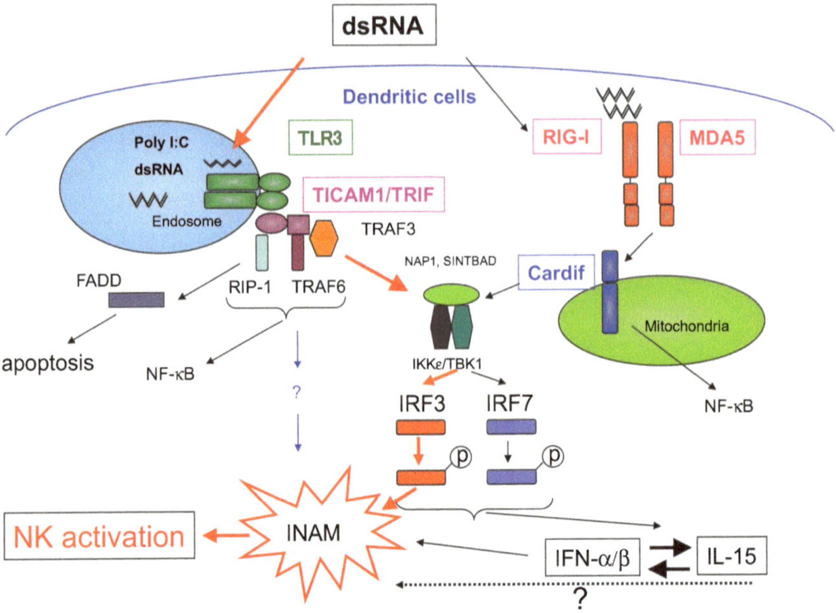


**Fig. 16.3** The molecular mechanism of dendritic cell maturation by polyI:C. NK cell activation by polyI:C. TLR3 is localized in the endosome of dendritic cells and activates IRF3 in response to polyI:C. TLR3-TICAM-1 signal induces to express membrane proteins, including INAM on the dendritic cell surface. INAM also expressed in NK cells, by promoting synapse formation and NK cells and promoting NK activation. PolyI:C also activates the MAVS pathway, which causes endotoxin-like toxicity. It is desirable to activate a single adapter (TICAM-1 or MAVS) for the development of nontoxic RNA derivatives. TICAM-1 selective activation is feasible for this purpose. Monophospholipid A (MPLA), a TLR4 agonist, barely activates the MyD88 pathway, which is an alternative candidate for the adjuvant. Indeed, MPLA is a TLR4 agonist, but it preferentially activates TICAM-1 without robust activation of MyD88

## 16.6 DC-Mediated CTL Induction by Adjuvant

Adjuvants usually target dendritic cells (DC) for immune enhancing. Human CD141+ DC specifically express TLR2 and TLR3 but do not express TLR4, TLR5, TLR7, and TLR9 (Fig. 16.1). TLR2 recognizes bacterial lipopeptides and peptidoglycan and activates the MyD88 pathway [1]. TLR3 recognizes the stem-structured RNA and activates the TICAM-1 pathway [20]. Therefore, we explain the differences in cross-priming response of these two pathways in dendritic cells. Some adjuvants primarily promote antibody production, while others evoke cellular immunity in antitumor immunity. The latter adjuvants are preferable when tumor antigens are taken up in DC. Proteins and long-chain peptide are good as tumor-associated antigens (TAAs), since they have multivalent epitopes involving CD4 activation. It is TLR2 and TLR3 to strongly promote the antigen presentation [21].

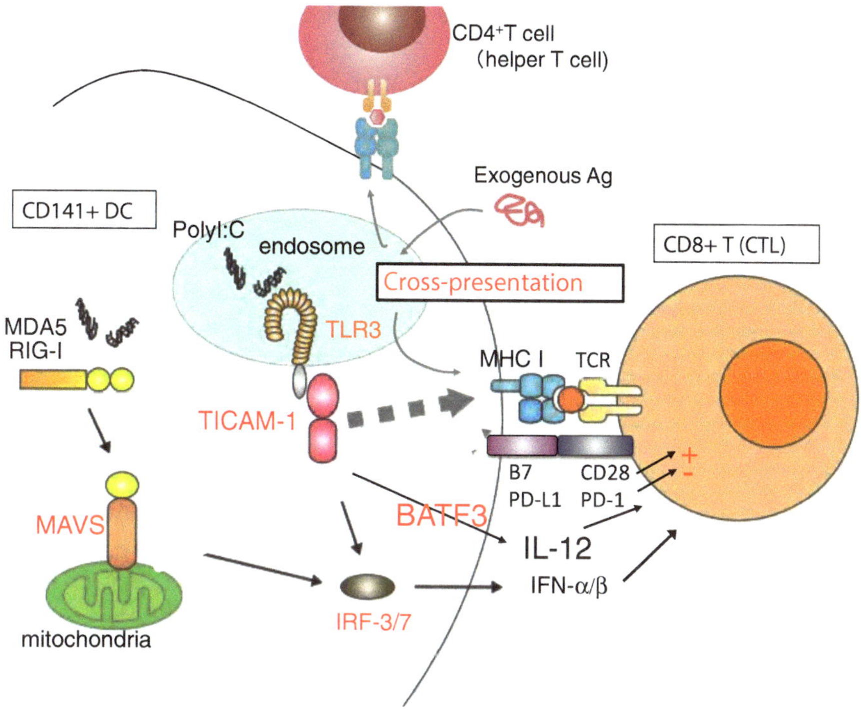


**Fig. 16.4** CD141+ DC mature in response to polyI:C. CD141+ DC possess cytoplasmic sensors (RIG-I/MDA5) and TLR3 in endosome. Viral RNA or polyI:C is recognized intracellularly in cytoplasm, whereas extracellular RNA is recognized by TLR3. TLR3 mainly participates in cross-presentation and IL-12 production, where BATF3 is required. Efficient MHC class I presentation occurs in DC to cross-prime T cells. These responses link the CTL proliferation. CD4+ T cells are activated in response to exogenous antigens presented on MHC class II. Production of type I IFN and upregulation of MHC and B7 molecules are also induced. Robust inflammatory cytokines are produced via MAVS in response to RNA

The immunostimulatory function of TLR3 adjuvant is to induce inflammatory cytokines/chemokines, high expression of MHC, upregulation of costimulatory molecules, promotion of cross-presentation, production of type I interferon (IFN), and production of IL-12 (Fig. 16.4). IFN induces T cell proliferation and releases the exhaustion of CD8 T cell to confer long live on T cells. Type I IFN further activates CD4 helper and NK cells [17]. These lymphocytes generally maintain the activity by type I IFN or IL-12, and IL-12 is important for the exertion of cytotoxicity in tumor [22]. A good activation marker of lymphocytes is IFN-γ. IFN-γ reflects the active behaviors of multiple lymphocytes, which is influenced by the type of adjuvant. IL-12 is produced depending on the BATF3-TLR3 signaling (TICAM-1 pathway) [21, 22].

TLR2 evokes cross-presentation secondary to activation of the MyD88 pathway. The MyD88 pathway is a fundamental pathway involved in inflammation. Thus, TLR2 ligand induces inflammation, including inflammatory cytokines with maturation of dendritic cells (Fig. 16.1). A typical ligand of TLR2 is Pam2 lipopeptides including MALP-2 [23]. This adjuvant does not induce IL-12 or type I IFN but induce high levels of inflammatory cytokines, as well as activation of IRAK. It has been reported that an effective example of clinical trials using MALP-2 is pancreatic cancer [24].

PD-1 is expressed in CD8 T cells. Notably, PD-1 is upregulated by IL-12 but not by type I IFN. Effective cases of PD-1/PD-L1 are nearly 30 % in the solid tumors [25]. In case of tumor regression, lymphocytes with low PD-1 expressions infiltrate in tumor nests [26]. It was shown from the ineffective cases that tumor regression cannot be expected in patients without lymphocyte infiltration in the tumor. A question is whether the combination of chemokines or adjuvants resolves the properties of tumor-infiltrating lymphocytes.

## 16.7 Perspectives for Adjuvant Immunotherapy

We have analyzed the mechanism about how adjuvant-mediated dendritic cell maturation is necessary to separately drive immune effector cells with a focus on innate immunity. The pattern recognition is essential for the maturation of dendritic cells, while tumor-infiltrating macrophages become a trigger to convert precancerous cells to malignant cells [27]. Some examples include that BCG is highly effective in superficial cancer that has no basal layer invasion, such as bladder cancer (transitional cell carcinoma) [28]. However, a fundamental reason why tumor immunity is not so effective in solid cancer would be an issue of the myeloid cell ambivalence in tumor microenvironment [27]. This tumor-immune cell abnormality has neither been dissolved nor in general been made even a grasp of this basic molecular situation. In addition, the tumor-bearing state is a special immune modulatory state. When the tumor is surgically excised from the patients, many manifestations are diminished as the reflection [29]. Currently, proving that the cause of these anomalies is due to the innate immune-modulating molecules known collectively as DAMP from cancer cells, many researchers want to identify DAMPs in patients with cancer (Fig. 16.2).

So far, antitumor immunotherapy has been diagnosed the prognosis from regression effect of cancer mainly through the peptide vaccine therapy. According to Rosenberg's report, the effective rate of the peptide vaccine therapy was about 2.6 % against melanoma [30]; there is a need to develop highly effective adjuvant and therapeutic way for raising immune potential. Since inflammation sometimes promotes carcinogenesis and tumor cell invasion, a method for selective stimulation of dendritic cells has been adopted. However, this is not convenient and not amenable to health care. On the other hand, you can develop a molecular targeting therapy if you identify a pathway and molecules that are specifically expressed in tumor-infiltrating macrophages and dendritic cells. This kind of therapy will reduce side effects and contribute to establishment of evidence-based treatment. By considering the orientation of the dendritic cells, you could selectively use an appropriate adjuvant that promotes immune cell activation without carcinogenesis or inflammatory signals [31]. If you identify functional molecules related to inducing antitumor effector in the dendritic cells, the research results could be immediately applicable to cancer treatment. What you need for patients is a simple immunotherapy cure.

**Acknowledgments** We are grateful to our lab members for invaluable discussions. This work was supported in part by the Grants-in-Aid from the Ministry of Education, Culture, Sports, Science and Technology (MEXT); "the Carcinogenic Spiral" a MEXT Grant-in-Project; the Ministry of Health, Labour and Welfare of Japan; the Takeda Foundation; the Yasuda Cancer Research Foundation; and the Kato Memorial Bioscience Foundation.

## References

1. Iwasaki A, Medzhitov R (2004) Toll-like receptor control of the adaptive immune responses. Nat Immunol 5(10):987–995
2. Franchi L et al (2009) The inflammasome: a caspase-1-activation platform that regulates immune responses and disease pathogenesis. Nat Immunol 10(3):241–247
3. Nikoopour E et al (2008) Therapeutic benefits of regulating inflammation in autoimmunity. Inflamm Allergy Drug Targets 7(3):203–210
4. Medzhitov R et al (1997) A human homologue of the drosophila toll protein signals activation of adaptive immunity. Nature 388(6640):394–397
5. Medzhitov R, Janeway CA Jr (1997) Innate immunity: the virtues of a nonclonal system of recognition. Cell 91(3):295–298
6. Akira S (2003) Toll-like receptor signaling. J Biol Chem 278(40):38105–38108
7. Hoshino K et al (2006) IkappaB kinase-alpha is critical for interferon-alpha production induced by Toll-like receptors 7 and 9. Nature 440(7086):949–953
8. Rathinam VA, Vanaja SK, Waggoner L, Sokolovska A, Becker C, Stuart LM, Leong JM, Fitzgerald KA (2012) TRIF licenses caspase-11-dependent NLRP3 inflammasome activation by gram-negative bacteria. Cell 150(3):606–619
9. Matsumoto M, Seya T (2008) TLR3: interferon induction by double-stranded RNA including poly(I:C). Adv Drug Deliv Rev 60(7):805–812
10. Duthie MS, Windish HP, Fox CB, Reed SG (2011) Use of defined TLR ligands as adjuvants within human vaccines. Immunol Rev 239(1):178–196
11. Heil F, Hemmi H, Hochrein H, Ampenberger F, Kirschning C, Akira S, Lipford G, Wagner H, Bauer S (2004) Species-specific recognition of single-stranded RNA via toll-like receptor 7 and 8. Science 303(5663):1526–1529
12. Reynolds JM, Dong C (2013) Toll-like receptor regulation of effector T lymphocyte function. Trends Immunol 34(10):511–519
13. Yamazaki S et al (2003) Direct expansion of functional CD25+ CD4+ regulatory T cells by antigen-processing dendritic cells. J Exp Med 198(2):235–247
14. Miyake T et al (2009) Poly I:C-induced activation of NK cells by CD8alpha+ dendritic cells via the IPS-1 and TRIF-dependent pathways. J Immunol 183(4):2522–2528
15. Tezuka H et al (2007) Regulation of IgA production by naturally occurring TNF/iNOS-producing dendritic cells. Nature 448(7156):929–933
16. Atarashi K et al (2008) ATP drives lamina propria T(H)17 cell differentiation. Nature 455 (7214):808–812
17. Akazawa T et al (2007) Antitumor NK activation induced by the Toll-like receptor 3-TICAM-1 (TRIF) pathway in myeloid dendritic cells. Proc Natl Acad Sci U S A 104(1):252–2527

18. Ebihara T et al (2008) Hepatitis C virus-infected hepatocytes extrinsically modulate dendritic cell maturation to activate T cells and natural killer cells. Hepatology 48(1):48–58
19. Kasamatsu J, Azuma M, Oshiumi H, Morioka Y, Okabe M, Ebihara T, Matsumoto M, Seya T (2014) INAM plays a critical role in IFN-γ production by NK cells interacting with polyinosinic-polycytidylic acid-stimulated accessory cells. J Immunol 193(10):5199–5207
20. Tatematsu M, Nishikawa F, Seya T, Matsumoto M (2013) Toll-like receptor 3 recognizes incomplete stem structures in single-stranded viral RNA. Nat Commun 4:1833
21. Jongbloed SL, Kassianos AJ, McDonald KJ, Clark GJ, Ju X, Angel CE, Chen CJ, Dunbar PR, Wadley RB, Jeet V, Vulink AJ, Hart DN, Radford KJ (2007) Human CD141+(BDCA-3)+ dendritic cells (DCs) represent a unique myeloid DC subset that cross-presents necrotic cell antigens. J Exp Med 207(6):1247–1260
22. Azuma M, Takeda Y, Nakajima H, Sugiyama H, Ebihara T, Oshiumi H, Matsumoto M, Seya T (2015) BATF3 fundamentally supports TLR3-derived IL-12 induction in CD8α$^+$ dendritic cell, which promotes antitumor T cell responses by poly(I:C). Cancer Res (in Press)
23. Colonna M, Cella M (2007) Crosspresentation: plasmacytoid dendritic cells are in the business. Immunity 27(3):419–421
24. Schmidt J, Welsch T, Jäger D, Mühlradt PF, Büchler MW, Märten A (2007) Intratumoural injection of the toll-like receptor-2/6 agonist 'macrophage-activating lipopeptide-2' in patients with pancreatic carcinoma: a phase I/II trial. Br J Cancer 97(5):598–604. Alexandroff AB et al (1999) BCG immunotherapy of bladder cancer: 20 years on. Lancet 353(9165):1689–1694
25. Herbst RS, Soria JC, Kowanetz M, Fine GD, Hamid O et al (2014) Predictive correlates of response to the anti-PD-L1 antibody MPDL3280A in cancer patients. Nature 515:563–567
26. Gerner MY, Heltemes-Harris LM, Fife BT, Mescher MF (2013) Cutting edge: IL-12 and type I IFN differentially program CD8 T cells for programmed death 1 re-expression levels and tumor control. J Immunol 191:1011–1015
27. Shime H, Matsumoto M, Oshiumi H, Tanaka S, Nakane A et al (2011) Toll-like receptor 3 signaling converts tumor-supporting myeloid cells to tumoricidal effectors. Proc Natl Acad Sci USA 109:2066–2071
28. Alexandroff AB et al (1999) BCG immunotherapy of bladder cancer: 20 years on. Lancet 353 (9165):1689–1694
29. Kodama K et al (2009) Innate immune therapy with a Bacillus Calmette-Guérin cell wall skeleton after radical surgery for non-small cell lung cancer: a case-control study. Surg Today 39(3):194–200
30. Rosenberg SA et al (2004) Cancer immunotherapy: moving beyond current vaccines. Nat Med 10(9):909–915
31. Akazawa T et al (2004) Adjuvant-mediated tumor regression and tumor-specific cytotoxic response are impaired in MyD88-deficient mice. Cancer Res 64(2):757–764

# Chapter 17
# Novel Adjuvants

**Burcu Temizoz, Etsushi Kuroda, Kouji Kobiyama, Taiki Aoshi, and Ken J. Ishii**

**Abstract** Several clinical trials suggested that one promising immunotherapeutic approach is cancer vaccines, containing novel adjuvants capable of stimulating innate immunity to result in breakage of immunotolerance in the tumor microenvironment and development of potent antitumor immune responses. In particular, agonists for TLR and STING are actively investigated adjuvants due to their high potential for induction of antitumor immune responses. Moreover, recent efforts to improve the efficacy of TLR9 agonist as adjuvants by coupling with delivery molecules and nanoparticle and/or by mixing with other innate immune stimuli such as STING agonists revealed novel cancer vaccine adjuvants with high efficacy. In this review, we introduce recent advances in the development of novel adjuvants for cancer immunotherapy.

**Keywords** Innate immunity • TLR9 • CpG ODN • K3-SPG • STING • DMXAA

B. Temizoz • E. Kuroda
Laboratory of Vaccine Science, WPI Immunology Frontier Research Center (iFReC), Osaka University, Osaka, Japan

K. Kobiyama
Laboratory of Adjuvant Innovation, National Institutes of Biomedical Innovation, Health and Nutrition (NIBIOHN), Osaka, Japan

T. Aoshi
Laboratory of Vaccine Science, WPI Immunology Frontier Research Center (iFReC), Osaka University, Osaka, Japan

Laboratory of Adjuvant Innovation, National Institutes of Biomedical Innovation, Health and Nutrition (NIBIOHN), Osaka, Japan

K.J. Ishii (✉)
Laboratory of Vaccine Science, WPI Immunology Frontier Research Center (iFReC), Osaka University, Osaka, Japan

Laboratory of Adjuvant Innovation, National Institutes of Biomedical Innovation, Health and Nutrition (NIBIOHN), Osaka, Japan

6F IFReC Research Building, Osaka University, 3-1 Yamada-oka, Suita, Osaka 565-0871, Japan
e-mail: kenishii@biken.osaka-u.ac.jp


Y. Yamaguchi (ed.), *Immunotherapy of Cancer*,
DOI 10.1007/978-4-431-55031-0_17

## 17.1 Introduction

Cancer immunotherapy aims at modulating the immune system so that it becomes capable of recognizing and destroying the tumor cells. Tumors usually interfere with the development of antitumor immune responses by providing an immunosuppressive microenvironment via several different mechanisms. Therefore, the challenge for cancer immunotherapy is to find the optimal approaches to overcome this immunosuppression for generating effective antitumor immune responses without serious side effects.

With the expanding knowledge of various tumor-associated antigens, cancer immunotherapy has become one of the most promising approaches for treating cancer, being used as an alternative or together with the well-known treatment approaches of surgery, chemotherapy, and radiotherapy [1]. Among the cancer immunotherapy approaches, including cell-based therapies, antibody therapies, and cytokine therapies, cancer vaccines have attracted great attention, especially after US Food and Drug Administration (FDA) approved the first therapeutic cancer vaccine Provenge, which was designed by using the dendritic cells from the self-peripheral blood to fight against the cancerous cells in prostate cancer patients, in 2010 [2]. Despite the promising results using the cancer vaccine Provenge, according to the results from large-scale clinical trials using cancer peptide vaccines, such as the Rosenberg et al.'s cancer vaccine trials, effectiveness rates were as low as 2.6 %, due to the lack of potent adjuvants or improper selection of the antigens [3]. Thus, one key component of the cancer vaccines for establishing cancer immunotherapy as an efficient treatment is a potent adjuvant, which is strong enough to overcome the immunosuppression provided by the tumor microenvironment. In this review, we will focus on the novel adjuvants which are used either in the therapeutic cancer vaccines or as immunotherapeutic agents for cancer.

## 17.2 Innate Immunity and Tumor Immunity

Innate immune cells, such as natural killer (NK) cells, dendritic cells (DCs), and macrophages, provide the first line of defense against pathogens and other types of threats faced by the host [4]. Detection of the infection or danger by the innate immune cells is accomplished by the sensing of damage-associated molecular patterns (DAMPs) or pathogen-associated molecular patterns (PAMPs), such as viral/bacterial nucleic acids and bacterial cell wall components (e.g., lipopolysaccharide), via the various kinds of pattern-recognition receptors (PRRs) expressed on innate immune cells [5]. PRRs include toll-like receptors (TLRs), RIG-1-like receptors (RLRs), C-type lectin receptors (CLRs), AIM2-like receptors (ALRs), and NOD-like receptors (NLRs) (Table 17.1) [4, 5]. Once the PAMPs are detected by innate immune cells, in addition to acting directly on the infected or stressed cells, innate immune cells also interact with adaptive immune cells to generate robust immune responses against intracellular pathogens as well as cancer [4, 5]. Immune system can also destroy tumor cells by recognizing tumor-specific antigens [6]. However, formation of potent antitumor immune responses requires antigen-presenting cells that can induce development of T-helper 1 (Th1) cells, which can produce the tumoricidal cytokine (also Th1 cytokine) IFNγ and aid in effector functions and activation of $CD8^+$ cytotoxic T lymphocytes (CTLs) [6, 7]. Moreover, NK cells contribute to antitumor immunity by producing the tumoricidal cytokines IFNγ, TNF-α, in addition to exerting natural or antibody-dependent cytotoxic activities via the mechanisms, such as antibody-dependent cell-mediated cytotoxicity (ADCC) [8]. Therefore, one reasonable approach for enhancing the efficacy of cancer vaccines would be to include adjuvants, which can function either as an immunostimulatory agent or as a drug delivery system that can enhance antigen-specific immune responses through efficient delivery of the antigens into APCs (Table 17.2).

## *17.2.1 Cancer Vaccine Adjuvants*

### 17.2.1.1 QS-21

QS-21 is a saponin-based adjuvant with low toxicity and the ability to stimulate antigen-specific Th1, CTL, and antibody responses. Clinical trials using QS-21 as a cancer vaccine adjuvant revealed that QS-21 provided immunogenicity in several patients with different types of tumors [9, 10]. Currently, QS-21 or combinations of QS-21 with different adjuvants are under investigation as potential vaccine adjuvants for different types of vaccines [11].

### 17.2.1.2 Immunostimulating Complex (ISCOM)

ISCOM is another saponin-based adjuvant composed of saponin, phospholipid, and cholesterol. ISCOMs form 40-nm cage-like particles, in which the antigen is captured, allowing efficient delivery of the antigen into the cells and promoting antigen-specific humoral and cellular immune responses [12]. Furthermore, clinical trials in patients with NY-ESO-1-positive tumors (including melanoma) showed that the vaccine, composed of ISCOMATRIX adjuvant and recombinant NY-ESO-1, is safe and potently immunogenic [13, 14].

### 17.2.1.3 Liposomes

Liposomes are synthetic vesicles, are composed of a phospholipid bilayer, and can be used as antigen or adjuvant delivery agents [15]. Although they are shown to promote antigen-specific humoral and cellular immune responses in experimental

**Table 17.1** Pattern-recognition receptors (PRRs) and their ligands

| Innate immune receptors (PRRs) | | Ligands (PAMPs) | Adjuvants binding to these receptors | Cellular localization | Cytokine profile | Type of immune response |
|---|---|---|---|---|---|---|
| TLRs | TLR1/2 | Triacyl lipopeptide | Pam3CSK4 | Membrane | Inflammatory cytokines | Ab, Th1, NK [49–51] |
| | TLR2/6 | Diacyl lipopeptide | Macrophage-activating lipopeptide 2 (MALP-2) | Membrane | Inflammatory cytokines, type I IFN | Ab, Th2 [52, 53] |
| | TLR3 | dsRNA | Poly I:C | Endosome | Inflammatory cytokines, type I IFN | Ab, Th1, CTL, NK [54–57] |
| | TLR4 | LPS | Monophosphoryl lipid A (MPL) | Membrane | Inflammatory cytokines, type I IFN | Ab, Th1/Th2 [58, 59] |
| | TLR5 | Bacterial flagellin | Flagellin-protein fusions | Membrane | Inflammatory cytokines | Ab, Th2, CTL [60–62] |
| | TLR7, TLR8 | ssRNA | Imiquimod (R-837), resiquimod (R-848) | Endosome | Inflammatory cytokines, type I IFN | Ab, Th1, CTL [63–65] |
| | TLR9 | Unmethylated CpG DNA | CpG ODNs (type A, type B, type C, type P) | Endosome | Inflammatory cytokines, type I IFN | Ab, Th1, CTL, NK [36, 37] |
| | TLR11 | Profilin-like protein (T. gondii) | Unknown | Membrane | Inflammatory cytokines | Unknown |
| RLRs | RIG-I | 5′-PPP ssRNA or short (~1 kb) dsRNA | Unknown | Cytosol | Inflammatory cytokines, type I IFN | Unknown |
| | MDA5 | Long (>2 kb) dsRNA | Poly I:C | Cytosol | Inflammatory cytokines, type I IFN | Th1, CTL [66] |
| NLRs | NOD1 | Peptideglycans, diaminopimelic acid (iE-DAP) | FK156, FK565 | Cytosol | Inflammatory cytokines, type I IFN | Th2 [67] |
| | NOD2 | Peptideglycans, muramyl dipeptides (MDP) | Muramyl dipeptides (MDP) | Cytosol | Inflammatory cytokines, type I IFN | Th2 [68] |
| | NLRP3 | Cellular stress, lysosomal damage | Aluminum salts, MSU, silica | Cytosol | Inflammatory cytokines | Th2 [69] |
| | NAIP5 | Bacterial flagellin | Flagellin-protein fusions | Cytosol | Inflammatory cytokines | Unknown |

| | | | | | | |
|---|---|---|---|---|---|---|
| CLRs | Dectin-1 | β1,3-Glucan | Curdlan, lentinan, schizophyllan | Membrane | Inflammatory cytokines | Th1, Th17, CTL [70, 71] |
| | Dectin-2 | High-mannose structures | Man9GlcNAc2 | Membrane | Inflammatory cytokines | Th2, Th17 [72, 73] |
| | Mincle | Trehalose-6,6-dimycolate (TDM) | Trehalose-6,6-dibehenate (TDB) | Membrane | Inflammatory cytokines | Th1, Th17 [74] |
| ALRs | AIM-2 | dsDNA | Unknown | Cytosol | Inflammatory cytokines | Th2 [75] |
| | IFI16 | dsDNA | Unknown | Cytosol | Type I IFN | Th2 [76] |

**Table 17.2** Adjuvants with their modes of action

| Adjuvants | Mode of action | Type of immune response |
|---|---|---|
| Saponins: Quil-A, QS-21, tomatine, ISCOM, ISCOMATRIX | Immunostimulants | Ab, Th1, Th2, CTL [77, 78] |
| TLR ligands: CpG ODN, poly I:C, MPLA, imiquimod | Immunostimulants (via TLR receptors) | Ab, Th1, Th2, CTL, NK [23, 36] |
| Mineral salt: alum, AS04 | Drug delivery systems (depot formation) | Th1, Th2 [20] |
| Emulsions: IFA, AS02, MF59, Montanide, QS-21 | Drug delivery systems (antigen delivery to APCs) | Th1, Th2 [22] |
| Liposomes | Drug delivery systems (antigen delivery to APCs) | Th1 [15, 16] |
| Virosomes | Drug delivery systems (antigen delivery to APCs) | Th1, Th2 [79] |

vaccines, concerns about the stable production of vaccine-grade liposomal adjuvants limited their use for human applications [16, 17].

#### 17.2.1.4 Mineral Salt

Alum is a widely used vaccine adjuvant in many different human vaccines, such as vaccines against hepatitis A virus, diphtheria, pertussis, tetanus, polio virus, human papilloma virus (HPV), or *Haemophilus influenzae* type B [18]. Nevertheless, the mechanisms mediating the adjuvant effect of alum are not fully understood. It is believed that at the injection site, aluminum salts form a depot, which allows gradual release of the antigen to provide long-term exposure of immune cells, which results in enhanced antigen-specific T- and B-cell responses to provide long-term protection. Alum is capable of enhancing antigen-specific antibody production [19], and alum-containing combination adjuvants, like AS04, have been reported to induce a mixed Th1/Th2 response against protein antigens in humans [20].

In addition, our group previously showed that adjuvant activity of alum is mediated by the host DNA release, which occurs upon alum-induced cell death. Our studies also showed that subsequent host DNA signaling induces interferon response factor 3 (IRF3)-dependent IgE and IRF3-independent IgG1-type antibody responses, which are Th2-type antibody responses. Thus, alum-induced cell death causes the release of host DNA, which mediates the adjuvant activity of alum by acting as a DAMP [21]. However, as it usually fails to induce potent cellular immune responses, which are considered protective against cancer, the use of alum as a cancer vaccine adjuvant is limited [18].

#### 17.2.1.5 Emulsions

Emulsion adjuvants, such as CFA, Montanide, and MF59, involve both water-in-oil and oil-in-water emulsion adjuvants, and, similar to alum, they function by forming a depot at the site of injection, allowing gradual release of the antigen over a long period of time to enhance antibody production by plasma cells [22]. On the other hand, some emulsion adjuvants, like CFA, cause severe inflammatory reactions at the injection site in humans, thereby limiting their application to animal vaccines, only [23].

#### 17.2.1.6 Montanide

Montanide adjuvants are emulsion adjuvants, consisting of various different types of emulsion adjuvants, like ISA 51 VG and ISA720, which are water-in-oil adjuvants prepared by using mannide monooleate family surfactants [24, 25]. Although Montanide adjuvants, like ISA 206 and 50 V, have been used only as animal vaccine adjuvants, ISA 720 and 51 have been used in clinical trials, which reported that Montanide is an efficacious adjuvant for many cancer vaccines [26, 27].

#### 17.2.1.7 MF59

MF59 is another oil-in-water emulsion adjuvant, prepared on the basis of squalene by using Tween 80 and Span 85 as surfactants for the emulsification. It forms stable nanodroplets of less than 250 nm diameter, and it has been used as an adjuvant for flu vaccines in Europe (Fluad) [23]. MF59 was shown to enhance antigen-specific antibody and balanced Th1/Th2 responses, providing protection against flu both in children and elderly [28]. Although it is rarely tested in cancer vaccines because it can also induce Th2-type responses in addition to Th1-type responses, an experimental cancer vaccine using a combination of MF59 with the TLR9 ligand, CpG oligodeoxynucleotide (CpG ODN), as an adjuvant was shown to confer protection against melanoma in explanted mouse tumor model [29].

#### 17.2.1.8 TLR Ligands

TLRs function as the PRRs of the innate immune system, recognizing conserved microbial structures and danger signals to start an immune response for elimination of intracellular pathogens or tumors [5]. TLR stimulation leads to the breakage of the immunotolerance in the APCs, to the tumor antigens by promoting the production of proinflammatory cytokines and upregulating costimulatory molecules, resulting in the generation of innate as well as adaptive immune responses against tumor [30, 31]. Especially, type I IFN production, resulting from TLR stimulation

(TLR3, TLR4, TLR7, TLR8, TLR9), has been shown to enhance antitumor immunity [32, 33]. Several TLR ligands demonstrated promising immunotherapeutic potential as a potent inducer of antitumor immune responses [6, 33].

## 17.3 Impact of TLR9 Ligand on Tumor Immunotherapy

TLR9 ligand, CpG ODN, is a synthetic single-stranded DNA molecule, resembling to microbial genomes due to its unmethylated CpG motifs, making it immunostimulatory [34, 35]. Once the TLR9 binds to CpG ODN, a signal is conveyed through the adaptor molecule MyD88 to induce production of type I IFNs in an IRF7-dependent manner while inducing proinflammatory cytokines in an NF-κB-dependent manner [36]. Moreover, in vivo, CpG ODNs have been shown to trigger a Th1-type response, being potential Th1 vaccine adjuvants for cancer vaccines [36]. Particularly, D-type CpG ODN has the ability to induce type I and type II IFN production but not B-cell activation [36, 37]. K-type CpG ODN (e.g., K3 CpG) is a weak inducer of type I and type II IFNs, but it is a potent inducer of B-cell activation to result in IL-6 and antibody production. Furthermore, CpG ODN that is available for the clinical use is K-type CpG ODN as D-type CpG ODN forms aggregates [36, 37].

CpG ODNs have shown some promising results by suppressing tumors and extending survival in clinical trials using peptide vaccines, cell vaccines, and chemotherapy [38, 39]. Despite these promising results, it is not known yet whether CpG ODNs can outperform the immunosuppression in cancer patients.

## 17.4 Modified CpG

Recently, efforts have been made to increase the efficacy of CpG ODN both as a vaccine adjuvant for various types of vaccines and as an immunotherapeutic agent for cancer. In addition to combinatorial use of CpG ODNs with other adjuvants, such efforts include chemical conjugation of CpG ODNs to the antigens or nanoparticles in order to achieve efficient delivery of both the antigen and the adjuvant to APCs. For instance, mouse studies showed that conjugation of CpG ODN to tumor antigen or nanoparticles showed superior efficacy as a cancer vaccine compared to non-modified CpG ODN [40, 41]. Furthermore, Gungor et al. reported that CpG ODN nanorings, prepared by using $Tat_{(47–57)}$ peptide of HIV origin in order to form multimerized K-type ODN nanorings, are potential cancer vaccine adjuvants with high efficacy in mouse tumor models [42].

### 17.4.1 CpG ODN + Cyclic Guanosine Monophosphate (cGAMP)

Cyclic dinucleotides, like cyclic guanosine monophosphate (cGAMP), known as bacterial second messengers, are ligands for the ER resident adaptor molecule stimulator of IFN gene (STING), which activates TBK1-IRF3 signaling axis to stimulate type I IFN production upon ligand binding [43, 44]. Studies in mice demonstrated that cyclic dinucleotides serve as potent vaccine adjuvants to enhance antigen-specific antibody and T-cell responses [45]. However, according to our previous studies, STING ligand, 5,6-dimethylxanthenone-4-acetic acid (DMXAA), induces type 2 immune responses via the mechanisms involving STING-IRF3-type I IFN pathway [46]. Since type 2 immune responses are considered undesirable for induction of antitumor immunity, therapeutic potential of cyclic dinucleotides as cancer vaccine adjuvants is limited. On the other hand, K-type CpG ODN (K3 CpG) is a Th1 adjuvant but also a weak IFN inducer, thereby limiting its immunotherapeutic applications. Thus, in order to overcome the limitations of K3 CpG and cyclic dinucleotide, cGAMP, we combined these two adjuvants, simply by mixing them, and found that TLR9 and STING agonists, K3 CpG and cGAMP, synergistically induce innate and adaptive type II IFN (IFN$\gamma$), becoming a potent type 1 adjuvant and an antitumor agent. Our in vitro studies using human PBMCs and several different mouse cells suggested that synergistic effect between K3 CpG and cGAMP culminated in IFN$\gamma$ production by NK cells and this synergistic effect is mediated by the cooperative action of IL-12 and type I IFNs. Our in vivo immunization studies in mice revealed that combination of K3 CpG and cGAMP functions as a potent type 1 adjuvant that can induce strong type 1 immune (IgG2c from B cells and IFN$\gamma$ from T cells) and CTL responses while suppressing cGAMP-induced type 2 immune responses (IgG1 from B cells and IL-13 from T cells). In addition, in mouse tumor models of thymoma (EG-7) and melanoma (B16 F10), we showed that our combination is a strong antigen-free immunotherapeutic agent for cancer. Thus, our study suggests that combination of CpG ODN and cGAMP is better than the singular use, as not only an advantageous type 1 adjuvant for vaccines requiring strong cellular immunity but also an antigen-free antitumor agent, being able to activate not only mouse cells but also human NK cells for synergistic IFN$\gamma$ production [47].

### 17.4.2 K3-SPG

Recently, our group also produced a novel nanoparticle, K3-SPG, by wrapping the nonagonistic dectin-1 ligand around K3 CpG. Our in vitro studies showed that K3-SPG became a strong inducer of type I and type II IFNs in human peripheral blood mononuclear cells. Moreover, it became a potent vaccine adjuvant capable of inducing robust antigen-specific cellular and humoral immune responses, especially

CTL responses. In addition, its adjuvant activity as an influenza vaccine adjuvant was also observed in murine and nonhuman primate models [48]. Although its efficacy as a cancer vaccine adjuvant or immunotherapeutic agent has not been tested yet, based on the type of immune responses that it induces, we believe that it may also be a useful immunotherapeutic agent for cancer.

In conclusion, studies using modified CpG ODNs, such as K3-SPG and CpG ODN nanorings, suggested that particulate forms of CpG ODN have superior adjuvant and/or immunotherapeutic potentials over CpG ODN alone due to the formation of nanoparticle structures that cause more efficient APC activation or maybe more efficient delivery of the adjuvant to the tumor site to result in the generation of potent antitumor immune responses.

## 17.5 Future Perspectives

In this review, we provide an overview of the novel adjuvants used for cancer immunotherapy. During the past years, reports from several clinical trials using adjuvanted therapeutic cancer vaccines showed promising results in several types of cancers, thereby proving the key role of adjuvants in cancer immunotherapy. Adjuvants contribute to the generation of antitumor immune responses usually by stimulating PRRs of the innate immune system and subsequently initiating an adaptive immune response against tumors. However, they can also stimulate immune responses that may contribute to tumor formation. Thus, it is critical to clarify the mechanisms of action of these adjuvants in addition to their efficacy and safety. Furthermore, elucidation of the interplay between tumor-promoting signals and innate signals may provide insights into development of novel therapeutic cancer vaccine adjuvants that can overcome the immunosuppressive microenvironment of tumors.

## References

1. Rosenberg SA (2001) Progress in human tumour immunology and immunotherapy. Nature 411:380–384
2. Cheever MA, Higano CS (2011) PROVENGE (Sipuleucel-T) in prostate cancer: the first FDA-approved therapeutic cancer vaccine. Clin Cancer Res 17:3520–3526
3. Rosenberg SA, Yang JC, Restifo NP (2004) Cancer immunotherapy: moving beyond current vaccines. Nat Med 10:909–915
4. Takeuchi O, Akira S (2010) Pattern recognition receptors and inflammation. Cell 140:805–820
5. Kawai T, Akira S (2010) The role of pattern-recognition receptors in innate immunity: update on Toll-like receptors. Nat Immunol 11:373–384
6. Vesely MD, Kershaw MH, Schreiber RD, Smyth MJ (2011) Natural innate and adaptive immunity to cancer. Annu Rev Immunol 29:235–271
7. Ossendorp F, Offringa R, Melief CJM (1999) CD4 T cells and their role in antitumor immune responses. J Exp Med 189:753–756

8. Pedroza-Pacheco I, Madrigal A, Saudemont A (2013) Interaction between natural killer cells and regulatory T cells: perspectives for immunotherapy. Cell Mol Immunol 10:222–229
9. Gilewski TA, Ragupathi G, Dickler M, Powell S, Bhuta S, Panageas K et al (2007) Immunization of high-risk breast cancer patients with clustered sTn-KLH conjugate plus the immunologic adjuvant QS-21. Clin Cancer Res 13:2977–2985
10. Galonic DP, Gin DY (2009) Chemical glycosylation in the synthesis of glycoconjugate antitumor vaccines. Nature 446:1000–1007
11. Ragupathi G, Gardner JR, Livingston PO, Gin DY (2011) Natural and synthetic saponin adjuvant QS-21 for vaccines against cancer. Expert Rev Vaccines 10:463–470
12. Sanders MT, Brown LE, Deliyannis G, Pearse MJ (2005) ISCOM-based vaccines: the second decade. Immunol Cell Biol 83:119–128
13. Chen Q, Jackson H, Parente P, Luke T, Rizkalla M, Tai TY et al (2004) Immunodominant CD4 + responses identified in a patient vaccinated with full-length NY-ESO-1 formulated with ISCOMATRIX adjuvant. Proc Natl Acad Sci U S A 101:9363–9368
14. Ian DD, Weisan C, Heather J, Phillip P, Mark S, Wendie H et al (2004) Recombinant NY-ESO-1 protein with ISCOMATRIX adjuvant induces broad integrated antibody and CD4+ and CD8+ T cell responses in humans. Proc Natl Acad Sci U S A 102:10697–10702
15. Saupe A, Mcburney W, Rades T, Hook S (2006) Immunostimulatory colloidal delivery systems for cancer vaccines. Expert Opin Drug Deliv 3:345–354
16. Shek PN, Yung BY, Stanacev NZ (1983) Comparison between multilamellar and unilamellar liposomes in enhancing antibody formation. Immunology 49:37–44
17. Gregoriadis G (1990) Immunological adjuvants: a role for liposomes. Immunol Today 11: 89–97
18. HogenEsch H (2013) Mechanism of immunopotentiation and safety of aluminum adjuvants. Front Immunol 3:1–13
19. Gavin AL, Hoebe K, Duong B, Ota T, Martin C, Beutler B et al (2006) Adjuvant-enhanced antibody responses occur without Toll-like receptor signaling. Science 314:1936–1938
20. Didierlaurent AM, Morel S, Lockman L, Giannini SL, Bisteau M, Carlsen H et al (2009) AS04, an aluminum salt- and TLR4 agonist-based adjuvant system, induces a transient localized innate immune response leading to enhanced adaptive immunity. J Immunol 183:6186–6197
21. Marichal T, Ohata K, Bedoret D, Mesnil C, Sabatel C, Kobiyama K et al (2011) DNA released from dying host cells mediates aluminum adjuvant activity. Nat Med 8:996–1002
22. Tritto E, Mosca F, De Gregorio E (2009) Mechanism of action of licensed vaccine adjuvants. Vaccine 27:3331–3334
23. Guy B (2007) The perfect mix: recent progress in adjuvant research. Nat Rev Microbiol 5: 505–517
24. Aucouturier J, Dupuis L, Deville S, Ascarateil S, Ganne V (2002) Montanide ISA 720 and 51: a new generation of water in oil emulsions as adjuvants for human vaccines. Expert Rev Vaccines 1:111–118
25. Miles AP, McClellan HA, Rausch KM, Zhu D, Whitmore MD, Singh S et al (2005) Montanide ISA 720 vaccines: quality control of emulsions, stability of formulated antigens, and comparative immunogenicity of vaccine formulations. Vaccine 23:2530–2539
26. Lawrence GW, Pye D, Saul A, Giddy AJ, Kemp R (1997) Phase I trial in humans of an oil-based adjuvant SEPPIC MONTANIDE ISA. Vaccine 15:176–178
27. Chianese-Bullock KA, Pressley J, Garbee C, Hibbitts S, Murphy C, Yamshchikov G et al (2005) MAGE-A1-, MAGE-A10-, and gp100-derived peptides are immunogenic when combined with granulocyte-macrophage colony-stimulating factor and montanide ISA-51 adjuvant and administered as part of a multipeptide vaccine for melanoma. J Immunol 174: 3080–3086
28. Podda A (2001) The adjuvanted influenza vaccines with novel adjuvants: experience with the MF59-adjuvanted vaccine. Vaccine 19:2673–2680

29. Yang M, Yan Y, Fang M, Wan M, Wu X, Zhang X et al (2012) MF59 formulated with CpG ODN as a potent adjuvant of recombinant HSP65-MUC1 for inducing anti-MUC1+ tumor immunity in mice. Int Immunopharmacol 13:408–416
30. Watts C, West MA, Zaru R (2010) TLR signalling regulated antigen presentation in dendritic cells. Curr Opin Immunol 22:124–130
31. Iwasaki A, Medzhitov R (2010) Regulation of adaptive immunity by the innate immune system. Science 327:291–295
32. Takaoka A, Tamura T, Taniguchi T (2008) Interferon regulatory factor family of transcription factors and regulation of oncogenesis. Cancer Sci 99:467–478
33. Jinushi M (2012) The role of innate immune signals in antitumor immunity. Oncoimmunology 1:189–194
34. Hartmann G, Krieg AM (2000) Mechanism and function of a newly identified CpG DNA motif in human primary B cells. J Immunol 164:944–953
35. Wagner H (2004) The immunobiology of the TLR9 subfamily. Trends Immunol 25:381–386
36. Krieg AM (2006) Therapeutic potential of Toll-like receptor 9 activation. Nat Rev Drug Discov 5:471–484
37. Klinman DM (2004) Immunotherapeutic uses of CpG oligodeoxynucleotides. Nat Rev Immunol 4:1–10
38. Pashenkov M, Goëss G, Wagner C, Hörmann M, Jandl T, Moser A et al (2006) Phase II trial of a toll-like receptor 9-activating oligonucleotide in patients with metastatic melanoma. J Clin Oncol 24:5716–5724
39. Manegold C, Gravenor D, Woytowitz D, Mezger J, Hirsh V, Albert G et al (2008) Randomized phase II trial of a toll-like receptor 9 agonist oligodeoxynucleotide, PF-3512676, in combination with first-line taxane plus platinum chemotherapy for advanced-stage non-small-cell lung cancer. J Clin Oncol 26:3979–3986
40. Cho HJ, Takabayashi K, Cheng P, Nguyen M, Corr M, Tuck S et al (2000) Immunostimulatory DNA-based vaccines induce cytotoxic lymphocyte activity by a T-helper cell-independent mechanism. Nat Biotechnol 18:509–514
41. De Titta A, Ballester M, Julier Z, Nembrini C, Jeanbart L, Van Der Vlies AJ (2013) Nanoparticle conjugation of CpG enhances adjuvancy for cellular immunity and memory recall at low dose. Proc Natl Acad Sci U S A 110:19902–19907
42. Gungor B, Yagci FC, Tincer G, Bayyurt B, Alpdundar E, Yildiz S et al (2014) CpG ODN nanorings induce IFNα from plasmacytoid dendritic cells and demonstrate potent vaccine adjuvant activity. Sci Transl Med 6:1–11
43. Burdette DL, Monroe KM, Sotelo-Troha K, Iwig JS, Eckert B, Hyodo M et al (2011) STING is a direct innate immune sensor of cyclic di-GMP. Nature 478:515–518
44. McWhirter SM, Barbalat R, Monroe KM, Fontana MF, Hyodo M, Joncker NT et al (2009) A host type I interferon response is induced by cytosolic sensing of the bacterial second messenger cyclic-di-GMP. J Exp Med 206:1899–1911
45. Li X-D, Wu J, Gao D, Wang H, Sun L, Chen ZJ (2013) Pivotal roles of cGAS-cGAMP signaling in antiviral defense and immune adjuvant effects. Science 341:1390–1394
46. Tang CK, Aoshi T, Jounai N, Ito J, Ohata K, Kobiyama K et al (2013) The chemotherapeutic agent DMXAA as a unique IRF3-dependent type-2 vaccine adjuvant. PLoS One 8:1–6
47. Temizoz B, Kuroda E, Ohata K, Jounai N, Ozasa K, Kobiyama K, Aoshi T, Ishii KJ (2015) TLR9 and STING agonists synergistically induce innate and adaptive type II IFN. Eur J Immunol 45(4):1159–1169
48. Kobiyama K, Aoshi T, Narita H, Kuroda E, Hayashi M, Tetsutani K et al (2014) Nonagonistic Dectin-1 ligand transforms CpG into a multitask nanoparticulate TLR9 agonist. Proc Natl Acad Sci U S A 111:3086–3091
49. Chassin C, Picardeau M, Goujon J-M, Bourhy P, Quellard N, Darche S et al (2009) TLR4- and TLR2-mediated B cell responses control the clearance of the bacterial pathogen, Leptospira interrogans. J Immunol 183:2669–2677

50. Taylor RC, Richmond P, Upham JW (2006) Toll-like receptor 2 ligands inhibit TH2 responses to mite allergen. J Allergy Clin Immunol 117:1148–1154
51. Szomolanyi-Tsuda E, Liang X, Welsh RM, Kurt-Jones EA, Finberg RW (2006) Role for TLR2 in NK cell-mediated control of murine cytomegalovirus in vivo. J Virol 80:4286–4291
52. Borsutzky S, Kretschmer K, Becker PD, Mühlradt PF, Kirschning CJ, Weiss S et al (2005) The mucosal adjuvant macrophage-activating lipopeptide-2 directly stimulates B lymphocytes via the TLR2 without the need of accessory cells. J Immunol 174:6308–6313
53. Rharbaoui F, Drabner B, Borsutzky S, Winckler U, Morr M, Ensoli B et al (2002) The mycoplasma-derived lipopeptide MALP-2 is a potent mucosal adjuvant. Eur J Immunol 32: 2857–2865
54. Schmidt KN, Leung B, Kwong M, Zarember KA, Satyal S, Navas TA et al (2004) APC-independent activation of NK cells by the Toll-like receptor 3 agonist double-stranded RNA. J Immunol 172:138–143
55. Navabi H, Jasani B, Reece A, Clayton A, Tabi Z, Donninger C et al (2009) A clinical grade poly I: C-analogue (Ampligen®) promotes optimal DC maturation and Th1-type T cell responses of healthy donors and cancer patients in vitro. Vaccine 27:107–115
56. Fujimoto C, Nakagawa Y, Ohara K, Takahashi H (2004) Polyriboinosinic polyribocytidylic acid [poly(I:C)]/TLR 3 signaling allows class I processing of exogenous protein and induction of HIV-specific CD8+ cytotoxic T lymphocytes. Int Immunol 16:55–63
57. Stahl-Hennig C, Eisenblätter M, Jasny E, Rzehak T, Tenner-Racz K, Trumpfheller C et al (2009) Synthetic double-stranded RNAs are adjuvants for the induction of t helper 1 and humoral immune responses to human papillomavirus in rhesus macaques. PLoS Pathog 5:1–15
58. Tan AM, Chen H-C, Pochard P, Eisenbarth SC, Herrick CA, Bottomly HK (2010) TLR4 signaling in stromal cells is critical for the initiation of allergic Th2 responses to inhaled antigen. J Immunol 184:3535–3544
59. Hayashi EA, Granato A, Paiva LS, Bertho AL, Bellio M, Nobrega A (2010) TLR4 promotes B cell maturation: independence and cooperation with B lymphocyte-activating factor. J Immunol 184:4662–4672
60. Nguyen CT, Hong SH, Sin JI, Vu HVD, Jeong K, Cho KO et al (2013) Flagellin enhances tumor-specific CD8+ T cell immune responses through TLR5 stimulation in a therapeutic cancer vaccine model. Vaccine 31:3879–3887
61. Vijay-Kumar M, Carvalho FA, Aitken JD, Fifadara NH, Gewirtz AT (2010) TLR5 or NLRC4 is necessary and sufficient for promotion of humoral immunity by flagellin. Eur J Immunol 40: 3528–3534
62. Didierlaurent A, Ferrero I, Otten LA, Dubois B, Reinhardt M, Carlsen H et al (2004) Flagellin promotes myeloid differentiation factor 88-dependent development of Th2-type response. J Immunol 172:6922–6930
63. Marin-Esteban V, Abdul M, Charron D, Haziot A, Mooney N (2008) Dendritic cells differentiated in the presence of a single-stranded viral RNA sequence conserve their ability to activate CD4 T lymphocytes but lose their capacity for Th1 polarization. Clin Vaccine Immunol 15: 954–962
64. Rechtsteiner G, Warger T, Osterloh P, Schild H, Radsak MP (2005) Priming of CTL by transcutaneous peptide immunization with imiquimod. J Immunol 174:2476–2480
65. Johnston D, Bystryn JC (2006) Topical imiquimod is a potent adjuvant to a weakly-immunogenic protein prototype vaccine. Vaccine 24:1958–1965
66. Trumpfheller C, Caskey M, Nchinda G, Longhi MP, Mizenina O, Huang Y et al (2008) The microbial mimic poly IC induces durable and protective CD4+ T cell immunity together with a dendritic cell targeted vaccine. Proc Natl Acad Sci U S A 105:1–6
67. Fritz JH, Le Bourhis L, Sellge G, Magalhaes JG, Fsihi H, Kufer TA et al (2007) Nod1-mediated innate immune recognition of peptidoglycan contributes to the onset of adaptive immunity. Immunity 26:445–459
68. Magalhaes JG, Fritz JH, Le Bourhis L, Sellge G, Travassos LH, Selvanantham T et al (2008) Nod2-dependent Th2 polarization of antigen-specific immunity. J Immunol 181:7925–7935

69. Besnard AG, Guillou N, Tschopp J, Erard F, Couillin I, Iwakura Y et al (2011) NLRP3 inflammasome is required in murine asthma in the absence of aluminum adjuvant. Eur J Allergy Clin Immunol 66:1047–1057
70. Zenaro E, Donini M, Dusi S (2009) Induction of Th1/Th17 immune response by mycobacterium tuberculosis: role of dectin-1, mannose receptor, and DC-SIGN. J Leukoc Biol 86:1393–1401
71. Agrawal S, Gupta S, Agrawal A (2010) Human dendritic cells activated via dectin-1 are efficient at priming th17, cytotoxic CD8 T and B cell responses. PLoS One 5:1–8
72. Saijo S, Ikeda S, Yamabe K, Kakuta S, Ishigame H, Akitsu A et al (2010) Dectin-2 recognition of alpha-mannans and induction of Th17 cell differentiation is essential for host defense against Candida albicans. Immunity 32:681–691
73. Barrett NA, Rahman OM, Fernandez JM, Parsons MW, Xing W, Austen KF et al (2011) Dectin-2 mediates Th2 immunity through the generation of cysteinyl leukotrienes. J Exp Med 208:593–604
74. Desel C, Werninghaus K, Ritter M, Jozefowski K, Wenzel J, Russkamp N et al (2013) The mincle-activating adjuvant TDB induces MyD88-dependent Th1 and Th17 responses through IL-1R signaling. PLoS One 8:1–9
75. Dombrowski Y, Peric M, Koglin S, Kaymakanov N, Schmezer V, Reinholz M et al (2012) Honey bee (Apis mellifera) venom induces AIM2 inflammasome activation in human keratinocytes. Allergy 67:1400–1407
76. Unterholzner L, Keating SE, Baran M, Horan KA, Jensen SB, Sharma S et al (2010) IFI16 is an innate immune sensor for intracellular DNA. Nat Immunol 11:997–1004
77. Sjölander A, van't Land B, Lövgren BK (1997) Iscoms containing purified Quillaja saponins upregulate both Th1-like and Th2-like immune responses. Cell Immunol 177:69–76
78. Duewell P, Kisser U, Heckelsmiller K, Hoves S, Stoitzner P, Koernig S et al (2011) ISCOMATRIX adjuvant combines immune activation with antigen delivery to dendritic cells in vivo leading to effective cross-priming of CD8+ T cells. J Immunol 187:55–63
79. Stegmann T, Kamphuis T, Meijerhof T, Goud E, de Haan A, Wilschut J (2010) Lipopeptide-adjuvanted respiratory syncytial virus virosomes: a safe and immunogenic non-replicating vaccine formulation. Vaccine 28:5543–5550

# Part VI
# Immunocheckpoints

# Chapter 18
# Anti-CTLA-4 Ab

**Takuto Tokudome**

**Abstract** Ipilimumab (MDX-010, BMS-734016) is a fully human monoclonal immunoglobulin (IgG1) specific for human cytotoxic T lymphocyte-associated antigen 4 (CTLA-4, CD152), which is expressed on a subset of activated T cells as a negative regulator of T-cell activation. Two phase III clinical studies (MDX010-20 and CA184-024) of ipilimumab have demonstrated a clinically meaningful and statistically significant survival benefit in pretreated advanced melanoma and previously untreated advanced melanoma, respectively (Hodi FS et al., N Engl J Med 363:711–723, 2010; Robert C et al., N Engl J Med 364:2517–2526, 2011). Ipilimumab (Yervoy™) has been approved for clinical use in advanced melanoma in over 40 countries as the first immune checkpoint inhibitor to show overall survival benefit in patients with advanced melanoma. From the experiences in both clinical development and clinical use of ipilimumab in more than 18,000 patients, some unique features of ipilimumab such as response patterns, durability of response, long-term survival benefit, immune-related adverse events (irAEs), and their management have been recognized. Challenges that contribute to the further development of ipilimumab are currently underway, including combination therapies and biomarker research.

**Keywords** Ipilimumab • CTLA-4 • Immune checkpoint inhibitor • Advanced melanoma • Durability of response • Long-term survival benefit • Immune-related adverse events (irAE)

## 18.1 Introduction

In 1970, Bretscher et al. proposed the two-signal model in which activation of T cells requires both a signal involving antigen-specific stimulation via T-cell receptor (TCR) (signal 1) and a costimulatory signal (signal 2) for the first time [1]. In subsequent decades, the engagement of CD28 by B7 (CD80 or CD86) molecules became widely understood as one of the dominant costimulatory signals as signal

T. Tokudome (✉)
Bristol-Myers K.K. Research and Development, 6-5-1 Nishi-Shinjuku, Shinjuku-ku, Tokyo 163-1328, Japan
e-mail: takuto.tokudome@bms.com



Y. Yamaguchi (ed.), *Immunotherapy of Cancer*,
DOI 10.1007/978-4-431-55031-0_18

2, and, in addition, the presence of negative costimulatory (co-inhibitory) signals that inhibit T-cell activation such as human cytotoxic T lymphocyte-associated antigen 4 (CTLA-4 or CD152) and programmed death-1 (PD-1 or CD279) were established [2, 3].

In 2011, an anti-CTLA-4 monoclonal antibody (mAb), ipilimumab (Yervoy™), was approved for clinical use in advanced melanoma as the first immune checkpoint inhibitor based on the two phase III clinical studies [4, 5]. Other immune checkpoint inhibitors such as PD-1 are currently being developed for various types of cancer. Advances in understanding the mechanisms regulating T-cell activation have allowed the development of better strategies for the immunotherapy of cancers.

## 18.2 Cytotoxic T Lymphocyte-Associated Antigen 4 (CTLA-4)

CTLA-4 was discovered as the fourth in a series of gene products identified in a subtractive cDNA library produced from activated CTLs in 1987 (hence CTL activation gene number 4, or CTLA-4) [6]. CTLA-4 is an activation-induced T-cell surface molecule that also binds B7, but with greater affinity than CD28 [7].

CTLA-4 ligation downregulates T-cell responses. Several studies have demonstrated that, in vitro, soluble anti-CTLA-4 mAb enhanced T-cell responses, whereas directly cross-linking CTLA-4 results in blockade of cell cycle progression, diminished cytokine expression, and decreased proliferation [8–11]. Blockade of CTLA-4/B7 interactions prevents induction of peripheral T-cell tolerance upon vaccination with peptides under tolerogenic conditions, suggesting that CTLA-4 is involved in the induction of anergy [12].

The observation that CTLA-4 knockout mice suffer a fatal lymphoproliferative disorder supports the idea that CTLA-4 functions as a key negative regulator of T-cell responses [13–15]. However, blockade of CTLA-4 function by the antibody does not lead to any detectable nonspecific T-cell activation or proliferation, although the antibody can augment autoimmune responses in mice prone to specific autoimmune disease [16]. Using anti-CTLA-4 mAb, CTLA-4 blockade enhanced rejection of B7-transfected tumors and induced rejection of unmodified tumor cells and immunity to rechallenge in a T-cell-dependent mechanism [17].

Blockade of CTLA-4 interaction with its ligands also enhances host responses against bacteria and parasites and limits viral spread in human immunodeficiency virus-infected T cells in vitro [18–20].

In addition to being expressed on activated effector T cells, CTLA-4 is constitutively expressed on the surface of regulatory T cells. CTLA-4 blockade can also reduce regulatory T-cell function, which may lead to an increase in antitumor immune response [21, 22]. Anti-CTLA-4 mAb may selectively deplete regulatory T cells at the tumor site, leading to an increase in the intratumoral effector/regulatory T-cell ratio which drives tumor cell death [23–25].

## 18.3 Anti-CTLA-4 Antibodies

### *18.3.1 Ipilimumab (Yervoy™)*

Ipilimumab (MDX-010, BMS-734016) is a fully human monoclonal immunoglobulin (IgG1) antibody with a half-life of approximately 14 days. The mechanism of action for ipilimumab is interference of the interaction of CTLA-4, expressed on a subset of activated T cells, with B7 molecules on antigen-presenting cells (APCs). This results in tumor antigen-specific T-cell proliferation and activation due to blockade of the inhibitory modulation of T-cell activation and thereby is believed to inhibit tumor growth (Fig. 18.1) [26].

Currently, ipilimumab (Yervoy™) has been approved for clinical use in advanced melanoma in over 40 countries as the first agent to show overall survival

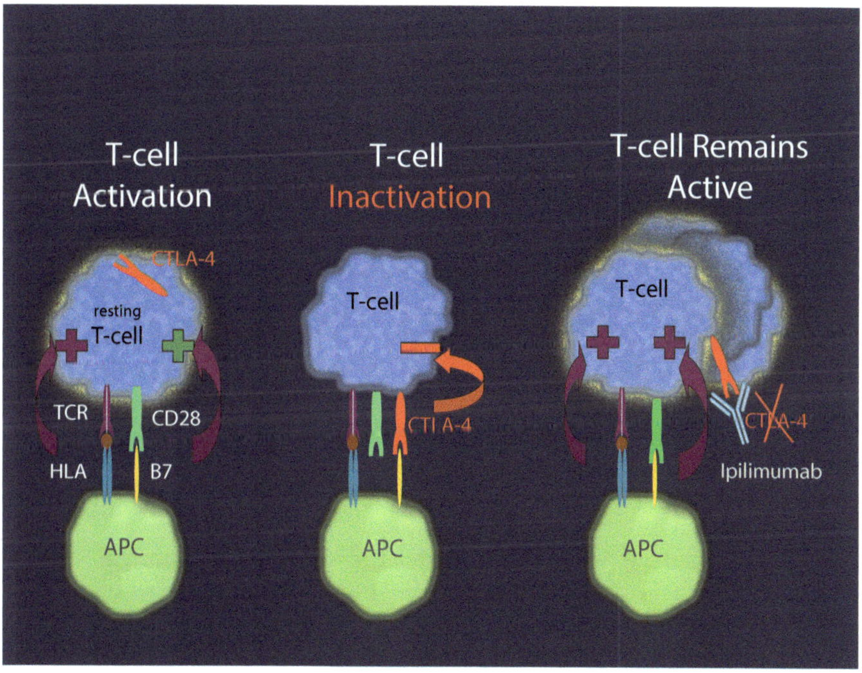


**Fig. 18.1** Ipilimumab MOA. The two key signals between APCs and T cells that are required for T-cell activation are (1) the tumor-specific antigen is presented (as a peptide on major histocompatibility complex [MHC] molecules) to the T-cell receptor and (2) a B7-costimulatory signal is delivered to the CD28 receptor. This leads to proliferation of activated T cells with the capacity to attack and kill antigen-bearing tumor cells. Subsequently, as part of a negative feedback loop, CTLA-4, a high-affinity inhibitory receptor, is expressed on activated T cells and blocks the B7-costimulatory signal, which disrupts the integrity of the immunological synapse, reduces cytokine production, and slows T-cell proliferation. With CTLA-4 blockade by ipilimumab, the negative feedback loop is interrupted, and tumor-specific T-cell activation and proliferation are potentiated and thereby are believed to inhibit tumor growth

(OS) benefit in patients with advanced melanoma. As a CTLA-4 immune checkpoint inhibitor, ipilimumab is being developed for use in the treatment of various types of cancer, including prostate cancer and lung cancer.

### *18.3.2 Tremelimumab*

Tremelimumab (CP-675,206) is another CTLA-4 immune checkpoint inhibitor (a fully monoclonal immunoglobulin [IgG2] antibody with a half-life of approximately 22 days) that is being investigated for several tumor types including advanced melanoma. In the early phase studies, tremelimumab showed promising antitumor activity in patients with advanced melanoma [27]. However, a phase III study of tremelimumab was halted after interim analysis failed to show OS benefit compared with standard therapy although the results showed favorable outcomes with tremelimumab therapy [28].

## 18.4 Clinical Development of Ipilimumab

The clinical development of ipilimumab was initiated in 2000 by Medarex Inc. (MDX), which started a joint development program with Bristol-Myers Squibb (BMS) in 2004. BMS and MDX (acquired by BMS in 2009) have cosponsored an extensive clinical development program for ipilimumab, encompassing more than 18,000 patients in several cancer types in completed and ongoing studies, as well as a compassionate use program. The focus of the clinical program is in melanoma, prostate cancer, and lung cancer, with advanced melanoma being the most comprehensively studied indication. Ipilimumab is being investigated both as monotherapy and in combination with other modalities such as chemotherapy, radiation therapy, and other immunotherapies.

In melanoma, two completed phase III studies (MDX010-20 and CA184-024) have demonstrated a clinically meaningful and statistically significant survival benefit in pretreated advanced melanoma and previously untreated advanced melanoma, respectively (data will be showed later in this chapter) [4, 5]. In 2010, a biologics license application (BLA) for ipilimumab was filed with the US Food and Drug Administration (FDA) and European Medical Agency (EMA) for approval in patients with advanced melanoma, primarily based on the MDX010-20 results (ipilimumab 3 mg/kg) on efficacy and safety. Ipilimumab (Yervoy™) has been approved for clinical use in advanced melanoma in over 40 countries including the USA (March, 2011), the EU (July, 2011), and Australia (July, 2011) as the first agent to show OS benefit in patients with advanced melanoma. Currently, ipilimumab is designated as category 1 anticancer treatment option for advanced melanoma in the National Comprehensive Cancer Network (NCCN) guideline and used regardless of BRAFV600 mutation. Also, both the NCCN and European

Society for Medical Oncology (ESMO) recommend ipilimumab for use in advanced melanoma, regardless of whether the patients have received treatment in the past or are treatment naïve [29, 30].

For prostate cancer, a completed phase III study (CA184-043) evaluated ipilimumab in patients with metastatic castration-resistant prostate cancer (mCRPC) who had progressed during or following docetaxel. Eligible patients were randomized to a single dose of bone-directed radiotherapy, followed by either ipilimumab 10 mg/kg or placebo. This study did not meet its primary endpoint of OS although the hazard ratio (HR) of 0.85 showed a favorable trend for ipilimumab [31]. A second phase III study evaluating ipilimumab 10 mg/kg versus placebo in patients with chemotherapy-naïve mCRPC with no visceral metastases is underway (CA184-095, NCT01057810).

For lung cancer, a completed large phase II study (CA184-041) has investigated the addition of ipilimumab to carboplatin and paclitaxel using two different schedules (concurrent and phased) in patients with non-small cell lung cancer (NSCLC) or small cell lung cancer (SCLC). A concurrent group consisted of four cycles of chemotherapy with ipilimumab followed by two chemotherapy cycles with a placebo. A phased group consisted of two chemotherapy cycles followed by four chemotherapy cycles with ipilimumab. The phased, but not the concurrent schedule, demonstrated activity in both NSCLC and SCLC, including significant improvement of immune-related progression-free survival (irPFS) and a favorable trend for OS improvement [32, 33]. Currently, the efficacy and safety of ipilimumab in a phased schedule with carboplatin and paclitaxel is being investigated in a phase III study in patients with squamous NSCLC (CA184-104, NCT01285609). The efficacy and safety of ipilimumab in a phased schedule with etoposide and platinum in patients with extensive disease (ED) SCLC are also being investigated in an ongoing phase III study (CA184-156, NCT01450761).

In Japan, clinical development of ipilimumab started in 2010 with a phase I study (CA184-113) to evaluate the safety of ipilimumab combined with carboplatin and paclitaxel in Japanese patients with NSCLC. The study confirmed that ipilimumab 3 and 10 mg/kg doses administered in combination with carboplatin and paclitaxel were tolerable in Japanese patients, and safety and pharmacokinetics were similar compared to non-Japanese patients [34]. For melanoma, a Japanese phase II study of ipilimumab at 10 mg/kg in combination with DTIC in chemotherapy-naïve patients with advanced melanoma (CA184-202) was conducted; however, this study was discontinued due to high incidence of severe liver toxicity (currently under publication). Another phase II study of ipilimumab monotherapy at 3 mg/kg in patients with advanced melanoma (CA184-396, NCT01990859) is underway. Except for melanoma, ipilimumab is currently being developed for NSCLC, SCLC, and gastric cancer in Japan.

## 18.5 Clinical Studies on Melanoma

### *18.5.1 Phase III Study in Previously Treated Advanced Melanoma (MDX010-20)*

The first phase III study (MDX010-20) was conducted in 676 patients with melanoma previously treated with chemotherapy. The primary endpoint of this study was to compare the OS of the groups of ipilimumab (3 mg/kg) plus peptide vaccine, gp100 ($n = 403$), ipilimumab alone ($n = 137$), and gp100 alone ($n = 136$) in a 3:1:1 ratio. Median survival was 10 months in the combination group and 10.1 months in the ipilimumab-alone group, as compared with 6.4 months in the gp100-alone group, indicating a statistically significant prolongation of OS in both comparisons (HR 0.68 and 0.66, respectively) (Fig. 18.2) [4]. No difference was observed in OS between the combination group and the ipilimumab-alone group, which suggests that it is appropriate to administer ipilimumab alone instead of coadministering gp100.

The 1-year survival rate in the combination group, the ipilimumab-alone group, and the gp100-alone group was 44 %, 46 %, and 25 %, respectively, and the 2-year survival rate 22 %, 24 %, and 14 %, respectively. Of responders in the ipilimumab-alone group, 60 % (9/15) showed response duration of more than 2 years, and there were patients in whom best overall response (BOR) improved from partial response (PR) or stable disease (SD) to complete response (CR), or from SD to PR, after 24 weeks of the first administration of ipilimumab. The survival benefit of ipilimumab in this study was observed across all relevant subgroups, including age, gender, race, metastasis stage, Eastern Cooperative Oncology Group (ECOG) performance status (PS), baseline LDH level, prior use of immunotherapy, prior use of IL-2, response to prior systemic therapy, and demographic region.

Immune-related adverse events (irAEs) occurred in approximately 56.8–59.5 % in the ipilimumab groups (the combination group and the ipilimumab-alone group) compared with 31.8 % in the gp100-alone group. Common irAEs in the combination group, the ipilimumab-alone group, and the gp100-alone group, respectively, were gastrointestinal (GI) tract (28.2 %, 31.1 %, 14.4 %), skin (42.0 %, 38.9 %, 16.7 %), liver (3.1 %, 2.1 %, 3.8 %), and endocrine (7.6 %, 3.4 %, 1.5 %). Common grade $\geq$3 irAEs were GI irAE (colitis and diarrhea), which were reported in 3–5 % in the ipilimumab groups. Most frequent drug-related AEs leading to discontinuation were diarrhea (1.5 %, 2.6 %, 0 %) and colitis (2.3 %, 2.4 %, 0 %). Of the 12 drug-related deaths in the ipilimumab groups, seven were associated with an irAE, of which four were due to GI perforation [35].

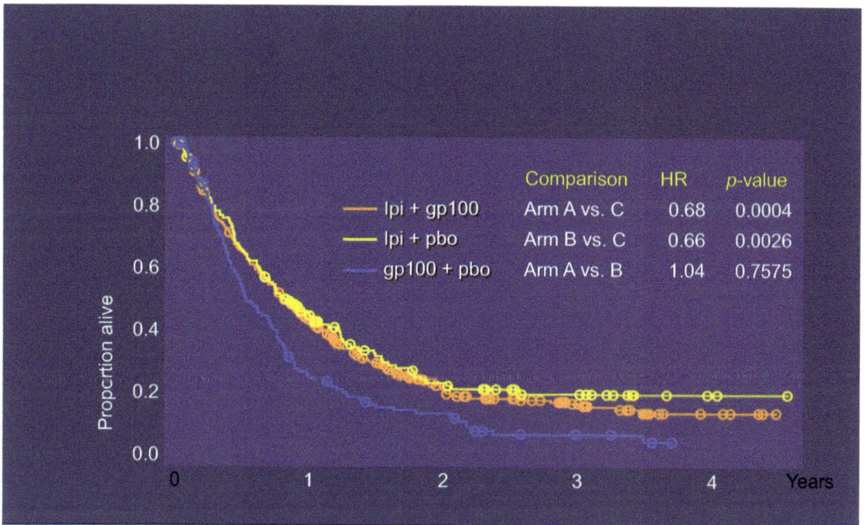


| Survival Rate | Ipi + gp100 N=403 | Ipi + pbo N=137 | gp100 + pbo N=136 |
|---|---|---|---|
| 1 year | 44% | 46% | 25% |
| 2 year | 22% | 24% | 14% |

**Fig. 18.2** Overall survival study MDX010-20. Kaplan-Meier survival curves were similar among the three groups during approximately 4 months after the treatment start, after which the curves started to divert from one another, showing a more favorable OS in ipilimumab 3 mg/kg + gp100 group and in ipilimumab 3 mg/kg group compared with gp100 group. Compared with the risk of death in gp100 group, the risk decreased by 32 % in the ipilimumab 3 mg/kg + gp100 group (hazard ratio = 0.68 [95 % CI: 0.55, 0.85], $p = 0.0004$) and by 34 % in the ipilimumab 3 mg/kg group (hazard ratio = 0.66 [95 % CI: 0.51, 0.87], $p = 0.0026$), with differences being statistically significant in both treatment groups. In contrast, no difference in the risk of death was observed between the ipilimumab 3 mg/kg + gp100 group and ipilimumab 3 mg/kg group (hazard ratio = 1.04 [95 % CI: 0.83, 1.30] $p = 0.7575$). The median OS was 9.95 months (95 % CI: 8.48, 11.50) in ipilimumab 3 mg/kg + gp100 group, 10.12 months (95 % CI: 8.02, 13.80) in ipilimumab 3 mg/kg group, and 6.44 months (95 % CI: 5.49, 8.71) in gp100 group

### *18.5.2 Phase III Study in Untreated Advanced Melanoma (CA184-024)*

Another phase III study (CA184-024) was conducted in 502 chemotherapy-naïve patients with melanoma. The primary endpoint of this study was to compare the OS in the combination group (ipilimumab 10 mg/kg plus DTIC, $n = 250$) and the DTIC-alone group ($n = 252$). Median survival was 11.2 months in the combination group and 9.1 months in the DTIC-alone group (HR 0.72; 95 % CI = 0.59–0.87), indicating 28 % decrease in the risk of death with combined use of ipilimumab. The best overall response rate (BORR) was 15.2 % (38/250) in the combination group and 10.3 % (26/252) in the DTIC-alone group. The median duration of response in

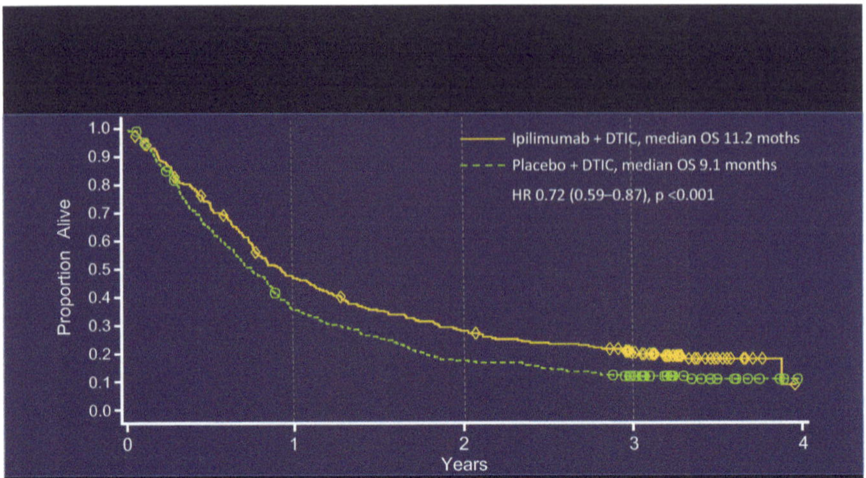


| Estimated Survival Rate | 1 Year | 2 Year | 3 Year | *4 Year | *5 Year |
|---|---|---|---|---|---|
| Ipilimumab + DTIC n=250 | 47.3 | 28.5 | 20.8 | 19.0 | 18.2 |
| Placebo + DTIC n=252 | 36.3 | 17.9 | 12.2 | 9.6 | 8.8 |

**Fig. 18.3** Overall survival study CA184-024. The hazard ratio between the two groups was 0.72 (95 % CI: 0.59, 0.87, $p = 0.0009$), showing a significant hazard reduction (by 28 %) of death in ipilimumab + DTIC group compared with DTIC monotherapy group. Kaplan-Meier survival curves were similar between the two groups up to approximately 4 months after the treatment start, after which the curves started to divert from each other, showing a significantly beneficial effect of ipilimumab + DTIC on OS compared with DTIC monotherapy. Median OS was 11.2 months (95 % CI: 9.4, 13.6) in ipilimumab + DTIC group and 9.1 months (95 % CI: 7.8, 10.5) in DTIC monotherapy group

those patients who achieved an objective response (CR and/or PR) was 19.3 months in the combination group ($n = 38$) and 8.1 months in the DTIC-alone group ($n = 26$). In the combination group and the DTIC-alone group, the 1-year survival rate was 47.3 % and 46 %, the 2-year survival rate was 28.5 % and 17.9 %, the 3-year survival rate was 20.8 % and 12.2 %, and the 4-year survival rate was 19.0 % and 9.6 %, respectively (Fig. 18.3) [5, 36].

IrAEs were reported in 75.7 % in the combination group compared with 30.7 % in the DTIC-alone group. Grade ≥3 irAEs were reported for 37.2 % in the combination group compared with 2.4 % in the DTIC-alone group. Common irAEs in the combination group and the DTIC-alone group, respectively, were the GI (35.6 % vs. 16.7 %), skin (42.9 % vs. 10.4 %), liver (36.8 % vs. 6.0 %), and endocrine (2.8 % vs. 0.8 %). Common grade ≥3 irAEs were liver irAEs (ALT/AST increased), which were reported in 27.9 % in the ipilimumab group and 2.0 % in DTIC-alone group. Grade ≥3 GI irAEs were reported in 5.7 % in the combination group and 0 % in DTIC-alone group. No GI perforation was reported in this study.

Common toxicities associated with DTIC (e.g., nausea, vomiting, and myelosuppression) were not increased in the combination group compared to the DTIC-alone group. Most frequent drug-related AEs leading to discontinuation were AST increased (17.0 %) and AST increased (16.6 %). The incidence of drug-related deaths was 0.4 % ($n = 1$) in the DTIC-alone group, and no drug-related deaths were observed in the combination group [35].

### *18.5.3 Adjuvant Therapy*

For patients with earlier stage melanoma, two phase III studies are currently being conducted.

One phase III study (CA184-029) demonstrated that ipilimumab 10 mg/kg ($n = 475$) significantly improved recurrence-free survival (RFS) compared with placebo ($n = 476$) for patients with stage III melanoma who are at high risk of recurrence following complete surgical resection. A 25 % reduction in the risk of recurrence or death was observed (HR 0.75; 95 % CI = 0.64–0.90). At 3 years, an estimated 46.5 % of patients treated with ipilimumab were free of disease recurrence compared to an estimated 34.8 % of patients on placebo. The median RFS was 26.1 months for ipilimumab vs. 17.1 months for placebo, with a median follow-up of 2.7 years. Grade ≥3 irAEs in the ipilimumab and placebo groups, respectively, were the GI (15.9 % vs. 0.8 %), liver (10.6 % vs. 0.2 %), endocrine (8.5 % vs. 0 %), and skin (4.5 % vs. 0 %). The incidence of drug-related death in the ipilimumab group was 1.1 % ($n = 5$, GI perforation in two patients), and no drug-related deaths were observed in the placebo group. Of the patients who began treatment with ipilimumab, 48.8 % discontinued treatment due to drug-related AEs as compared with 1.7 % in the placebo group [37].

Another phase III study (NCT01274338) in the adjuvant setting is underway to investigate ipilimumab at doses of 3 mg/kg and 10 mg/kg, or high-dose interferon alfa-2b in patients with high-risk stage III or resectable stage IV melanoma.

## 18.6 Unique Features of Ipilimumab

### *18.6.1 Patterns of Response*

The unique immune-based mechanism of action of ipilimumab is reflected in the clinical patterns of antitumor activity in some patients.

Ipilimumab impacts tumor cells indirectly, and measurable clinical effects emerge after the immunological effects. Tumor infiltration with lymphocytes and the associated inflammation is likely the cornerstone of the effect of ipilimumab and can manifest in various patterns of clinical activity leading to tumor control. In some cases, inflammation may not be noted by radiological examination, and objective response is observed with the first tumor assessment in a manner seen in patients receiving other types of anticancer treatments. In other cases, response may be preceded by an apparent increase in initial tumor volume and/or the appearance of new lesions, which may be mistaken for tumor progression on radiological evaluations [38]. Notably, the effects of immune activation appear to persist after discontinuation of treatment, leading to continued tumor shrinkage in some cases, durable response or stable disease, and long-term survival.

Therefore, in patients who are not experiencing rapid clinical deterioration, confirmation of progression is recommended, at the physician's discretion, to better understand the prognosis as well as to avoid unnecessarily initiating potentially toxic alternative therapies in patients who might be benefiting from treatment. Immune-related response criteria (irRC) were developed based on these observations to systematically categorize novel patterns of clinical activity and are currently being prospectively evaluated in clinical studies [39].

### 18.6.2 Durability of Response and Long-Term Survival Benefit

One of the hallmarks of ipilimumab efficacy is durability of response.

In the phase III study (MDX010-20), response duration was longer than 2 years in 60.0 % (9/15) of responders in the ipilimumab-alone group and 17.4 % (4/23) of responders in the ipilimumab plus gp100 group. Twelve out of these 13 responders had ongoing responses at the time of the primary analysis, with their response duration ranging from 26.5 to 44.4 months at censoring. A total of three patients in the ipilimumab groups maintained the response for more than 3 years (all ongoing at the primary analysis). None of the patients in the gp100-alone group remained in response at the 2-year time point [4].

In another phase III study (CA184-024), the response rate was 15.2 % in the combination group (ipilimumab plus DTIC) compared with 10.3 % in the DTIC-alone group, indicating that tumor reduction in the former group was not much greater than in the latter group. However, the duration of response in the combination group was 19.3 months, which was more than double the duration in the DTIC-alone group (8.1 months) [5].

Five-year survival rates from this study showed further long-term benefit of ipilimumab in treatment-naïve patients with advanced melanoma. The 5-year OS rates were 18.2 % for combination and 8.8 % for DTIC alone. The rates are similar to the previously reported 3-year OS rates (20.8 % in the combination group, 12.2 % in DTIC-alone group) and 4-year OS rates (19.0 % in the combination group, 9.6 % in the DTIC-alone group), suggesting that OS plateaus at the 3-year mark and the antitumor effect of ipilimumab may persist for one to several years [40].

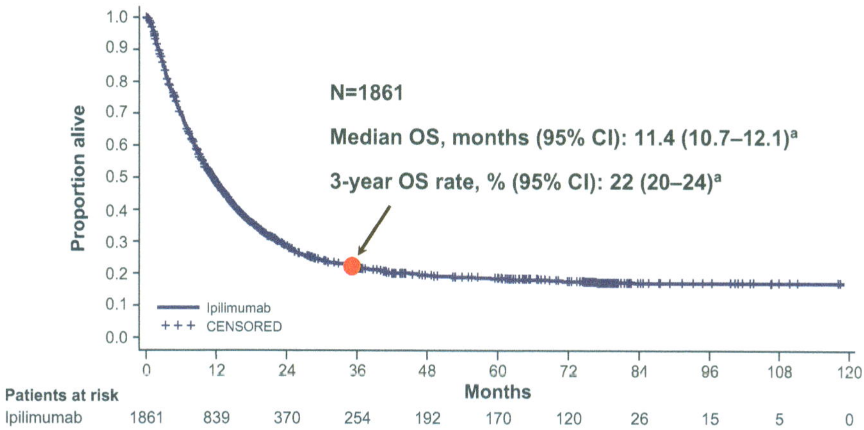


**Fig. 18.4** Pooled OS data from melanoma. In a pooled analysis of 12 studies, an OS plateau starts at approximately 3 years with follow-up of up to 10 years in some patients

The long-term survival benefit with ipilimumab beyond 3 years is also supported by a long-term follow-up from a pooled analysis of 12 prospective and retrospective ipilimumab melanoma studies for which OS data are available ($N = 1{,}861$). A total of 254 patients have a minimum follow-up of 3 years. The OS plateau appears at year 3 in previously untreated ($N = 604$) and treated ($N = 1{,}257$) patients (26 % and 20 %, respectively) with longest OS up to year 7 and 10, respectively (Fig. 18.4) [41]. The durability of ipilimumab survival benefit against melanoma has also been confirmed in other clinical studies [42].

### *18.6.3 Immune-Related Adverse Events (irAEs) and Management of irAEs*

The unique immune-based mechanism of action of ipilimumab is also reflected in the safety profile.

The safety profile of ipilimumab has been described by immune-related AEs (irAEs), which are defined as (1) AEs that are related to ipilimumab, (2) are consistent with an inflammatory process, and (3) alternative etiologies (e.g., tumor progression, infections, and other medications) can be excluded.

IrAEs primarily involve the GI tract (e.g., diarrhea, colitis), skin (e.g., pruritus, rash), and less frequently, the liver (e.g., transaminase elevations), endocrine glands (e.g., hypophysitis with hypopituitarism, hypothyroidism, or adrenal insufficiency), and nervous system (e.g., motor neuropathy, sensory neuropathy). The majority of these irAEs initially manifested during treatment; however, a minority occurred weeks to months after discontinuation of ipilimumab.

IrAEs are generally manageable using symptomatic or immunosuppressive therapy as recommended through management algorithm which was developed based on the irAE safety experience across the ipilimumab clinical program. According to the algorithm, irAEs are managed with either symptomatic therapy for mild to moderate irAEs (grades 1–2), systemic corticosteroids for severe irAEs (grade 3 or higher), or other immunosuppressants (e.g., infliximab, mycophenolate mofetil [MMF]) for steroid-unresponsive GI or liver irAEs, as appropriate. Upon irAE improvement, corticosteroids should be tapered gradually over at least 1 month. In general, moderate irAEs are managed by withholding ipilimumab, while ipilimumab should be permanently discontinued for severe irAEs [35, 43, 44].

Early diagnosis and treatment intervention for inflammatory events can help prevent the occurrence of complications, such as GI perforation. Patients should be assessed for signs and symptoms of enterocolitis, dermatitis, neuropathy, and endocrinopathy, and clinical chemistries (including liver and thyroid function tests) should be evaluated at baseline and before each dose of ipilimumab. Serological, immunological, imaging, and biopsy with histology data should be used to support the diagnosis of irAEs.

### 18.6.4 Skin irAE

The most common skin irAEs by ipilimumab are rash and pruritus with a highest incidence of approximately 50 % at all grades. Most cases are mild to moderate in severity, and the incidence of grade 3 or higher skin irAEs based on the pooled data of the monotherapy with ipilimumab at a dose of 10 mg/kg was 3 % [42]. Skin irAEs usually resolve with symptomatic therapy (topical emollients, antihistamines, etc.) or topical steroids. Two cases of fatal drug-related toxic epidermal necrolysis (TEN) was reported in clinical studies of ipilimumab [35].

### 18.6.5 Gastrointestinal (GI) irAE

The most common site for ipilimumab-induced GI irAE is the lower GI tract, and the most common presentation is mild to severe diarrhea or colitis with occasional bloody stools. In some cases, diarrhea occurs as mild and then worsens. The incidence of grade 3 or higher GI irAEs based on the pooled data was 12 % [42]. GI irAEs generally resolve by systemic corticosteroids; however, during the early phase of clinical development when steroid therapy was not adequately recommended and used, fatal cases of GI perforation were reported in melanoma studies [35]. Delay in corticosteroid treatment may be associated with a poor outcome for patients with high-grade diarrhea.

### 18.6.6 Liver irAE

Patients receiving ipilimumab may develop elevations in liver function tests (LFTs), mainly ALT/AST increased (T-Bil elevation is rare), generally in the absence of clinical symptoms. Most of inflammatory hepatitis responded to high-dose corticosteroids (IV route recommended). The incidence of grade 3 or higher liver irAEs based on the pooled data of ipilimumab monotherapy was 7 % [45]; however, grade 3 or higher ALT/AST increased was observed in approximately 30 % of the patients in the phase III study in combination with DTIC (CA184-024) [5]. Also, one phase I combination study with vemurafenib (simultaneous concomitant therapy) was discontinued due to the high incidence of liver toxicity (CA184-161, NCT01400451) [46]. LFTs should be routinely assessed and reviewed prior to administration of each dose of ipilimumab.

### 18.6.7 Endocrine irAE

The most common endocrine irAEs are hypophysitis and hypopituitarism. Secondary adrenal insufficiency, hypothyroidism or thyroiditis, and, less commonly, other endocrinopathies such as diabetes mellitus may occur. Most patients with hypopituitarism presented with nonspecific complaints such as appetite loss, fatigue, headache, hypotension, etc. Some patients with hypopituitarism can demonstrate enlarged pituitary glands based on brain MRI. Low adrenocorticotropic hormone (ACTH), low cortisol, abnormal (mostly low) thyroid-stimulating hormone (TSH), free thyroxine (fT4), and free triiodothyronine (fT3) are the most common abnormalities in clinical laboratory test. Symptoms of hypopituitarism and other endocrine toxicities were generally controlled with corticosteroid and appropriate hormone replacement; however, some laboratory abnormalities (TSH, ACTH) can be persisted for long periods of time. The endocrine irAEs are least common (6 % at any grade based on the pooled data) and slower onset, but require more time for resolution than other irAEs [45].

### 18.6.8 Neurological irAE

Neurological manifestations in patients treated with ipilimumab may include motor and/or sensory neuropathy. Fatal Guillain-Barre syndrome (GBS) and cases of myasthenia gravis (MG) were reported in clinical studies of ipilimumab [35].

Approximate onset time and course of each irAE are shown in Fig. 18.5 [45].

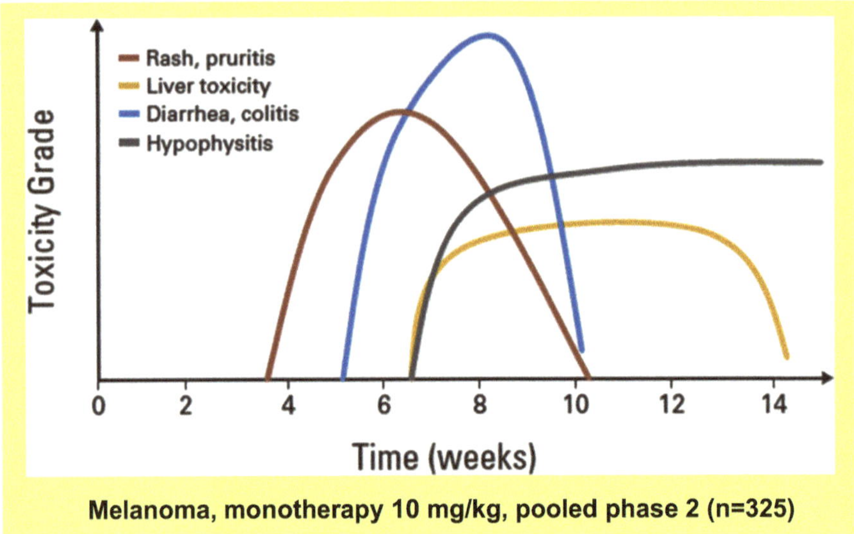


**Fig. 18.5** irAE onset time and course

# 18.7 Challenges for the Future

## *18.7.1 Optimum Dose of Ipilimumab*

The two pivotal phase III studies (MDX010-20, CA184-024) showed comparable median OS and long-term OS outcomes (1- and 2-year survival rates); however, the combination study (CA184-024, ipilimumab 10 mg/kg plus DTIC) has not been approved due to high incidence rates of severe liver toxicities (grade 3 or higher) [4, 5].

The current approval dose of ipilimumab is 3 mg/kg monotherapy. Three doses of ipilimumab (0.3 mg/kg, 3 mg/kg and 10 mg/kg) as a monotherapy were compared in a phase II study (CA184-022), and this study demonstrated dose-dependent efficacy (BORR, 0 %, 4.2 %, 11.1 %) and safety (grade 3 or higher irAEs, 0 %, 7 %, 25 %), suggesting that 10 mg/kg monotherapy was tolerable and more efficacious than 3 mg/kg monotherapy [47].

For the purpose of determining the optimum dose of ipilimumab monotherapy for advanced melanoma, one phase III study requested by FDA to compare ipilimumab 3 mg/kg vs. 10 mg/kg monotherapies in patients with advanced melanoma is ongoing (CA184-169, NCT01515189).

### 18.7.2 Combination Therapy

In the clinical development of ipilimumab for the treatment of advanced melanoma, several combination studies have been investigated.

As described earlier, the combination of ipilimumab with DTIC in the phase III study (CA184-024) developed approximately 30 % of severe liver toxicities, and the combination with peptide vaccine (gp100) in another phase III study (MDX010-20) failed to show the superiority to ipilimumab monotherapy [4, 5].

For patients with BRAF-mutated advanced melanoma, a phase I combination study with vemurafenib discontinued due to ALT/AST increased (CA184-161, NCT01400451), whereas a phase I combination study with dabrafenib did not show liver toxicity [47, 48]. The Society for Immunotherapy of Cancer (SITC) has recently described the sequential use of ipilimumab and BRAF inhibitors in the consensus statement, suggesting that ipilimumab should be given first for BRAF-mutated patients with good PS, and a BRAF inhibitor should be considered when the disease is progressing rapidly or when PS is poor [49].

At present, combined use with a PD-1 immune checkpoint inhibitor (nivolumab) is most likely to become the best combination partner for ipilimumab for the treatment of advanced melanoma. A phase I combination study demonstrated remarkable synergistic antitumor effect with tolerable safety profile in advanced melanoma (CA209-004, NCT01024231). The ORR of the initial 53 patients who received concurrent therapy was 41 % ($n = 22$). Long-term follow-up showed that 42 % of the patients had ≥80 % tumor reduction by week 36, and the 1-year and 2-year OS rates were 85 % and 79 %, respectively, with a median OS of 40 months and a median PFS of 27 weeks [50, 51]. Currently, two late-stage studies are underway to investigate the combination therapy of ipilimumab plus nivolumab vs. either agent alone in patients with advanced melanoma (NCT01844505, NCT01927419). This combination therapy has also shown promising antitumor activity in other tumor types, including renal cell carcinoma [52].

Combinations of ipilimumab with several forms of immunotherapy such as granulocyte macrophage colony-stimulating factor (GM-CSF) [53], oncolytic viral vaccines [54], dendritic cells (DCs) [55, 56], and indoleamine 2,3-dioxygenase (IDO) [57] for advanced melanoma have been recently reported. Some clinical case reports of ipilimumab combined with radiation therapy for melanoma have been recently reviewed [58, 59].

### 18.7.3 Biomarkers

Although the two phase III studies (MDX010-20 and CA184-024) indicated that ipilimumab contributes to prolongation of OS in patients with advanced melanoma, only 20–30 % of patients can enjoy the survival benefit. In addition, time of onset of antitumor effect is relatively long for ipilimumab. It is essential to find predictive biomarkers that can identify patients for whom clinical efficacy of ipilimumab can be expected at the initiation of therapy.

Retrospective analyses of several studies have suggested that there is significant correlation between safety (irAEs) and efficacy [60, 61]. Several biomarkers, including absolute lymphocyte count (ALC) [62, 63], sustained inducible T-cell co-stimulator (ICOS) [64], T-cell responses to tumor antigen NY-ESO-1 [65], myeloid-derived suppressor cells (MDSC) [66], and vascular endothelial growth factor (VEGF) [67], have been reported to be associated with clinical benefit from ipilimumab. Further prospective studies will be needed to establish the significance of these biomarker candidates. By biopsy evaluation in the tumor microenvironment, forkhead box P3 (FOXP3) and indoleamine 2,3-dioxygenase (IDO) have been reported to be correlated with clinical efficacy [68]. Expression of immune-related genes has also been reported to be a predictor of clinical efficacy in tumor microenvironment [69].

More recently, immunogenic neoantigens identified by tumor exome sequencing have been suggested to be a potentially important predictive biomarker for ipilimumab [70, 71].

## 18.8 Conclusion

An anti-CTLA-4 monoclonal antibody (mAb), ipilimumab (Yervoy™), was approved for clinical use in advanced melanoma as the first immune checkpoint inhibitor. From the abundant clinical experiences, unique features of ipilimumab such as response patterns, durability of response, long-term survival, irAEs, and its management have been identified. Future challenges including combination therapies and biomarker research are ongoing to maximize clinical benefit of ipilimumab.

## References

1. Bretscher P et al (1970) A theory of self-nonself discrimination. Science 169:1042–1049
2. Lenschow DJ et al (1996) CD28/B7 system of T-cell costimulation. Annu Rev Immunol 14:233–258
3. Ishida Y, Agata Y, Shibahara K et al (1992) Induced expression of PD-1, a novel member of the immunoglobulin gene superfamily, upon programmed cell death. EMBO J 11:3887–3895
4. Hodi FS et al (2010) Improved survival with ipilimumab in patients with metastatic melanoma. N Engl J Med 363:711–723
5. Robert C et al (2011) Ipilimumab plus dacarbazine for previously untreated metastatic melanoma. N Engl J Med 364:2517–2526
6. Brunet JF, Denizot F, Luciani MF et al (1987) A new member of the immunoglobulin superfamily – CTLA-4. Nature 328:267–270
7. Collins AV et al (2002) The interaction properties of costimulatory molecules revisited. Immunity 17:201–210

8. Kearney ER, Walunas TL, Karr RW et al (1995) Antigen-dependent clonal expansion of a trace population of antigen- specific CD4+ T cells in vivo is dependent on CD28 costimulation and inhibited by CTLA-4. J Immunol 155(3):1032–1036
9. Krummel MF et al (1995) CD28 and CTLA-4 have opposing effects on the response of T cells to stimulation. J Exp Med 182(2):459–465
10. Krummel MF et al (1996) Superantigen responses and co-stimulation: CD28 and CTLA-4 have opposing effects on T cell expansion *in vitro* and *in vivo*. Int Immunol 8(4):519–523
11. Walunas TL et al (1994) CTLA-4 can function as a negative regulator of T cell activation. Immunity 1(5):405–413
12. Perez VL, Van Parijs L, Biuckians A et al (1997) Induction of peripheral T cell tolerance in vivo requires CTLA-4 engagement. Immunity 6:411–417
13. Chambers CA et al (1997) Lymphoproliferation in CTLA-4-deficient mice is mediated by costimulation-dependent activation of CD4+ T cells. Immunity 7(6):885–895
14. Tivol EA et al (1995) Loss of CTLA-4 leads to massive lymphoproliferation and fatal multiorgan tissue destruction, revealing a critical negative regulatory role of CTLA-4. Immunity 3(5):541–547
15. Waterhouse P et al (1995) Lymphoproliferative disorders with early lethality in mice deficient in CTLA-4. Science 270(5238):985–988
16. Egen JG, Kuhns MS, Allison JP (2002) CTLA-4: new insights into its biological function and use in tumor immunotherapy. Nat Immunol 3:611–618
17. Yang YF, Zou JP, Mu J et al (1997) Enhanced induction of antitumor T-cell responses by cytotoxic T lymphocyte-associated molecule-4 blockade: the effect is manifested only at the restricted tumor-bearing stages. Cancer Res 57(18):4036–4041
18. McGaha T, Murphy JW (2000) CTLA-4 down-regulates the protective anticryptococcal cell-mediated immune response. Infect Immun 68(8):4624–4630
19. Gomes NA, Barreto-de-Souza V, Wilson ME et al (1998) Unresponsive CD4+ T lymphocytes from Leishmania chagasi-infected mice increase cytokine production and mediate parasite killing after blockade of B7-1/CTLA-4 molecular pathway. J Infect Dis 178(6):1847–1851
20. Riley JL, Schlienger K (2000) Modulation of susceptibility to HIV-1 infection by the cytotoxic T lymphocyte antigen 4 costimulatory molecule. J Exp Med 191(11):1987–1997
21. Read S et al (2006) Blockage of CTLA-4 on $CD4^{+}$ $CD25^{+}$ regulatory T cells abrogates their function in vivo. J Immunol 177(7):4376–4383
22. Wing K (2008) CTLA-4 control over $Foxp^{3+}$ regulatory T cell function. Science 322:271–275
23. Selby et al (2013) Anti CTLA 4 antibodies of IgG2a isotype enhance antitumor activity through reduction of intratumoral regulatory T. cells. Cancer Immunol Res 1:32–42
24. Simpson et al (2013) Fc-dependent depletion of tumor-infiltrating regulatory T cells co-defines the efficacy of anti-CTLA-4 therapy against melanoma. J Exp Med 210:1695
25. Liakou et al (2008) CTLA-4 blockade increases IFNγ-producing $CD4^{+}ICOS^{hi}$ cells to shift the ratio of effector to regulatory T cells in cancer patients. Proc Natl Acad Sci U S A 105:14987–14992
26. Korman AJ, Peggs KS, Allison JP (2006) Checkpoint blockade in cancer immunotherapy. Adv Immunol 90:297–339
27. Camacho LH, Antonia S, Sosman J et al (2009) Phase I/II trial of tremelimumab in patients with metastatic melanoma. J Clin Oncol 27:1075–1081
28. Ribas A, Kefford R, Marshall MA et al (2013) Phase III randomized clinical trial comparing tremelimumab with standard-of-care chemotherapy in patients with advanced melanoma. J Clin Oncol 31:616–622
29. National comprehensive cancer network clinical practice guidelines in oncology melanoma, version 3.2014
30. Dummer R, Hauschild A, Guggenheim M et al (2012) Cutaneous melanoma: ESMO clinical practice guidelines for diagnosis, treatment and follow-up. Ann Oncol 23(Supplement 7): vii86–vii91

31. Kwon ED et al (2014) Ipilimumab versus placebo after radiotherapy in patients with metastatic castration-resistant prostate cancer that had progressed after docetaxel chemotherapy (CA184-043): a multicentre, randomised, double-blind, phase 3 trial. Lancet Oncol 14:700–712
32. Lynch TJ et al (2046) Ipilimumab in combination with paclitaxel and carboplatin as first-line treatment in stage IIIB/IV non–small-cell lung cancer: results from a randomized, double-blind, multicenter phase II study. J Clin Oncol 30(17):2012
33. Reck M et al (2013) Ipilimumab in combination with paclitaxel and carboplatin as first-line therapy in extensive disease small-cell lung cancer: results from a randomized, double-blind, multicenter phase 2 trial. Ann Oncol 24:75–83
34. Nokihara H Phase 1 study of ipilimumab in combination with paclitaxel/carboplatin in patients with non-small cell lung cancer. Presented at: IASLC 15th world conference on lung cancer
35. Ipilimumab Investigator Brochure Ver.16.
36. Maio M, Bondarenko I, Robert C et al Four-year survival update for metastatic melanoma patients treated with ipilimumab plus dacarbazine on phase III study CA184-024. ESMO 2012, Abstract 1127
37. Eggermont AM et al (2014) Ipilimumab versus placebo after complete resection of stage III melanoma: initial efficacy and safety results from the EORTC 18071 phase III trial. ASCO 2014, LBA9008
38. Saenger YM et al (2008) The heterogeneity of the kinetics of response to ipilimumab in metastatic melanoma: patient cases. Cancer Immun 8:1
39. Wolchok JD et al (2009) Guidelines for the evaluation of immune therapy activity in solid tumors: immune-related response criteria. Clin Cancer Res 15:7412–7420
40. Maio M et al (2013) Survival analysis with 5 years of follow-up in a phase III study of ipilimumab and dacarbazine in metastatic melanoma. Oral presentation ESMO 2013, Abstract 3704
41. Schadendorf D, Hodi FS, Robert C et al (2013) Late breaking abstract: pooled analysis of long-term survival data from phase II and phase III trials of ipilimumab in metastatic or locally advanced, unresectable melanoma. ECCO Amsterdam, LBA24
42. Prieto PA et al (2012) CTLA-4 blockade with ipilimumab: long term follow-up of 177 patients with metastatic melanoma. Clin Cancer Res 18:2039–2047
43. YERVOY™ (ipilimumab) immune-mediated adverse reaction management guide. Available at: https://www.hcp.yervoy.com/pages/index.aspx. Accessed 9 Oct 2014
44. Giuseppina DVS et al (2014) Onco Targets Ther 7:203–209
45. Weber JS et al (2012) Management of immune-related adverse events and kinetics of response with ipilimumab. J Clin Oncol 30:2691–2697
46. Ribas A, Hodi FS, Callahan M et al (2013) Hepatotoxicity with combination of vemurafenib and ipilimumab. N Engl J Med 368:1365–1366
47. Wolchok JD et al (2010) Ipilimumab monotherapy in patients with pretreated advanced melanoma: a randomised, double-blind, multicenter, phase II, dose-ranging study. Lancet Oncol 11:155–164
48. Puzanov I, Callahan MK, Linette GP et al (2014) 1 study of the BRAF inhibitor dabrafenib (D) with or without the MEK inhibitor trametinib (T) in combination with ipilimumab (Ipi) for V600E/K mutation-positive unresectable or metastatic melanoma (MM). J Clin Oncol 32 (suppl 5S):abstr 2511
49. Kaufman HL, Kirkwood JM, Hodi FS et al (2013) The Society for Immunotherapy of Cancer consensus statement on tumour immunotherapy for the treatment of cutaneous melanoma. Nat Rev Clin Oncol 10:588–598
50. Wolchok JD et al (2013) Nivolumab plus ipilimumab in advanced melanoma. N Engl J Med 369:122–133
51. Sznol M, Kluger HM, Callahan MK et al (2014) Survival, response duration, and activity by BRAF mutation (MT) status of nivolumab (NIVO, anti-PD-1, BMS-936558, ONO 4538) and ipilimumab (IPI) concurrent therapy in advanced melanoma (MEL). J Clin Oncol 32(suppl 5S):abstr LBA9003

52. Hammers HJ, Plimack ER, Infante JR et al (2014) Phase I study of nivolumab in combination with ipilimumab in metastatic renal cell carcinoma (mRCC). J Clin Oncol 32(suppl 5S):abstr 4504
53. Hodi FS, Lee SJ, McDermott DF et al (2014) Ipilimumab plus sargramostim vs ipilimumab alone for treatment of metastatic melanoma: a randomized clinical trial. JAMA 312 (17):1744–1753
54. Puzanov I, Milhem MM, Andtbacka RHI et al (2014) Primary analysis of a phase 1b multicenter trial to evaluate safety and efficacy of talimogene laherparepvec (T-VEC) and ipilimumab (ipi) in previously untreated, unresected stage IIIB–IV melanoma. J Clin Oncol 32 (suppl 5S):abstr 9029
55. Dhodapkar MV, Sznol M, Zhao B et al (2014) Induction of antigen-specific immunity with a vaccine targeting NY-ESO-1 to the dendritic cell receptor DEC-205. Sci Transl Med 6:232ra51
56. Neyns B, Wilgenhof S, Corthals J et al (2014) Phase II study of autologous mRNA electroporated dendritic cells (TriMixDC-MEL) in combination with ipilimumab in patients with pretreated advanced melanoma. J Clin Oncol 32(suppl 5S):abstr 3014
57. Gibney GT, Hamid O, Gangadhar TC et al (2014) Preliminary results from a phase 1/2 study of INCB024360 combined with ipilimumab (ipi) in patients (pts) with melanoma. J Clin Oncol 32 (suppl 5s):abstr 3010
58. Barker CA, Postow MA, Khan SA et al (2013) Concurrent radiotherapy and ipilimumab immunotherapy for patients with melanoma. Cancer Immunol Res 1:92–98
59. Barker CA et al (2014) Combinations of radiation therapy and immunotherapy for melanoma: a review of clinical outcomes. Int J Radiat Oncol Biol Phys 88:986–997
60. Lutzky J, Wolchok J, Hamid O et al (2009) Association between immune-related adverse events and disease control or overall survival in patients with advanced melanoma treated with 10 mg/kg ipilimumab in three phase II clinical trials. J Clin Oncol 27:abstr 9034
61. Downey SG, Klapper JA, Smith FO et al (2007) Prognostic factors related to clinical response in patients with metastatic melanoma treated by CTL-associated antigen-4 blockade. Clin Cancer Res 13:6681–6688
62. Berman DM et al (2009) Association of peripheral blood absolute lymphocyte count (ALC) and clinical activity in patients with advanced melanoma treated with ipilimumab. J Clin Oncol 27:15s
63. Postow MA, Chasalow SD, Yuan J et al (2013) Pharmacodynamic effect of ipilimumab on absolute lymphocyte count (ALC) and association with overall survival in patients with advanced melanoma. J Clin Oncol 31(suppl):abstr 9052
64. Tang DN, Shen Y, Yuan J et al (2013) Increased frequency of ICOSt CD4 T cells as a pharmacodynamic biomarker for anti-CTLA-4 therapy. Cancer Immunol Res 1:229–234
65. Yuan J et al (2011) Integrated NY-ESO-1 antibody and CD8+ T-cell responses correlate with clinical benefit in advanced melanoma patients treated with ipilimumab. Proc Natl Acad Sci U S A 108:16723–16728
66. Kitano S, Postow M, Yuan J et al (2012) Myeloid derived suppressor cell quantity prior to treatment with ipilimumab at 10 mg/kg predicts for clinical benefit and improved overall survival in patients with metastatic melanoma. J Clin Oncol 30, (suppl; abstr 2518)
67. Yuan J, Zhou J, Dong Z et al (2014) Pretreatment serum VEGF is associated with clinical response and overall survival in advanced melanoma patients treated with ipilimumab. Cancer Immunol Res 2:127–132
68. Hamid O et al (2011) A prospective phase II trial exploring the association between tumor microenvironment biomarkers and clinical activity of ipilimumab in advanced melanoma. J Transl Med 9:204
69. Ji RR et al (2012) An immune-active tumor microenvironment favors clinical response to ipilimumab. Cancer Immunol Immunother 61:1019–1031

70. van Rooij N, van Buuren MM, Philips D et al (2013) Tumor exome analysis reveals neoantigen-specific T-cell reactivity in an ipilimumab-responsive melanoma. J Clin Oncol 31:e439–e442
71. Charen AS, Makarov V, Merghoub T et al (2014) The neoantigen landscape underlying clinical response to ipilimumab. J Clin Oncol 32(suppl 5S):abstr 3003

# Chapter 19
# Anti-PD-1 and Anti-PD-L1 mAbs

**Yoshimasa Tanaka, Craig T. Morita, and Haruki Okamura**

**Abstract** Programmed death-1 (PD-1) is a co-receptor molecule expressed on immune effector cells and plays a pivotal role in the down-modulation of the immune system. Upon engagement with PD-L1 or PD-L2 ligands, PD-1 delivers an inhibitory signal to immune effector cells. In animal models, the blockade of the PD-1/PD-L1 checkpoint by anti-PD-1 or anti-PD-L1 monoclonal antibodies (mAbs) is an effective strategy for reversing immunosuppression of effector T cells significantly enhancing tumor immunity in vivo. In humans, the expression of PD-1 ligands on tumor cells has been shown to correlate with poor prognosis in a wide spectrum of tumors. More recently, clinical trials have been carried out to examine the effect of inhibiting the PD-1/PD-L1 checkpoint in patients with advanced tumors. Blocking either PD-1 or PD-L1 with specific mAbs effectively treats patients with a variety of cancers including melanoma, renal cell carcinoma, non-small-cell lung cancer, and others, in some cases inducing durable remissions. Although their use is still under study to determine which cancers respond to treatment and which mAb combinations might be the most effective, blocking mAbs specific for the PD-1/PD-L1 immune checkpoint promise to revolutionize cancer therapy.

**Keywords** Co-inhibitory receptor • Monoclonal antibody • PD-1 • PD-L1 • Immune effector cells

---

Y. Tanaka (✉)
Center for Therapeutic Innovation, Graduate School of Biomedical Sciences, Nagasaki University, 1-14 Bunkyo-machi, Nagasaki 852-8521, Japan
e-mail: ystanaka@nagasaki-u.ac.jp

C.T. Morita
Division of Immunology, Department of Internal Medicine and the Interdisciplinary Graduate Program in Immunology, University of Iowa Carver College of Medicine, Iowa City, IA, USA

H. Okamura
Department of Tumor Immunology and Cell Therapy, Hyogo College of Medicine, Hyogo, Japan



Y. Yamaguchi (ed.), *Immunotherapy of Cancer*,
DOI 10.1007/978-4-431-55031-0_19

## 19.1 PD-1/PD-L1, Co-inhibitory Receptor/Ligand

T lymphocytes require signaling by T-cell receptors (TCRs) and by nonclonotypic cell surface immune co-receptors. Co-receptors such as CD28, inducible T-cell co-stimulator (ICOS), cytotoxic T-lymphocyte-associated protein-4 (CTLA-4), and programmed death-1 (PD-1) regulate the course of immune responses by amplifying or reducing the transcriptional effects of TCR triggering, which is critical for activation of immune responses and tolerance. PD-1 was originally identified by subtractive hybridization in a T-cell line undergoing activation-induced cell death [1]. This molecule is a type I transmembrane glycoprotein and one of the co-inhibitory immune receptors belonging to immunoglobulin superfamily that contains a single V-set extracellular domain, a transmembrane segment, and a cytoplasmic tail. There are two tyrosine residues in the cytoplasmic tail that could deliver a co-inhibitory signal [2, 3]. An N-terminal tyrosine residue in the immunoreceptor tyrosine-based inhibitory motif (ITIM)-like stretch is, however, not involved in the delivery of co-inhibitory signal. Instead, another tyrosine residue in the C-terminal immunoreceptor tyrosine-based switch motif (ITSM)-like region plays a pivotal role in the execution of signal cascade through recruitment of src homology 2-domain-containing tyrosine phosphatase-2 (SHP-2) [4]. Cognate receptors for PD-1 are PD-L1 (CD274, also known as B7-H1) and PD-L2 (CD273, also termed B7-DC), both of which are type I transmembrane glycoproteins that consist of tandem V-set and C1-set immunoglobulin superfamily extracellular domains, a transmembrane segment, and a cytoplasmic tail. PD-L1 is expressed on a variety of lymphohematopoietic cells including a minor population of T and B cells in the spleen, the majority of pre-B cells and myeloid cells in the bone marrow, and some subsets of thymocytes. In contrast, PD-L2 expression is restricted to dendritic cells and monocytes, but not on lymphohematopoietic cells, suggesting that the ligands function in a nonredundant manner [5–10].

Although other immune co-receptor molecules have specific motifs such as an MYPPPY motif for CD28 and CTLA-4 and a FDPPPF motif for ICOS for interaction with their cognate ligands, PD-1 lacks such motifs in its extracellular domains [11]. Our X-ray crystallographic analysis shows that PD-1/PD-L1 forms a 1:1 complex of monomeric PD-1 and PD-L1. The PD-1/PD-L1 interface consists of the side chains of residues on the β-strands (CC'FG) of PD-1 and the β-strands (GFCC') of PD-L1 [12]. The binding surface of PD-1/PD-L1 is thus significantly different from that of other co-receptor/ligand complexes and is similar to the interaction between the V domains of immunoglobulins and T-cell receptors. The dissociation constant of PD-1/PD-L1 is ~8,000 nM based on binding experiments using surface plasmon resonance, suggesting that the interaction between PD-1 and PD-L1 is weaker than the interactions between other stimulatory or inhibitory co-receptors and their ligands (2,500 nM for CD28/CD80, 2,300 nM for CD28/CD86, 200 nM for CTLA-4/CD80, and 2,200 nM for CTLA-4/CD86) [13].

## 19.2 The PD-1/PD-L1 Pathway and Autoimmune Disease

PD-1-deficient mice develop moderate, strain-dependent autoimmune diseases, such as a late-onset, progressive arthritis and a lupus-like glomerulonephritis in B6 mice [14] and cardiomyopathy in Balb/c mice [15, 16]. The autoimmune diseases can be exacerbated by the introduction of the *lpr* gene deficiency. In PD-L1-deficient mice, the responsiveness of CD4 and CD8 T cells is markedly enhanced and the cytokine production of CD4 T cells is significantly augmented, compared to T cells from wild-type mice, although no autoimmune manifestations are observed [17]. In contrast, CTLA-4-deficient mice develop massive lymphoaccumulation in secondary organs and T-cell infiltration of different tissues shortly after birth, leading to their death before 4 weeks of age [18, 19]. This dichotomy could be explained by the higher co-receptor/ligand affinity of CTLA-4 for CD80 (200 nM) compared with the affinity of PD-1 for PD-L1 (~8,000 nM). Perhaps more likely is differences in the phase of the immune response that they regulate. As noted above, PD-1 and PD-L1 deficiency does not lead to severe autoimmune disorders, probably because this co-inhibitory pathway is primarily involved in regulating the effector phase of the disease rather than the priming phase such that autoimmune cells are not generated. Thus, the major physiological role of the PD-1/PD-L1 pathway is to suppress inflammatory responses and unwanted autoimmune responses to self in the periphery.

## 19.3 PD-L1 Expression and Cancer Prognosis

Although the PD-1 signaling pathway is essential for the maintenance of peripheral tolerance and as a defense against pathogenic self-reactive cytotoxic T cells in tissues and organs, this function can be usurped by cancer cells. Expression of PD-L1 and/or PD-L2 by cancer cells can aid in their escape from immunosurveillance, immunologic recognition, and elimination. To determine the prognostic value of PD-L1/PD-L2 expression in ovarian cancer, we examined the correlation between PD-L1 expression levels on ovarian cancer cells and the patient's clinical outcome by staining tissue samples with the 27A2 monoclonal antibody (mAb) that recognizes PD-L1 in formalin-fixed, paraffin-embedded specimens. When PD-L1 expression was evaluated by immunohistochemical staining, 22 specimens (31.4 %) were scored as negative or with very weak expression and 48 specimens (68.5 %) with moderate or high expression. The overall survival rate of patients with high expression of PD-L1 was $52.6 \pm 7.7$ %, whereas patients with negative/low expression had survival rates of $80.2 \pm 8.9$ % ($p = 0.016$). The progression-free survival rate of patients with high expression of PD-L1 was $43.5 \pm 7.2$ %, whereas patients with negative/low expression had rates of $68.2 \pm 9.9$ % ($p = 0.038$). The overall survival period of patients with high expression was $6.48 \pm 0.62$ years, whereas patients with low expression survived for $9.56 \pm 0.82$ years. Thus, ovarian cancer patients whose tumors had moderate or high expression of PD-L1 had a markedly poorer prognosis than those with tumors with absent or low expression. In addition, a significant inverse correlation was observed between PD-L1 expression levels and CD8 T-cell infiltration, strongly suggesting that tumor cells expressing PD-L1 could escape from the cytotoxic activity of killer CD8 T cells [20].

Similar findings have been reported in patients with other malignancies. In patients with renal cell carcinoma, patients with higher levels (≥10 %) of PD-L1 expression on their tumors were almost three times more likely to die than those with lower expression levels (<10 %). This again suggests that PD-L1 expression on tumor cells impairs the functions of host immune cells through interaction with PD-1 to foster tumor progression [21]. Of 41 patients with esophageal cancer, 18 had tumors that expressed PD-L1 and/or PD-L2, while 23 had tumors that did not. The overall survival rate of patients whose tumors expressed PD-L1 and/or PD-L2 was significantly worse than that of negative patients, especially for patients with more advanced disease. PD-L1/PD-L2 status was shown by multivariate analysis to be an independent prognostic factor for patients with esophageal cancer [22]. Tumor expression of PD-L1 in patients with gastric carcinoma was also significantly associated with enhanced risk for death [23].

In patients with urothelial cancer, all surgically resected specimens of urothelial cancer were positive for PD-L1 expression with a mean proportion of PD-L1-positive cancer cells of 21.1 ± 11.0 %. A significant association was found between PD-L1 expression and tumor progression based on WHO grade. When the cutoff point was set at 12.2 % (which was the mean of the median percentage of PD-L1 expression), the overall survival was significantly worse in patients with higher levels of PD-L1 expression than those with lower levels. In fact, the 5-year survival rate of patients with higher PD-L1 expression levels was 55 % compared with 100 % survival for patients with lower expression. The 5-year postoperative recurrence-free survival rate for the PD-L1-high expression group was 42 %, much worse than the 81 % rate for the low expression group [24].

Expression of PD-L1 also helped to predict survival of patients with pancreatic cancer. Thirty-nine percent of pancreatic cancers (20 out of 51) were positive for PD-L1. The 1-year postoperative survival rate for these PD-L1-positive patients was 33.5 % compared with 60.5 % for PD-L1-negative patients. In addition, a significant inverse correlation was observed between PD-L1 expression on tumor cells and the proportion of CD8 T cells among tumor-infiltrating lymphocytes, strongly suggesting that PD-L1 expression on pancreatic carcinoma cells directly suppresses the numbers of infiltrating cytotoxic CD8 T cells [25].

PD-L1 levels also correlated with the vertical growth of malignant melanomas. High levels of PD-L1 were observed on melanomas from 25 out of 59 patients, and high PD-L1 levels were associated with the increased vertical growth of the melanomas. Moreover, the overall survival of patients with high PD-L1 expression was significantly lower than that of patients with low expression, indicating that, again, tumor PD-L1 expression is associated with a poorer prognosis [26].

In breast cancer patients, 152 out of 650 (23.4 %) breast cancer specimens expressed PD-L1. In univariate survival analyses, PD-L1-positive patients had a significantly lower overall survival rate (HR = 4.430, $p < 0.0001$). Additionally, breakdown of the data by breast cancer subtype showed that PD-L1 expression was associated with decreased overall survival rate in the luminal B HER2$^-$ subtype (HR = 3.888, $p < 0.0001$), the luminal B HER2$^+$ subtype (HR = 5.127, $p < 0.0001$), the HER2 subtype (HR = 2.834, $p = 0.0131$), and the basal-like subtype (HR = 4.973, $p < 0.0001$). Multivariate analyses demonstrated that PD-L1 expression in breast cancer was an independent negative prognostic factor for overall survival (HR = 3.063, $p < 0.0001$) [27].

PD-L1 and HLA class I expression was also assessed on hepatocellular carcinoma cells from 80 patients who underwent hepatectomy. Tumors from the patients could be divided into four groups: high HLA class I expression/low PD-L1 expression ($n = 21$), low HLA class I/low PD-L1 ($n = 22$), high HLA class I/high PD-L1 ($n = 23$), and low HLA class I/high PD-L1 ($n = 14$). The 10-year recurrence-free survival ($p = 0.0252$) and overall survival ($p = 0.0415$) of the high HLA class I/low PD-L1 expression group was markedly higher than those of the other three groups. Multivariate analyses demonstrated that high HLA class I/low PD-L1 expression was an independent prognostic factor in both recurrence-free survival (HR = 3.38, $p = 0.0095$) and overall survival (HR = 4.67, $p = 0.0128$) [28].

PD-L1 expression was also determined for 109 lung cancer specimens, which included 46 adenocarcinomas and 63 squamous cell carcinomas. The proportions of PD-L1-positive specimens were 65.2 and 44.4 % ($p = 0.032$) for the adenocarcinoma and squamous cell carcinoma specimens, respectively. Multivariate analyses showed that high PD-L1 expression was a negative prognostic factor in non-small-cell lung cancer [29].

In addition to measuring PD-L1 expression on the surface of tumor cells, a recent study reported high levels of soluble PD-L1 in the blood of some patients with aggressive diffuse large B-cell lymphoma. When soluble PD-L1 levels were measured in plasma samples from 288 patients, patients with plasma PD-L1 levels of 1.52 ng/ml or greater had a poorer prognosis with a 3-year overall survival rate of 76 %, compared to 89 % ($p < 0.0001$) for those with low soluble PD-L1 levels. If this is the case in other malignancies, plasma PD-L1 level could help predict which cancer patients would respond to therapy with PD-1/PD-L1 checkpoint blockade without the requirement for a tumor biopsy [30]. In summary, these studies on a broad spectrum of tumor types clearly show that elevated PD-L1 expression by a tumor is associated with a poorer prognosis.

## 19.4 Animal Models of Cancer Immunotherapy

Given that the expression of PD-L1 on tumors was a negative prognostic factor for tumor progression, these findings strongly suggested that blocking the PD-1/PD-L1 interaction could greatly enhance immune responses to tumors. We therefore examined the in vitro effect of PD-1/PD-L1 interaction on the cytotoxic activity of effector T cells. For this study, we derived a rat mAb, 1-111A, that is specific for mouse PD-L1. The 1-111A mAb was used to study the effect of blocking PD-1/PD-L1 interactions on the recognition of P815 mastocytoma cells by the 2C cytotoxic T-cell clone that expresses high levels of PD-1. Whereas the P815 cell line (that lacks PD-L1) was killed by alloreactive 2C cytotoxic T cells, P815 cells expressing PD-L1 by transfection were relatively resistant to killing. However, this was reversed by the addition of $F(ab)_2$ fragments of the 1-111A mAb such that killing was equivalent to that observed for untransfected P815 cells. These findings demonstrate that PD-1/PD-L1 engagement transduces a co-inhibitory signal to effector T cells.

To study the biological effect of PD-1/PD-L1 interactions in vivo, we used a syngeneic mouse model with P815 mastocytoma cells derived from DBA/2 mice. P815 and P815 transfectants expressing PD-L1 were injected into 7-week-old female DBA/2 mice. Whereas only 50 % of the mice injected with the parent P815 cells died by day 45, 100 % of the mice injected with PD-L1-expressing P815 cells were dead by day 27. In contrast, the growth of P815 and P815/PD-L1 cells was identical in Balb/c nu/nu mice that lack T cells. These findings clearly demonstrate that the PD-1/PD-L1 pathway negatively regulates the effector functions of immune cells in vivo allowing increased tumor growth. We then examined the effect of the blockade of PD-1/PD-L1 interactions. When PD-L1-expressing P815 cells were subcutaneously injected into DBA/2 mice, the administration of anti-PD-L1 mAb markedly inhibited local tumor growth, whereas control isotype-matched IgG had no effect. Four out of ten mice that were injected with PD-L1-expressing P815 cells and anti-PD-L1 mAb survived more than 100 days, whereas all mice that received PD-L1-expressing P815 cells and control IgG died by day 50.

This was evidence that anti-PD-L1 mAbs could be utilized as therapeutic drugs for cancer immunotherapy. To provide further supporting evidence for the use of anti-PD-L1 mAb, we examined the therapeutic effect of anti-PD-L1 mAb with other tumors. J558L myeloma cells derived from Balb/c mice naturally express high levels of PD-L1. Therefore, we subcutaneously injected J558L into Balb/c mice and treated them with an anti-PD-L1 mAb. The anti-PD-L1 mAb significantly reduced the growth of J558L cells compared to control IgG. Based on these results, we concluded that blockade of the PD-1/PD-L1 interaction by mAbs represented a promising approach for cancer immunotherapy [31].

Similar findings were observed using other murine tumors. After intravenous injection of CT26 colon cancer cells derived from Balb/c mice into syngeneic mice, tumor formation in the lung was significantly inhibited by an anti-PD-1 mAb but not by a control IgG. When B16 melanoma cells derived from C57BL/6 mice were intrasplenically injected into C57BL/6 mice, PD-1 blockade by anti-PD-1 mAb inhibited hematogenous dissemination of B16 cells to the liver. These findings clearly demonstrate that blockade of PD-1/PD-L1 interactions by anti-PD-1 mAb can also be an efficient therapeutic strategy for cancer [32]. In a different animal model using C3H/HeN mice, PD-L1-transfected mouse squamous cell carcinoma (SCC) cells were intraperitoneally injected into C3H/HeN mice. Then, T cells prepared from the syngeneic mice that had been preimmunized with SCC-pulsed dendritic cells were stimulated with an anti-CD3 mAb plus IL-2. Although

C3H/HeN mice injected with activated T cells failed to reject PD-L1-expressing SCC cells, the administration of a hamster mAb specific for mouse PD-L1 significantly prolonged the overall survival of the mice. This demonstrates that blocking PD-1/PD-L1 axis by mAb enhances the therapeutic effects of T-cell-based immunotherapy for SCC [33]. Thus, murine studies with tumors derived from a variety of tissues show that blockade of the PD-1/PD-L1 pathway with anti-PD-1 or anti-PD-L1 mAbs greatly enhances tumor immunity and prolongs survival of tumor-bearing mice.

## 19.5 Anti-PD-1 mAbs in Clinical Trials

### *19.5.1 Nivolumab*

Based on the promising results of PD-1/PD-L1 blockade in animal models, the safety and efficacy of several anti-PD-1 mAbs for cancer immunotherapy have been examined in humans. Nivolumab (MDX-1106/BMS-936568/ONO-4538) is a fully human $IgG_4$ mAb specific for human PD-1. To determine its safety and tolerability, 39 patients with advanced refractory tumors including melanoma, colorectal cancer, castration-resistant prostate cancer, non-small-cell lung cancer, and renal cell carcinoma were treated. The patients received a single intravenous infusion of nivolumab in dose-escalating 6-patient cohorts at 0.3, 1, 3, or 10 mg/kg, followed by a 15-patient cohort at 10 mg/kg. The regimen was well tolerated and associated with evidence of antitumor activity [34]. A larger phase I study was reported in 2012, in which patients with advanced melanoma, non-small-cell lung cancer, castration-resistant prostate cancer, renal cell cancer, or colorectal cancer received nivolumab at doses of 0.1–10 mg/kg every 2 weeks for up to 12 cycles until disease progression or a complete response occurred. Of 296 patients, 14 % experienced grade 3 or 4 treatment-related adverse events with three drug-related deaths due to pneumonitis. Objective responses rates (all doses) were 28 % (26/94) for patients with melanoma, 18 % (14/76) for patients with non-small-cell lung cancer, and 27 % (9/33) for patients with renal cell cancer. No responses were observed with patients with prostate cancer and colorectal cancer. PD-L1 expression could be assessed in tumors from 42 patients. Nine of the 25 (36 %) patients whose tumors expressed PD-L1 had objective responses, whereas none of the 17 patients whose tumors did not expressed PD-L1 responded [35]. A subsequent analysis of three patients from the trial was reported. A patient with colorectal cancer experienced a complete response, which was ongoing after 3 years. A patient with renal cell cancer achieved a partial response, which converted a complete response after 3 years off therapy and was ongoing at 12 months. A patient with melanoma experienced a partial response, which was stable for 16 months off therapy [36]. Further long-term follow-up analyses of 107 patients with advanced melanoma were reported. The mean overall survival rate was 16.8 months and 1- and

2-year survival rates were 62 % and 43 %, respectively [37]. PD-L1 expression on the tumor cells correlated well with objective responses to anti-PD-1 mAb therapy [38].

A combination therapy of nivolumab with peptide vaccine was performed as a phase I clinical trial. In this study, 90 patients with ipilimumab (an anti-CTLA-4 mAb)-refractory or ipilimumab-naive melanoma received nivolumab at 1, 3, or 10 mg/kg every 2 weeks for 24 weeks, then every 12 weeks for up to 2 years, with or without a multipeptide vaccine. The regimen was well tolerated and the RECIST 1.1 response rate was 25 %. These results strongly suggested the possibility that combining or sequencing therapy with nivolumab and ipilimumab for malignancies would be more effective [39]. A phase I clinical trial of nivolumab combined with ipilimumab was conducted in patients with advanced melanoma. A total of 53 patients received combined therapy with nivolumab and ipilimumab and 33 received sequenced treatment. The objective response rates of the combined and sequenced regimen groups were 40 % and 20 %, respectively, indicating that combined therapy was more effective than nivolumab alone or when used in sequenced therapy. Concurrent therapy had an acceptable side effect profile and resulted in rapid and deep tumor regression in a number of patients with several complete responses [40].

### *19.5.2 Pidilizumab*

Pidilizumab (CT-001) is a humanized $IgG_1$ mAb that binds to PD-1. In 1989, a mAb specific for Daudi, a human Burkitt's lymphoma cell line, was derived and shown to induce T-cell proliferation and increase cytotoxic activity in human peripheral blood cells [41]. The mAb had a potent antitumor effect and induced tumor regression in mice [42]. The mAbs were later shown to recognize PD-1 and were humanized for use in cancer immunotherapy. Seventeen patients with advanced stage hematologic malignancies, such as acute myeloid leukemia, chronic lymphocytic leukemia, Hodgkin lymphoma, multiple myeloma, and non-Hodgkin lymphoma, received escalating doses of pidilizumab ranging from 0.2 to 6 mg/kg. The regimen was well tolerated, and clinical benefit was observed in 33 % of the patients with one patient achieving a prolonged complete response longer than 68 weeks [43]. The safety and efficacy of pidilizumab in combination with rituximab (an anti-CD20 mAb) was examined in a phase II trial. Thirty-two patients with relapsed follicular lymphoma received pidilizumab and rituximab. The combination of pidilizumab and rituximab was well tolerated, and no autoimmune- or treatment-related adverse events of grade 3 or 4 were observed. Of 29 evaluable patients, 19 (66 %) achieved an objective response with complete responses noted in 15 (52 %) patients and partial responses in 4 (14 %) patients [44].

### *19.5.3 Pembrolizumab*

Pembrolizumab (Keytruda/lambrolizumab/MK-3475) is a humanized $IgG_4$-κ mAb specific for PD-1. A total of 135 patients with advanced melanoma received pembrolizumab at a dose of 10 mg/kg every 2 or 3 weeks or 2 mg/kg every 3 weeks, and tumor responses were assessed every 12 weeks. Common treatment-related adverse events were fatigue, rash, pruritus, and diarrhea, and thus the regimen was well tolerated. The confirmed response rate across all dose levels was 38 %. Responses were durable and the median progression-free survival was longer than 7 months [45]. The safety and efficacy of pembrolizumab was further determined in an open-label, international, multicenter expansion cohort of a phase I trial. A total of 173 patients with ipilimumab (anti-CTLA-4 mAb)-refractory advanced melanoma received pembrolizumab at 2 or 10 mg/kg every 3 weeks. Treatment was well tolerated and the response rate was 26 % at both doses [46].

## 19.6 Anti-PD-L1 mAb in Clinical Trials

BMS-936559/MDX-1105 is a fully human $IgG_4$ mAb specific for PD-L1. Because this mAb enhanced immune function in vitro and mediated antitumor activity in preclinical activity, a multicenter phase I trial was conducted. A total of 207 patients with advanced cancer including non-small-cell lung cancer, colorectal cancer, renal cell cancer, ovarian cancer, pancreatic cancer, gastric cancer, and breast cancer received escalating doses of BMS-936559 ranging from 0.3 to 10 mg/kg every 2 weeks in 6-week cycles for up to 16 cycles or until the patient had a complete response or confirmed disease progression. Treatment-related adverse events of grade 3 or 4 were observed in 9 % of patients. Of evaluable patients, 6–17 % showed objective responses, and the responses lasted for 1 year or more in 8 of 16 patients with at least 1 year of follow-up [47]. Additional anti-PD-L1 mAbs including MPDL3280A, MSB0010718C, and MED1473 are being tested in early phase clinical trials.

## 19.7 Conclusions

Cancer immunotherapy was selected by the editors of Science magazine as the breakthrough of the year in 2013 [48]. Initially, anti-CTLA-4 mAb was examined for its effects on the overall survival rate in patients with advanced melanoma, and objective responses were observed. CTLA-4 signaling is, however, primarily involved in blocking the initiation of T-cell responses in the lymph nodes, and anti-CTLA-4 mAbs therefore provoke relatively severe adverse reactions, which have been anticipated from the early lethality in mice deficient in CTLA-4 and the high affinity between CTLA-4 and CD80. By contrast, the PD-1/PD-L1 pathway is involved in the effector phase of responses to limit the activity of immune effector cells such as αβ T cells, γδ T cells [49], and NK cells in the tumor microenvironment. Thus, anti-PD-1 mAbs blocking the PD-1/PD-L1 pathway develop less adverse reactions than anti-CTLA-4 mAbs. The divergent roles of the PD-1 and CTLA-4 pathways suggest the potential for combination therapy using a high dose of anti-PD-1 mAb and a low dose of CTLA-4 mAb. Although much needs to be done, the development of immune checkpoint inhibitors has launched a new era of cancer immunotherapy.

## References

1. Ishida Y, Agata Y, Shibahara K, Honjo T (1992) Induced expression of PD-1, a novel member of the immunoglobulin gene superfamily, upon programmed cell death. EMBO J 11 (11):3887–3895
2. Shinohara T, Taniwaki M, Ishida Y, Kawaichi M, Honjo T (1994) Structure and chromosomal localization of the human PD-1 gene (PDCD1). Genomics 23(3):704–706
3. Finger LR, Pu J, Wasserman R, Vibhakar R, Louie E, Hardy RR et al (1997) The human PD-1 gene: complete cDNA, genomic organization, and developmentally regulated expression in B cell progenitors. Gene 197(1–2):177–187
4. Okazaki T, Maeda A, Nishimura H, Kurosaki T, Honjo T (2001) PD-1 Immunoreceptor inhibits B cell receptor-mediated signaling by recruiting src homology 2-domain-containing tyrosine phosphatase 2 to phosphotyrosine. Proc Natl Acad Sci U S A 98(24):13866–13871
5. Freeman GJ, Long AJ, Iwai Y, Bourque K, Chernova T, Nishimura H et al (2000) Engagement of the PD-1 immunoinhibitory receptor by a novel B7 family member leads to negative regulation of lymphocyte activation. J Exp Med 192(7):1027–1034
6. Dong H, Zhu G, Tamada K, Chen L (1999) B7-H1, a third member of the B7 family, co-stimulates T-cell proliferation and interleukin-10 secretion. Nat Med 5(12):1365–1369
7. Latchman Y, Wood CR, Chernova T, Chaudhary D, Borde M, Chernova I et al (2001) PD-L2 is a second ligand for PD-1 and inhibits T cell activation. Nat Immunol 2(3):261–268
8. Tseng SY, Otsuji M, Gorski K, Huang X, Slansky JE, Pai SI et al (2001) B7-DC, a new dendritic cell molecule with potent costimulatory properties for T cells. J Exp Med 193 (7):839–846
9. Ishida M, Iwai Y, Tanaka Y, Okazaki T, Freeman GJ, Minato N et al (2002) Differential expression of PD-L1 and PD-L2, ligands for an inhibitory receptor PD-1, in the cells of lymphohematopoietic tissues. Immunol Lett 84(1):57–62
10. Yamazaki T, Akiba H, Iwai H, Matsuda H, Aoki M, Tanno Y et al (2002) Expression of programmed death 1 ligands by murine T cells and APC. J Immunol 169(10):5538–5545
11. Agata Y, Kawasaki A, Nishimura H, Ishida Y, Tsubata T, Yagita H et al (1996) Expression of the PD-1 antigen on the surface of stimulated mouse T and B lymphocytes. Int Immunol 8 (5):765–772
12. Lin DY, Tanaka Y, Iwasaki M, Gittis AG, Su HP, Mikami B et al (2008) The PD-1/PD-L1 complex resembles the antigen-binding Fv domains of antibodies and T cell receptors. Proc Natl Acad Sci U S A 105(8):3011–3016
13. Greene JL, Leytze GM, Emswiler J, Peach R, Bajorath J, Cosand W et al (1996) Covalent dimerization of CD28/CTLA-4 and oligomerization of CD80/CD86 regulate T cell costimulatory interactions. J Biol Chem 271(43):26762–26771

14. Nishimura H, Nose M, Hiai H, Minato N, Honjo T (1999) Development of lupus-like autoimmune diseases by disruption of the PD-1 gene encoding an ITIM motif-carrying immunoreceptor. Immunity 11(2):141–151
15. Nishimura H, Okazaki T, Tanaka Y, Nakatani K, Hara M, Matsumori A et al (2001) Autoimmune dilated cardiomyopathy in PD-1 receptor-deficient mice. Science 291(5502):319–322
16. Okazaki T, Tanaka Y, Nishio R, Mitsuiye T, Mizoguchi A, Wang J et al (2003) Autoantibodies against cardiac troponin I are responsible for dilated cardiomyopathy in PD-1-deficient mice. Nat Med 9(12):1477–1483
17. Latchman YE, Liang SC, Wu Y, Chernova T, Sobel RA, Klemm M et al (2004) PD-L1-deficient mice show that PD-L1 on T cells, antigen-presenting cells, and host tissues negatively regulates T cells. Proc Natl Acad Sci U S A 101(29):10691–10696
18. Tivol EA, Borriello F, Schweitzer AN, Lynch WP, Bluestone JA, Sharpe AH (1995) Loss of CTLA-4 leads to massive lymphoproliferation and fatal multiorgan tissue destruction, revealing a critical negative regulatory role of CTLA-4. Immunity 3(5):541–547
19. Waterhouse P, Penninger JM, Timms E, Wakeham A, Shahinian A, Lee KP et al (1995) Lymphoproliferative disorders with early lethality in mice deficient in *Ctla-4*. Science 270 (5238):985–988
20. Hamanishi J, Mandai M, Iwasaki M, Okazaki T, Tanaka Y, Yamaguchi K et al (2007) Programmed cell death 1 ligand 1 and tumor-infiltrating $CD8^+$ T lymphocytes are prognostic factors of human ovarian cancer. Proc Natl Acad Sci U S A 104(9):3360–3365
21. Thompson RH, Gillett MD, Cheville JC, Lohse CM, Dong H, Webster WS et al (2004) Costimulatory B7-H1 in renal cell carcinoma patients: Indicator of tumor aggressiveness and potential therapeutic target. Proc Natl Acad Sci U S A 101(49):17174–17179
22. Ohigashi Y, Sho M, Yamada Y, Tsurui Y, Hamada K, Ikeda N et al (2005) Clinical significance of programmed death-1 ligand-1 and programmed death-1 ligand-2 expression in human esophageal cancer. Clin Cancer Res 11(8):2947–2953
23. Wu C, Zhu Y, Jiang J, Zhao J, Zhang XG, Xu N (2006) Immunohistochemical localization of programmed death-1 ligand-1 (PD-L1) in gastric carcinoma and its clinical significance. Acta Histochem 108(1):19–24
24. Nakanishi J, Wada Y, Matsumoto K, Azuma M, Kikuchi K, Ueda S (2007) Overexpression of B7-H1 (PD-L1) significantly associates with tumor grade and postoperative prognosis in human urothelial cancers. Cancer Immunol Immunother 56(8):1173–1182
25. Nomi T, Sho M, Akahori T, Hamada K, Kubo A, Kanehiro H et al (2007) Clinical significance and therapeutic potential of the programmed death 1 ligand/programmed death 1 pathway in human pancreatic cancer. Clin Cancer Res 13(7):2151–2157
26. Hino R, Kabashima K, Kato Y, Yagi H, Nakamura M, Honjo T et al (2010) Tumor cell expression of programmed cell death-1 ligand 1 is a prognostic factor for malignant melanoma. Cancer 116(7):1757–1766
27. Muenst S, Schaerli AR, Gao F, Daster S, Trella E, Droeser RA et al (2014) Expression of programmed death ligand 1 (PD-L1) is associated with poor prognosis in human breast cancer. Breast Cancer Res Treat 146(1):15–24
28. Umemoto Y, Okano S, Matsumoto Y, Nakagawara H, Matono R, Yoshiya S, et al (2015) Prognostic impact of programmed cell death 1 ligand 1 expression in human leukocyte antigen class I-positive hepatocellular carcinoma after curative hepatectomy. J Gastroenterol 50 (1):65–75; PMID: 24509608 Epub 2014-02-08
29. Mu CY, Huang JA, Chen Y, Chen C, Zhang XG (2011) High expression of PD-L1 in lung cancer may contribute to poor prognosis and tumor cells immune escape through suppressing tumor infiltrating dendritic cells maturation. Med Oncol 28(3):682–688
30. Rossille D, Gressier M, Damotte D, Maucort-Boulch D, Pangault C, Semana G, et al (2014) High level of soluble programmed cell death ligand 1 in blood impacts overall survival in aggressive diffuse large B-Cell lymphoma: results from a French multicenter clinical trial. Leukemia 28(12):2367–2375; PMID: 2432592 Epub 2014-09-05

31. Iwai Y, Ishida M, Tanaka Y, Okazaki T, Honjo T, Minato N (2002) Involvement of PD-L1 on tumor cells in the escape from host immune system and tumor immunotherapy by PD-L1 blockade. Proc Natl Acad Sci U S A 99(19):12293–12297
32. Iwai Y, Terawaki S, Honjo T (2005) PD-1 blockade inhibits hematogenous spread of poorly immunogenic tumor cells by enhanced recruitment of effector T cells. Int Immunol 17 (2):133–144
33. Strome SE, Dong H, Tamura H, Voss SG, Flies DB, Tamada K et al (2003) B7-H1 blockade augments adoptive T-cell immunotherapy for squamous cell carcinoma. Cancer Res 63 (19):6501–6505
34. Brahmer JR, Drake CG, Wollner I, Powderly JD, Picus J, Sharfman WH et al (2010) Phase I study of single-agent anti-programmed death-1 (MDX-1106) in refractory solid tumors: safety, clinical activity, pharmacodynamics, and immunologic correlates. J Clin Oncol 28 (19):3167–3175
35. Topalian SL, Hodi FS, Brahmer JR, Gettinger SN, Smith DC, McDermott DF et al (2012) Safety, activity, and immune correlates of anti-PD-1 antibody in cancer. N Engl J Med 366 (26):2443–2454
36. Lipson EJ, Sharfman WH, Drake CG, Wollner I, Taube JM, Anders RA et al (2013) Durable cancer regression off-treatment and effective reinduction therapy with an anti-PD-1 antibody. Clin Cancer Res 19(2):462–468
37. Topalian SL, Sznol M, McDermott DF, Kluger HM, Carvajal RD, Sharfman WH et al (2014) Survival, durable tumor remission, and long-term safety in patients with advanced melanoma receiving nivolumab. J Clin Oncol 32(10):1020–1030
38. Taube JM, Klein A, Brahmer JR, Xu H, Pan X, Kim JH et al (2014) Association of PD-1, PD-1 ligands, and other features of the tumor immune microenvironment with response to anti-PD-1 therapy. Clin Cancer Res 20(19):5064–5074
39. Weber JS, Kudchadkar RR, Yu B, Gallenstein D, Horak CE, Inzunza HD et al (2013) Safety, efficacy, and biomarkers of nivolumab with vaccine in ipilimumab-refractory or -naive melanoma. J Clin Oncol 31(34):4311–4318
40. Wolchok JD, Kluger H, Callahan MK, Postow MA, Rizvi NA, Lesokhin AM et al (2013) Nivolumab plus ipilimumab in advanced melanoma. N Engl J Med 369(2):122–133
41. Hardy B, Dotan D, Novogrodsky A (1989) A monoclonal antibody to human B lymphoblastoid cells activates human and murine T lymphocytes. Cell Immunol 118(1):22–29
42. Hardy B, Yampolski I, Kovjazin R, Galli M, Novogrodsky A (1994) A monoclonal antibody against a human B lymphoblastoid cell line induces tumor regression in mice. Cancer Res 54 (22):5793–5796
43. Berger R, Rotem-Yehudar R, Slama G, Landes S, Kneller A, Leiba M et al (2008) Phase I safety and pharmacokinetic study of CT-011, a humanized antibody interacting with PD-1, in patients with advanced hematologic malignancies. Clin Cancer Res 14(10):3044–3051
44. Westin JR, Chu F, Zhang M, Fayad LE, Kwak LW, Fowler N et al (2014) Safety and activity of PD1 blockade by pidilizumab in combination with rituximab in patients with relapsed follicular lymphoma: a single group, open-label, phase 2 trial. Lancet Oncol 15(1):69–77
45. Hamid O, Robert C, Daud A, Hodi FS, Hwu WJ, Kefford R et al (2013) Safety and tumor responses with lambrolizumab (anti-PD-1) in melanoma. N Engl J Med 369(2):134–144
46. Robert C, Ribas A, Wolchok JD, Hodi FS, Hamid O, Kefford R et al (2014) Anti-programmed-death-receptor-1 treatment with pembrolizumab in ipilimumab-refractory advanced melanoma: a randomised dose-comparison cohort of a phase 1 trial. Lancet 384(9948):1109–1117
47. Brahmer JR, Tykodi SS, Chow LQ, Hwu WJ, Topalian SL, Hwu P et al (2012) Safety and activity of anti-PD-L1 antibody in patients with advanced cancer. N Engl J Med 366 (26):2455–2465
48. Couzin-Frankel J (2013) Breakthrough of the year 2013. Cancer immunotherapy. Science 2013(342):1432–1433
49. Iwasaki M, Tanaka Y, Kobayashi H, Murata-Hirai K, Miyabe H, Sugie T et al (2011) Expression and function of PD-1 in human γδ T cells that recognize phosphoantigens. Eur J Immunol 41(2):345–355

# Chapter 20
# Novel Targets of Immune Inhibitory and Stimulatory Co-signals

**Koji Tamada**

**Abstract** Great success of anti-CTLA-4 and anti-PD-1 monoclonal antibodies (mAbs) has changed a landscape of cancer immunotherapy. Currently, there is no doubt about an importance of immune checkpoint molecules as one of the most promising targets in anticancer drugs. Thus, identification and characterization of novel checkpoint molecules other than CTLA-4 and PD-1 is a highly anticipated research subject. In addition, agonists of stimulatory co-signal molecules have a capability of enhancing antitumor immunity, rendering them attractive in anticancer drug development. From this perspective, this chapter introduces LAG-3, TIM-3, BTLA, 4-1BB, OX-40, and GITR, as representatives of potential targets which have been explored in cancer immunotherapy. Functions of these molecules in T cell immunity and antitumor effects in preclinical animal models as well as clinical trials, if available, are described here.

**Keywords** Immune checkpoints • T cell exhaustion • Stimulatory co-signal molecules

## 20.1 Introduction

In recent years, immune checkpoint blockade has demonstrated substantial advances and a striking success as a novel strategy in cancer immunotherapy. Anti-CTLA4 antibody (Ab) and anti-PD-1 Ab represent approaches of immune checkpoint blockade, which have been approved by FDA as drugs for advanced melanoma in 2011 and 2014, respectively. In future, application of these antibodies (Abs) is anticipated to expand through combinations with other methods of immunotherapies, e.g., tumor vaccine and adoptive T cell transfer, as well as non-immunotherapies including chemotherapeutic drugs, kinase inhibitors, and irradiation. At the same time, further efforts have been made to identify novel checkpoint molecules besides CTLA-4 and PD-1, so as to regulate the functions of

K. Tamada (✉)
Department of Immunology, Yamaguchi University Graduate School of Medicine, 1-1-1 Minami-Kogushi, Ube, Yamaguchi 755-8505, Japan
e-mail: ktamada@yamaguchi-u.ac.jp



Y. Yamaguchi (ed.), *Immunotherapy of Cancer*,
DOI 10.1007/978-4-431-55031-0_20

novel molecules for therapeutic purposes. In addition, agonistic Abs which deliver stimulatory co-signals to activate antitumor T cell responses have been also sought and tested by clinical trials as novel approaches in cancer immunotherapy. In this chapter, preclinical and clinical development of novel checkpoint molecules and stimulatory co-signal molecules is reviewed.

## 20.2 Novel Targets of Immune Checkpoint Molecules

As definition of immune checkpoint molecules, they deliver inhibitory co-signals into T cells and negatively regulate T cell responses. While they are expressed on T cells either constitutively on naïve status or inducibly in response to activation, the highest expression are often detected on nonfunctional status including exhausted T cells. Typically, checkpoint molecules possess unique intracellular motifs to deliver inhibitory signals, such as ITIM (immunoreceptor tyrosine-based inhibitory motif), which are crucial to render T cells that undergo functionally unresponsive status. Attenuation of immune checkpoint is capable of preventing and restoring the T cell unresponsiveness, providing the rationale for applying checkpoint-blocking Abs to cancer immunotherapy. According to the cells expressing ligands of checkpoint molecules, its blockade mediates the effect at two potential phases of T cell response, i.e., priming phase and effector phase. For instance, as CD80/CD86, ligands of CTLA-4, are expressed on professional APC including DC, blockade of CTLA-4 enhances T cell activation at the priming phase. On the other hand, PD-L1 (B7-H1), a ligand of PD-1, is expressed in the tumor microenvironment, e.g., tumor cells and tumor stromal cells, indicating that PD-1 blockade potentiates T cell functions at the effector phase. Collectively, immune checkpoint molecules for therapeutic targets should meet, at least in part, the following criteria: (1) capacity of delivering inhibitory signal to cause T cell unresponsiveness, (2) blockade of its functions to activate T cells by abrogating unresponsiveness, and (3) its expression on nonfunctional (e.g., exhausted) T cells and its ligand expression on APC or in the tumor microenvironment. LAG-3, TIM-3, and BTLA are among the promising and novel checkpoint molecules which meet these criteria.

### *20.2.1 LAG-3*

LAG-3 (lymphocyte activation gene-3, CD223), a molecule belonging to immunoglobulin superfamily, has structural homology to CD4 [1]. LAG-3 binds MHC class II via its D1 domain at 60 nM $K_d$, several orders higher affinity than that of CD4 for MHC class II [2]. Intracellular domain of LAG-3 contains a unique motif (KIEELE), which is essential for LAG-3 functions in T cell regulation [3, 4]. Expression of LAG-3 is detected on activated T cells, starting from 24 h after stimulation, peaking at 48 h and then gradually decreasing by day 8.

Immune-regulatory functions of LAG-3 were first revealed by experiments using anti-LAG-3 mAb, in which human CD4+ T cell clone exhibited persistent proliferation in vitro when LAG-3 was blocked [5]. Later, inhibitory function of LAG-3 was further consolidated by the studies that T cells in LAG-3 knockout (KO) animals augment proliferation, accumulation, and effector functions in response to mitogenic stimuli or cognate antigens [6, 7]. Regarding T cell inhibitory mechanism of LAG-3, transfection of LAG-3 gene lacking intracellular signaling domain lost its effects, indicating an intrinsic inhibitory mechanism [4]. On the other hand, LAG-3 expression on regulatory T cells (Treg) and its role in T cell suppression was also reported [8]. Anti-LAG-3 mAb abrogated suppressive effects of Treg, and Treg from LAG-3 KO mice reduced the suppressive activity. Ectopic expression of LAG-3 on CD4+ T cells confers them suppressive potential toward other T cells. These findings suggested extrinsic mechanisms of LAG-3 in T cell inhibition. As a cell surface marker, LAG-3 expression is associated with T cell exhaustion caused by chronic infection [9]. Recent studies further indicated that functionally impaired T cells in cancer also express LAG-3 simultaneously with PD-1 [10, 11].

Therapeutic application regulating LAG-3 functions for cancer immunotherapy has been attempted by means of LAG-3-Ig fusion proteins and anti-LAG-3 mAb. Administration of LAG-3-Ig induced growth retardation and regression of various types of tumor in mouse models [12]. It has been reported that mechanisms of antitumor effects by LAG-3-Ig are dependent on its binding to MHC class II and consequent maturation and activation of APC, including upregulated expression of co-stimulatory ligands and IL-12 production [13]. A potential role of LAG-3-Ig to block LAG-3 inhibitory signal in T cell activation remains largely unexplored. In clinical studies, LAG-3-Ig has been developed as IMP321 by Immutep and tested in renal cell carcinoma by a single agent and in breast cancer in combination with chemotherapy [14, 15]. Besides LAG-3-Ig, antagonistic anti-LAG-3 mAb has been shown to restore T cell exhaustion in mouse tumor model [11]. Accordingly, phase I clinical trial of anti-LAG-3 mAb (BMS-986016 developed by Bristol-Myers Squibb) with or without anti-PD-1 mAb in solid tumor as well as hematological malignancies has been initiated. Results of the clinical studies of LAG-3-Ig and anti-LAG-3 mAb are currently awaited with great expectations.

### *20.2.2 TIM-3*

TIM-3 belongs to TIM (T cell immunoglobulin) family molecules, type I membrane protein, which structurally consists of N-terminal IgV domain followed by a mucin domain, a transmembrane domain, and an intracellular domain [16]. In T cells, TIM-3 is uniquely expressed on those differentiated into IFN-γ-producing cells, such as Th1-type CD4+ and Tc1-type CD8+ T cells. Galectin-9, a soluble molecule that is upregulated by IFN-γ, was identified as a ligand of TIM-3 [17]. Binding of galectin-9 with TIM-3 triggers T cell death by dissociating Bat3

(HLA-B-associated transcript 3) from intracellular domain of TIM-3 [18]. Thus, TIM-3 plays an essential role in termination of IFN-γ-mediated inflammatory T cell responses. Consistent with this notion, blockade of TIM-3 by anti-TIM-3 or TIM-3-Ig fusion protein augments T cell responses, leading to exacerbation of autoimmune diseases and abrogation of T cell tolerance in animal models [19, 20]. Mice deficient of TIM-3 gene also demonstrated similar phenotypes [20].

In cancer immunotherapy, TIM-3 is a potential target as an immune checkpoint molecule to interfere with. TIM-3 expression is detected on tumor-infiltrating lymphocytes (TIL) in various types of cancer and associated with T cell exhaustion [21]. It should be noted that T cells expressing both PD-1 and TIM-3 represent the most deeply exhausted phenotype, in terms of proliferation and cytokine production of IL-2, TNF-α, and IFN-γ. Based on this finding, combined blockade of TIM-3 and PD-1 was tested and revealed a striking effect in tumor growth inhibition, more potent than a single blockade of either molecule [21, 22]. Restoration of T cell effector functions by dual blockade of TIM-3 and PD-1 has been reported in animal tumor models as well as T cells from melanoma patients [21, 23]. Besides direct effects on antitumor T cells, TIM-3 has been reported to promote granulocytic MDSC (myeloid-derived suppressor cells) via cognate interaction with galectin-9, which is expressed on $CD11b^+$ $Ly6G^+$ cells [24]. As MDSC expand in tumor-bearing hosts and facilitate immune suppression at tumor microenvironment, TIM-3 blockade could indirectly stimulate antitumor immunity by attenuating MDSC functions. In addition, recent intriguing studies discovered an increased expression of TIM-3 on leukemic cancer stem cells in patients with acute myeloid leukemia, suggesting a potential use of TIM-3 as a target for tumor killing [25, 26]. Collectively, TIM-3 could serve as a multifunctional molecule in tumor growth and antitumor immunity. Clinical trials to examine TIM-3-targeting reagents such as anti-TIM-3 mAb have yet to be initiated in cancer patients, and such studies are eagerly awaited.

### *20.2.3 BTLA*

BTLA (B and T lymphocyte attenuator, CD272) was cloned from activated T cells as a molecule structurally homologous to immunoglobulin superfamily [27]. Similar to PD-1 and CTLA-4, BTLA has one IgV domain in extracellular domain, followed by transmembrane domain and intracellular domain, where two ITIM motifs exist. The ligand of BTLA is HVEM (herpesvirus entry mediator, CD270), which belongs to TNF (tumor necrosis factor) receptor superfamily [28]. By interacting with HVEM, BTLA delivers inhibitory signal into activated T cells by recruiting SHP-1/2 via its intracellular ITIM motifs [28, 29]. Consistent with these findings, mice deficient of BTLA gene exhibited exacerbated autoimmune and inflammatory diseases [27, 30] and enhanced memory T cell responses [31]. While an increased expression of BTLA on anergic T cells was reported [32], another study indicated no correlation between BTLA expression level and a severity of T cell exhaustion [33].

Based on the findings described above, a role of HVEM-BTLA interaction in tumor immunity and its potential as a therapeutic target have been explored. In animal model, blockade of BTLA signal facilitated the effects of antitumor vaccine and inhibited tumor growth in vivo [34]. In melanoma patients, HVEM expression was detected on tumor cells, and tumor Ag-specific T cells persistently express high levels of BTLA [35]. $CD8^+$ T cells expressing BTLA were partially dysfunctional, and blockade of BTLA restored T cell proliferation and cytokine production in response to tumor Ag in vitro [33]. Thus, anti-BTLA mAb can be a novel approach of immune checkpoint blockade, although no clinical trial has initiated yet. It should be noted that HVEM-BTLA interaction can deliver bidirectional signal to both sides, where HVEM transmits stimulatory co-signal to T cells [36]. Thus, HVEM-BTLA pathway should be carefully manipulated for cancer immunotherapy, as simple blockade could diminish HVEM-mediated positive effects as well as BTLA negative signal.

## 20.3 Novel Targets of Immune Stimulatory Co-signal Molecules

Quality and quantity of T cell responses are determined by a fine balance between stimulatory and inhibitory co-signals. When stimulatory co-signals surmount inhibitory co-signals, T cells activate and generate productive responses. On the other hand, when inhibitory co-signals are dominant, T cells undergo dysfunctional state, such as anergy and exhaustion, leading to a termination of immune responses. Thus, in order to accelerate antitumor immunity, triggering stimulatory co-signals, in addition to blockade of inhibitory co-signals (=immune checkpoints), would be an important strategy. Accordingly, agonistic Abs against stimulatory co-signal molecules have been developed, and some of them are currently under clinical investigation. Abs against 4-1BB, OX-40, and GITR are among the most promising and advanced reagents in this strategy.

### *20.3.1 4-1BB*

4-1BB (CD137), a molecule of TNF receptor superfamily, is inducibly expressed on T cells along with their activation. Interaction with its ligand, 4-1BBL, triggers 4-1BB stimulatory co-signal, which activates NF-κB and MAPK via recruitment of TRAF [37]. 4-1BB signal enhances T cell activation and cytokine production and promotes their survival by inducing antiapoptotic molecules such as Bcl-$X_L$, especially in CD8+ T cells [38]. While mice deficient of 4-1BB gene exhibited a reduced number of memory CD8+ T cells in bone marrow, there is an accumulation of effector memory T cells in 4-1BB-overexpressing transgenic mice [39, 40]. Expression of 4-1BB is also detected on NK cells and DC, and stimulatory effects of 4-1BB on these cells have been also reported [41, 42].

In mouse tumor models, triggering 4-1BB stimulatory co-signal by agonistic Ab or gene transfection induced prominent effects of tumor regression [43, 44]. Mechanistically, these effects are dependent on activation of CD8+ T cells and NK cells and associated with an increased accumulation of TIL by IFN-$\gamma$ secretion [45]. Based on these studies, fully human anti-4-1BB mAbs with agonistic capacity have been developed by at least two pharmaceutical companies. Although early results from clinical trials indicated a substantial liver toxicity, more detailed examinations of anti-4-1BB mAbs as monotherapy or in combination with other mAbs are currently performed in patients with solid tumors and hematological malignancies [46].

### *20.3.2 OX-40*

OX-40 (CD134) is a member of TNF receptor superfamily and originally identified as an activation marker on rat CD4+ T cells [47]. Subsequent studies revealed that OX-40 is expressed on both CD4+ and CD8+ T cells upon activation, as well as NK cells, and OX-40 signal promotes proliferation, cytokine production, migration, and effector functions of these cells [48]. Mice deficient of OX-40 or OX-40L, a ligand of OX-40, exhibited impaired T cell responses in vivo, indicating a role of this pathway in providing a stimulatory co-signal to T cells [49, 50]. In animal experiments, administration of OX-40 agonists, including anti-OX-40 mAb and OX-40L-Ig fusion protein, prolonged the mouse survival in various tumor models [51]. In addition to direct effects in stimulating T cell activation, there is also evidence that OX-40 agonists dampen suppressive function of Treg, thus indirectly facilitate antitumor immunity [52, 53]. In cancer patients, the existence of OX-40-positive T cells in TIL and tumor-draining lymph nodes has been reported [54]. Phase I clinical trial using anti-OX-40 mAb demonstrated that the drug was tolerated, promoted T cell proliferation, and induced tumor shrinkage in some patients [55]. Further studies of OX-40 agonists are currently underway in clinical trials to evaluate its antitumor effects as monotherapy or in combination with other drugs.

### *20.3.3 GITR*

GITR (glucocorticoid-induced TNF receptor, CD357) is expressed on various immune cells including activated T cells. GITR signal delivers stimulatory co-signal into T cells and enhances their proliferation, cytokine production, and survival [56]. Compared to other stimulatory co-signal molecules, GITR has a unique feature that is constitutively expressed on Treg at high levels, and triggering GITR signal in Treg abrogates their suppressive function [57, 58]. As expected from these findings, treatment with anti-GITR agonistic mAb caused regression of tumor in animal models [59, 60]. Further studies suggested that GITR agonists decrease the number and suppressive function of Treg at the tumor microenvironment by causing Treg instability and depletion [61, 62]. A phase I clinical trial using humanized anti-GITR agonistic mAb in advanced melanoma and other solid tumors is currently ongoing.

## 20.4 Summary

Recent development of anti-CTLA-4 and anti-PD-1 mAbs represents magnificent success in cancer immunotherapy. Accordingly, approaches to manipulate inhibitory or stimulatory co-signal functions are considered to be a rising star in the field, and identification of novel targets with a potent therapeutic potential is eagerly anticipated. While this review focuses on several novel molecules which are among the most promising and progressive in clinical translation, there are many other intriguing targets which are not introduced here. Development of novel reagents to regulate these molecules as monotherapy or combined immunotherapy with current medical interventions including kinase inhibitors, chemotherapy, and radiotherapy will establish next generation of cancer treatment.

## References


1. Baixeras E, Huard B, Miossec C, Jitsukawa S, Martin M, Hercend T, Auffray C, Triebel F, Piatier-Tonneau D (1992) Characterization of the lymphocyte activation gene 3-encoded protein. A new ligand for human leukocyte antigen class II antigens. J Exp Med 176:327–337
2. Huard B, Prigent P, Tournier M, Bruniquel D, Triebel F (1995) CD4/major histocompatibility complex class II interaction analyzed with CD4- and lymphocyte activation gene-3 (LAG-3)-Ig fusion proteins. Eur J Immunol 25:2718–2721
3. Workman CJ, Vignali DA (2003) The CD4-related molecule, LAG-3 (CD223), regulates the expansion of activated T cells. Eur J Immunol 33:970–979
4. Workman CJ, Dugger KJ, Vignali DA (2002) Cutting edge: molecular analysis of the negative regulatory function of lymphocyte activation gene-3. J Immunol 169:5392–5395
5. Huard B, Tournier M, Hercend T, Triebel F, Faure F (1994) Lymphocyte-activation gene 3/major histocompatibility complex class II interaction modulates the antigenic response of CD4+ T lymphocytes. Eur J Immunol 24:3216–3221
6. Workman CJ, Cauley LS, Kim IJ, Blackman MA, Woodland DL, Vignali DA (2004) Lymphocyte activation gene-3 (CD223) regulates the size of the expanding T cell population following antigen activation in vivo. J Immunol 172:5450–5455
7. Grosso JF, Kelleher CC, Harris TJ, Maris CH, Hipkiss EL, De Marzo A, Anders R, Netto G, Getnet D, Bruno TC et al (2007) LAG-3 regulates CD8+ T cell accumulation and effector function in murine self- and tumor-tolerance systems. J Clin Invest 117:3383–3392

8. Huang CT, Workman CJ, Flies D, Pan X, Marson AL, Zhou G, Hipkiss EL, Ravi S, Kowalski J, Levitsky HI et al (2004) Role of LAG-3 in regulatory T cells. Immunity 21:503–513
9. Blackburn SD, Shin H, Haining WN, Zou T, Workman CJ, Polley A, Betts MR, Freeman GJ, Vignali DA, Wherry EJ (2009) Coregulation of CD8+ T cell exhaustion by multiple inhibitory receptors during chronic viral infection. Nat Immunol 10:29–37
10. Matsuzaki J, Gnjatic S, Mhawech-Fauceglia P, Beck A, Miller A, Tsuji T, Eppolito C, Qian F, Lele S, Shrikant P et al (2010) Tumor-infiltrating NY-ESO-1-specific CD8+ T cells are negatively regulated by LAG-3 and PD-1 in human ovarian cancer. Proc Natl Acad Sci U S A 107:7875–7880
11. Goding SR, Wilson KA, Xie Y, Harris KM, Baxi A, Akpinarli A, Fulton A, Tamada K, Strome SE, Antony PA (2013) Restoring immune function of tumor-specific CD4+ T cells during recurrence of melanoma. J Immunol 190:4899–4909
12. Prigent P, El Mir S, Dreano M, Triebel F (1999) Lymphocyte activation gene-3 induces tumor regression and antitumor immune responses. Eur J Immunol 29:3867–3876
13. Andreae S, Piras F, Burdin N, Triebel F (2002) Maturation and activation of dendritic cells induced by lymphocyte activation gene-3 (CD223). J Immunol 168:3874–3880
14. Brignone C, Escudier B, Grygar C, Marcu M, Triebel F (2009) A phase I pharmacokinetic and biological correlative study of IMP321, a novel MHC class II agonist, in patients with advanced renal cell carcinoma. Clin Cancer Res 15:6225–6231
15. Brignone C, Gutierrez M, Mefti F, Brain E, Jarcau R, Cvitkovic F, Bousetta N, Medioni J, Gligorov J, Grygar C et al (2010) First-line chemoimmunotherapy in metastatic breast carcinoma: combination of paclitaxel and IMP321 (LAG-3Ig) enhances immune responses and antitumor activity. J Transl Med 8:71
16. Monney L, Sabatos CA, Gaglia JL, Ryu A, Waldner H, Chernova T, Manning S, Greenfield EA, Coyle AJ, Sobel RA et al (2002) Th1-specific cell surface protein Tim-3 regulates macrophage activation and severity of an autoimmune disease. Nature 415:536–541
17. Zhu C, Anderson AC, Schubart A, Xiong H, Imitola J, Khoury SJ, Zheng XX, Strom TB, Kuchroo VK (2005) The Tim-3 ligand galectin-9 negatively regulates T helper type 1 immunity. Nat Immunol 6:1245–1252
18. Rangachari M, Zhu C, Sakuishi K, Xiao S, Karman J, Chen A, Angin M, Wakeham A, Greenfield EA, Sobel RA et al (2012) Bat3 promotes T cell responses and autoimmunity by repressing Tim-3-mediated cell death and exhaustion. Nat Med 18:1394–1400
19. Sanchez-Fueyo A, Tian J, Picarella D, Domenig C, Zheng XX, Sabatos CA, Manlongat N, Bender O, Kamradt T, Kuchroo VK et al (2003) Tim-3 inhibits T helper type 1-mediated auto- and alloimmune responses and promotes immunological tolerance. Nat Immunol 4:1093–1101
20. Sabatos CA, Chakravarti S, Cha E, Schubart A, Sanchez-Fueyo A, Zheng XX, Coyle AJ, Strom TB, Freeman GJ, Kuchroo VK (2003) Interaction of Tim-3 and Tim-3 ligand regulates T helper type 1 responses and induction of peripheral tolerance. Nat Immunol 4:1102–1110
21. Sakuishi K, Apetoh L, Sullivan JM, Blazar BR, Kuchroo VK, Anderson AC (2010) Targeting Tim-3 and PD-1 pathways to reverse T cell exhaustion and restore anti-tumor immunity. J Exp Med 207:2187–2194
22. Zhou Q, Munger ME, Veenstra RG, Weigel BJ, Hirashima M, Munn DH, Murphy WJ, Azuma M, Anderson AC, Kuchroo VK et al (2011) Coexpression of Tim-3 and PD-1 identifies a CD8+ T-cell exhaustion phenotype in mice with disseminated acute myelogenous leukemia. Blood 117:4501–4510
23. Fourcade J, Sun Z, Benallaoua M, Guillaume P, Luescher IF, Sander C, Kirkwood JM, Kuchroo V, Zarour HM (2010) Upregulation of Tim-3 and PD-1 expression is associated with tumor antigen-specific CD8+ T cell dysfunction in melanoma patients. J Exp Med 207:2175–2186
24. Dardalhon V, Anderson AC, Karman J, Apetoh L, Chandwaskar R, Lee DH, Cornejo M, Nishi N, Yamauchi A, Quintana FJ et al (2010) Tim-3/galectin-9 pathway: regulation of Th1 immunity through promotion of CD11b+Ly-6G+ myeloid cells. J Immunol 185:1383–1392

25. Jan M, Chao MP, Cha AC, Alizadeh AA, Gentles AJ, Weissman IL, Majeti R (2011) Prospective separation of normal and leukemic stem cells based on differential expression of TIM3, a human acute myeloid leukemia stem cell marker. Proc Natl Acad Sci U S A 108:5009–5014
26. Kikushige Y, Shima T, Takayanagi S, Urata S, Miyamoto T, Iwasaki H, Takenaka K, Teshima T, Tanaka T, Inagaki Y et al (2010) TIM-3 is a promising target to selectively kill acute myeloid leukemia stem cells. Cell Stem Cell 7:708–717
27. Watanabe N, Gavrieli M, Sedy JR, Yang J, Fallarino F, Loftin SK, Hurchla MA, Zimmerman N, Sim J, Zang X et al (2003) BTLA is a lymphocyte inhibitory receptor with similarities to CTLA-4 and PD-1. Nat Immunol 4:670–679
28. Sedy JR, Gavrieli M, Potter KG, Hurchla MA, Lindsley RC, Hildner K, Scheu S, Pfeffer K, Ware CF, Murphy TL et al (2005) B and T lymphocyte attenuator regulates T cell activation through interaction with herpesvirus entry mediator. Nat Immunol 6:90–98
29. Gavrieli M, Watanabe N, Loftin SK, Murphy TL, Murphy KM (2003) Characterization of phosphotyrosine binding motifs in the cytoplasmic domain of B and T lymphocyte attenuator required for association with protein tyrosine phosphatases SHP-1 and SHP-2. Biochem Biophys Res Commun 312:1236–1243
30. Miller ML, Sun Y, Fu YX (2009) Cutting edge: B and T lymphocyte attenuator signaling on NKT cells inhibits cytokine release and tissue injury in early immune responses. J Immunol 183:32–36
31. Krieg C, Boyman O, Fu YX, Kaye J (2007) B and T lymphocyte attenuator regulates CD8+ T cell-intrinsic homeostasis and memory cell generation. Nat Immunol 8:162–171
32. Hurchla MA, Sedy JR, Gavrieli M, Drake CG, Murphy TL, Murphy KM (2005) B and T lymphocyte attenuator exhibits structural and expression polymorphisms and is highly Induced in anergic CD4+ T cells. J Immunol 174:3377–3385
33. Fourcade J, Sun Z, Pagliano O, Guillaume P, Luescher IF, Sander C, Kirkwood JM, Olive D, Kuchroo V, Zarour HM (2012) CD8(+) T cells specific for tumor antigens can be rendered dysfunctional by the tumor microenvironment through upregulation of the inhibitory receptors BTLA and PD-1. Cancer Res 72:887–896
34. Han L, Wang W, Fang Y, Feng Z, Liao S, Li W, Li Y, Li C, Maitituoheti M, Dong H et al (2009) Soluble B and T lymphocyte attenuator possesses antitumor effects and facilitates heat shock protein 70 vaccine-triggered antitumor immunity against a murine TC-1 cervical cancer model in vivo. J Immunol 183:7842–7850
35. Derre L, Rivals JP, Jandus C, Pastor S, Rimoldi D, Romero P, Michielin O, Olive D, Speiser DE (2010) BTLA mediates inhibition of human tumor-specific CD8+ T cells that can be partially reversed by vaccination. J Clin Invest 120:157–167
36. Sakoda Y, Park JJ, Zhao Y, Kuramasu A, Geng D, Liu Y, Davila E, Tamada K (2011) Dichotomous regulation of GVHD through bidirectional functions of the BTLA-HVEM pathway. Blood 117:2506–2514
37. Wang C, Lin GH, McPherson AJ, Watts TH (2009) Immune regulation by 4-1BB and 4-1BBL: complexities and challenges. Immunol Rev 229:192–215
38. Lee HW, Park SJ, Choi BK, Kim HH, Nam KO, Kwon BS (2002) 4-1BB promotes the survival of CD8+ T lymphocytes by increasing expression of Bcl-xL and Bfl-1. J Immunol 169:4882–4888
39. Zhu Y, Zhu G, Luo L, Flies AS, Chen L (2007) CD137 stimulation delivers an antigen-independent growth signal for T lymphocytes with memory phenotype. Blood 109:4882–4889
40. Pulle G, Vidric M, Watts TH (2006) IL-15-dependent induction of 4-1BB promotes antigen-independent CD8 memory T cell survival. J Immunol 176:2739–2748
41. Wilcox RA, Tamada K, Strome SE, Chen L (2002) Signaling through NK cell-associated CD137 promotes both helper function for CD8+ cytolytic T cells and responsiveness to IL-2 but not cytolytic activity. J Immunol 169:4230–4236

42. Wilcox RA, Chapoval AI, Gorski KS, Otsuji M, Shin T, Flies DB, Tamada K, Mittler RS, Tsuchiya H, Pardoll DM et al (2002) Cutting edge: expression of functional CD137 receptor by dendritic cells. J Immunol 168:4262–4267
43. Melero I, Shuford WW, Newby SA, Aruffo A, Ledbetter JA, Hellstrom KE, Mittler RS, Chen L (1997) Monoclonal antibodies against the 4-1BB T-cell activation molecule eradicate established tumors. Nat Med 3:682–685
44. Ye Z, Hellstrom I, Hayden-Ledbetter M, Dahlin A, Ledbetter JA, Hellstrom KE (2002) Gene therapy for cancer using single-chain Fv fragments specific for 4-1BB. Nat Med 8:343–348
45. Wilcox RA, Flies DB, Wang H, Tamada K, Johnson AJ, Pease LR, Rodriguez M, Guo Y, Chen L (2002) Impaired infiltration of tumor-specific cytolytic T cells in the absence of interferon-gamma despite their normal maturation in lymphoid organs during CD137 monoclonal antibody therapy. Cancer Res 62:4413–4418
46. Croft M, Benedict CA, Ware CF (2013) Clinical targeting of the TNF and TNFR superfamilies. Nat Rev Drug Discov 12:147–168
47. Mallett S, Fossum S, Barclay AN (1990) Characterization of the MRC OX40 antigen of activated CD4 positive T lymphocytes – a molecule related to nerve growth factor receptor. EMBO J 9:1063–1068
48. Gramaglia I, Weinberg AD, Lemon M, Croft M (1998) Ox-40 ligand: a potent costimulatory molecule for sustaining primary CD4 T cell responses. J Immunol 161:6510–6517
49. Kopf M, Ruedl C, Schmitz N, Gallimore A, Lefrang K, Ecabert B, Odermatt B, Bachmann MF (1999) OX40-deficient mice are defective in Th cell proliferation but are competent in generating B cell and CTL Responses after virus infection. Immunity 11:699–708
50. Chen AI, McAdam AJ, Buhlmann JE, Scott S, Lupher ML Jr, Greenfield EA, Baum PR, Fanslow WC, Calderhead DM, Freeman GJ et al (1999) Ox40-ligand has a critical costimulatory role in dendritic cell: T cell interactions. Immunity 11:689–698
51. Weinberg AD, Rivera MM, Prell R, Morris A, Ramstad T, Vetto JT, Urba WJ, Alvord G, Bunce C, Shields J (2000) Engagement of the OX-40 receptor in vivo enhances antitumor immunity. J Immunol 164:2160–2169
52. Vu MD, Xiao X, Gao W, Degauque N, Chen M, Kroemer A, Killeen N, Ishii N, Li XC (2007) OX40 costimulation turns off Foxp3+ Tregs. Blood 110:2501–2510
53. Piconese S, Valzasina B, Colombo MP (2008) OX40 triggering blocks suppression by regulatory T cells and facilitates tumor rejection. J Exp Med 205:825–839
54. Vetto JT, Lum S, Morris A, Sicotte M, Davis J, Lemon M, Weinberg A (1997) Presence of the T-cell activation marker OX-40 on tumor infiltrating lymphocytes and draining lymph node cells from patients with melanoma and head and neck cancers. Am J Surg 174:258–265
55. Curti BD, Kovacsovics-Bankowski M, Morris N, Walker E, Chisholm L, Floyd K, Walker J, Gonzalez I, Meeuwsen T, Fox BA et al (2013) OX40 is a potent immune-stimulating target in late-stage cancer patients. Cancer Res 73:7189–7198
56. Tone M, Tone Y, Adams E, Yates SF, Frewin MR, Cobbold SP, Waldmann H (2003) Mouse glucocorticoid-induced tumor necrosis factor receptor ligand is costimulatory for T cells. Proc Natl Acad Sci U S A 100:15059–15064
57. Shimizu J, Yamazaki S, Takahashi T, Ishida Y, Sakaguchi S (2002) Stimulation of CD25(+) CD4(+) regulatory T cells through GITR breaks immunological self-tolerance. Nat Immunol 3:135–142
58. McHugh RS, Whitters MJ, Piccirillo CA, Young DA, Shevach EM, Collins M, Byrne MC (2002) CD4(+)CD25(+) immunoregulatory T cells: gene expression analysis reveals a functional role for the glucocorticoid-induced TNF receptor. Immunity 16:311–323
59. Cohen AD, Schaer DA, Liu C, Li Y, Hirschhorn-Cymmerman D, Kim SC, Diab A, Rizzuto G, Duan F, Perales MA et al (2010) Agonist anti-GITR monoclonal antibody induces melanoma tumor immunity in mice by altering regulatory T cell stability and intra-tumor accumulation. PLoS One 5:e10436

60. Turk MJ, Guevara-Patino JA, Rizzuto GA, Engelhorn ME, Sakaguchi S, Houghton AN (2004) Concomitant tumor immunity to a poorly immunogenic melanoma is prevented by regulatory T cells. J Exp Med 200:771–782
61. Schaer DA, Budhu S, Liu C, Bryson C, Malandro N, Cohen A, Zhong H, Yang X, Houghton AN, Merghoub T et al (2013) GITR pathway activation abrogates tumor immune suppression through loss of regulatory T cell lineage stability. Cancer Immunol Res 1:320–331
62. Bulliard Y, Jolicoeur R, Windman M, Rue SM, Ettenberg S, Knee DA, Wilson NS, Dranoff G, Brogdon JL (2013) Activating Fc gamma receptors contribute to the antitumor activities of immunoregulatory receptor-targeting antibodies. J Exp Med 210:1685–1693

# Part VII
# Regulation of Immunosuppression

# Chapter 21
# Regulatory T Cells

**Hideya Onishi, Takashi Morisaki, and Mitsuo Katano**

**Abstract** Regulatory T cells (Tregs) are $CD4^+$ T cells that inhibit autoreactive effector T cells to suppress antitumor immunity. Many anticancer therapeutics have limited efficacy, and it is thought that Tregs may, in part, be one of the reasons. From this viewpoint, Tregs may be a therapeutic target for cancer immunotherapy. Tregs also play a pivotal role in the induction of self-tolerance, and their dysfunction may lead to autoimmune disease. Promising results have recently been reported on the molecular targeting of drugs to Tregs. In the near future, the regulation of Tregs may be a central point for cancer immunotherapy. In this chapter, we focus on the immune-suppressing mechanism of Tregs and the development of strategies to modulate Tregs.

**Keywords** Regulatory T cells • Effector T cells • Foxp3 • Cancer immunotherapy

## 21.1 Subset of Regulatory T Cells (Tregs)

The concept of tumor suppressor T cells has drawn much attention since it was first reported in the 1980s that $CD4^+CD25^+$ T cells may suppress antitumor immunity [1]. In 1995, Sakaguchi et al. suggested that immunologic self-tolerance was maintained by activated T cells expressing the IL-2 receptor α chain (CD25) [2]. In 2003, the transcription factor forkhead box protein P3 (Foxp3) was reported to play a pivotal role in the differentiation, development, maintenance, and function of regulatory T cells (Tregs) [3]. Shortly thereafter, Sakaguchi defined naturally arising Foxp3-expressing $CD25^+CD4^+$ T cells and $Foxp3^+CD25^+CD4^+$ T cells as Tregs [4, 5].

H. Onishi (✉) • M. Katano
Department of Cancer Therapy and Research, Graduate School of Medical Sciences, Kyushu University, 3-1-1Maidashi, Higashi-ku, Fukuoka 812-8582, Japan
e-mail: ohnishi@surg1.med.kyushu-u.ac.jp

T. Morisaki
Department of Cancer Therapy and Research, Graduate School of Medical Sciences, Kyushu University, 3-1-1Maidashi, Higashi-ku, Fukuoka 812-8582, Japan

Fukuoka General Cancer Clinic, Fukuoka, Japan



Y. Yamaguchi (ed.), *Immunotherapy of Cancer*,
DOI 10.1007/978-4-431-55031-0_21

Generally, Tregs are divided into two principal subsets, naturally occurring Tregs (nTregs) which have differentiated in the thymus and inducible Tregs (iTregs) which differentiate in the periphery from naive $CD4^+$ T cells by VEGF, SDF-1, IL-10, and TGF-β [6, 7] and have recently received attention as a potential cancer immunotherapy. Myeloid-derived suppressor cells (MDSCs) which have the ability to inhibit T cell proliferation and effector function also play a role in inducing iTregs due in part to the expression of IL-10, TGF-β, and the inhibitory receptor cytotoxic T lymphocyte antigen-4 (CTLA-4) [8–11]. Type 1 Tregs (Tr1), T-helper 3 Tregs (Th3), and IL-35-inducible Tregs (iTr35) are also considered iTregs. Tr1 develop in response to IL-10, secrete IL-10 and TGF-β, and are expressed in $Foxp3^{low/-}CD25^{low/-}$ cells [12–14]. Th3 cells secrete elevated levels of TGF-β and express $Foxp3^+CD25^+$ [15, 16]. iTr35 cells rely on IL-35, which is a suppressive cytokine with the ability to inhibit T cell proliferation and antitumor activity [17]. iTr35 cells express mixed levels of Foxp3 and CD25 [17]. Although nTregs and iTregs express CD4, there are other Tregs that are not of the $CD4^+$ lineage. It is well established that $CD8^+$ Tregs exist [18]. Like $CD4^+$ Tregs, there are also naturally occurring $CD8^+$ Tregs and inducible $CD8^+$Tregs [8]. However, the nature of these $CD8^+$ Tregs remains poorly understood. Additional Treg subsets which are not of the $CD4^+$ or $CD8^+$ lineage, such as γδ-T cells, also seem to be important players of the immune system [19, 20].

Functionally, $Foxp3^+CD4^+$ cells are divided into three categories, $CD45RA^+$ resting Tregs (rTregs), $CD45RA^-$ activated Tregs (aTregs), and $CD45RA^-$ cytokine-secreting non-suppressive $Foxp3^+$ cells [21, 22]. Upon activation, rTregs begin to proliferate and are converted to aTregs while both rTregs and aTregs have similar T cell suppressive activity [22]. CD147 is a highly glycosylated type I transmembrane protein that is used to phenotypically distinguish rTregs ($CD25^+CD147^-$) from aTregs ($CD25^+CD147^+$) [21, 23].

## 21.2 Naturally Occurring Tregs and Inducible Tregs

Given that the function of nTregs and iTregs seem quite similar and the role of each population in tumor immunity is still controversial, how then are nTregs and iTregs distinguishable? Recently, it has been proposed that Helios, an Ikaros transcription factor family member expressed during embryonic hematopoietic development, plays an important role in Treg function [24, 25]. Thornton et al. have shown that Helios may be a marker for discriminating between nTregs and iTregs [26]. However, other studies appear to refute this hypothesis [27, 28], and the role for Helios remains controversial. There are other factors that may distinguish nTregs from iTregs, as it has been shown that iTregs express lower levels of *Nrp1*, *Plagl1*, *Swap70*, and *Ikzf2* mRNA and high levels of *Igfbp4* and *Dapl1* [29]. IL-6 inhibits the suppressive activity of nTregs but not of iTregs [30]. The vitamin A metabolite retinoic acid plays a role for tilting the balance toward iTreg differentiation [31].

The role of Foxp3 in mediating the suppressive function of Tregs remains unclear. However, Foxp3 intronic and promoter regions exhibit demethylated or hypomethylated structure in nTregs, while the same regions in iTregs have hypermethylated CpGs [32–35]. Understanding the difference between nTregs and iTregs may be important for immunotherapy and will require additional research.

## 21.3 Immunosuppressive Mechanism of Tregs

Four primary immunosuppressive mechanisms have been demonstrated for Tregs. First, cytokine production is a key factor, as Tregs secrete immunosuppressive cytokines such as IL-10, TGF-β, and IL-35 which regulate effector T cells [36]. Second, cytotoxic molecules such as perforin and granzyme B are secreted by Tregs and effector T cells and induce effector T cell apoptosis. A third mechanism is IL-2 deprivation [37]. Because Tregs express elevated levels of CD25, IL-2 in the local microenvironment is consumed by Tregs. Consequently, effector T cells cannot use IL-2 and may be induced to undergo apoptosis. In fact, it has been shown that the elimination of $CD25^+$ Tregs results in tumor regression [38]. However, some authors have demonstrated that IL-2 deprivation is not a primary immunosuppressive mechanism of Tregs [39, 40]. Fourth is the suppression of dendritic cell (DC) maturation. In this process, several possibilities are hypothesized. One is that the binding of CTLA-4 on Tregs and CD80/CD86 on DCs may deliver signals that suppress DC maturation [41]. Additionally, Tregs may upregulate the immunosuppressive enzyme indoleamine 2,3 dioxygenase (IDO) in DCs to inhibit effector T cell function [42]. Another potential mechanism is that Tregs physically remove CD80/CD86 molecules from the surface of DCs to reduce antigen-presenting capacity [43].

In addition, it has recently been shown that the NrP-1/sema-4 pathway is required to protect Tregs and prolong survival in the tumor microenvironment [44]. Adenosine, which is highly expressed on the surface of Tregs, also has a role. When Tregs contact effector T cells, cyclic adenosine monophosphate (cAMP) translocates to T cells via gap junctions, suppressing IL-2 gene expression and inhibiting effector T cell function [45, 46]. TLR8-MyD88-IRAK4-complexes may play a role in the functional regulation of Tregs [47]. Huber et al. have shown that p38MAP kinase signaling is required for the conversion of $CD4^+CD25^-$ T cells into iTregs [48].

To date, the study of Treg immunosuppression has focused on non-antigen-specific regulation. In the last decades, Tregs specific for many kinds of tumor-associated antigens (TAAs) such as gp100, NY-ESO-1, HER2/neu, and CEA have been identified [8, 49–51]. Better understanding of TAA-specific Tregs may contribute to the development of more effective immunotherapies to induce optimal effector T cell responses.

## 21.4 Cancer and Tregs

Tregs perform a key role in controlling effector T cells. Some investigators have shown that Tregs are more prevalent in peripheral blood mononuclear cells (PBMC) and/or cancer tissues in several types of advanced cancer, including ovarian, hepatocellular, prostate, gastric, esophageal, and colorectal [52–57]. A current challenge is that there is not a clear biomarker for use in immunotherapy. We have shown that patients with a high ratio of Tregs in PBMC exhibit a poor prognosis compared with those with reduced Treg levels following immunotherapy, suggesting that the PBMC Treg ratio might serve as a biomarker for immunotherapy response [52].

Treg infiltration of cancer tissue is also important. It has been shown that a reduced effector T cell/Treg ratio in cancer tissue is associated with poor prognosis in breast, ovarian, gastric, pancreatic, hepatocellular, and colorectal cancer [53, 58–62]. However, conflicting prognostic results have also been observed in B-cell lymphoma [63], suggesting additional research is needed to establish a better understanding of these observations.

A key question is how do Tregs infiltrate tissue? The interaction between CCL22, secreted by tumor cells or macrophages, and its ligand CCR4, produced by Tregs, plays a key role in Treg infiltration of cancer tissue [64]. Other chemokine receptors such as CCR4, CCR5, CCR7, CCR8, αE integrin chain, and CXCR4, which are expressed on Tregs, are also thought to induce Treg migration [36, 65].

## 21.5 Development of Cancer Immunotherapy Against Tregs

It may be effective to target Treg-specific surface markers for the development of effective immunotherapy. Common Treg markers include CD25, Foxp3, CD39, CD122, CD127, CTLA-4, LAG-3, and GITR [8, 66]. Among these, we focused on novel molecules that have recently gained attention in humans.

### *21.5.1 CTLA-4 and Programmed Death-1 (PD-1)*

CTLA-4 and PD-1 are recognized as inhibitory co-stimulatory molecules that act as key players in the balance and regulation of the adaptive immune response. CTLA-4 and PD-1 are expressed on T cells, including Tregs [67, 68]. Blocking CTLA-4 activation signals to CTLs inhibits antiproliferative signals that block the G0 to G1 cell cycle transition and reduce cytokine secretion [69, 70]. PD-1 inhibition induces the generation of CTLs and inhibits the suppressive function of Tregs [68]. Programmed death ligand-1 (PD-L1) is expressed on Tregs as well as cancer cells

[68]. Therefore, blockage of the CTLA-4 and PD-1/PD-L1 pathways may carry dual benefits, activation of effector T cells and inhibition of Tregs.

The anti-CTLA-4 mAb, ipilimumab, was approved by the FDA in March 2011 as a first- and second-line monotherapy for unresectable or metastatic melanoma [71, 72]. Ipilimumab improved overall survival in patients with advanced melanoma [73, 74]. The anti-PD-1 mAb, nivolumab, exhibited sustained and effective responses in patients with melanoma, renal cell cancer, and non-small-cell lung cancer [75]. There is substantial interest in nivolumab in large part owing to the low toxicity compared with ipilimumab [76]. Moreover, it has been reported that concurrent therapy with ipilimumab and nivolumab provided a rapid and deep tumor regression [77]. Ipilimumab and nivolumab are viewed as molecular-targeting drugs that may completely change the manner of cancer immunotherapy in the future.

### *21.5.2 Vascular Endothelial Growth Factor Receptor-2 (VEGFR2)*

We have demonstrated that VEGFR2 is selectively expressed on $FOXP3^{high}$ Tregs and that this Treg subpopulation acts as suppressive effector T cells [78]. We have also shown that elevated numbers of tumor-infiltrated $VEGFR2^{+}FOXP3^{high}$ Tregs correlate with poor prognosis in colorectal cancer [79]. These results suggest that VEGFR2 may be a therapeutic target in Tregs. Recently, others have shown that VEGF provides Tregs with a direct VEGFR2-dependent co-stimulatory proliferation signal [65, 80, 81] and that intratumoral Tregs produce elevated levels of VEGF. Thus, autocrine VEGF/VEGFR2 signaling might be important for Treg maintenance. Anti angiogenic drugs such as sunitinib and sorafenib are also shown to inhibit Treg function [82, 83]. It may be that these drugs act by inhibiting VEGF/VEGFR2 signaling.

Interestingly, under hypoxic conditions, Tregs are more able to suppress effector T cell function, presumably through the transcriptional factor hypoxia-inducible factor 1α (HIF-1α). For instance, HIF-1α increases Foxp3 expression and the number of functionally active Tregs [84]. It may be that Tregs secrete VEGF, which is downstream of HIF-1α and is upregulated under hypoxic conditions. However, the role of DCs may also be critical. Consistent with these results, we have shown that hypoxic DCs secrete more VEGF and produce more Tregs than those generated under normoxic conditions [85]. Given that the in vivo environment is thought to be hypoxic, immunotherapy targeting of Tregs through this angiogenic VEGF/VEGFR signaling may be an important approach.

### 21.5.3 Exosomes

Exosomes are microvesicles of 30–100 nm in diameter that are released from many cell types through an exocytosis pathway [86–88]. They contain a variety of cell-cell communication-related molecules such as MHC class I, class II, CD86, and heat-shock proteins [89, 90]. We have shown that malignant-effusion-derived exosomes (Eff-Ex) express TGF-β1 on the surface and that this TGF-β1 mediates Treg number and Foxp3 expression [91]. This suggests that Eff-Ex and/or TGF-β1 expressed on Eff-Ex may be a candidate target for Treg immunotherapy.

Others have also reported on Treg-related exosomes. Clayton et al. showed that human tumor-derived exosomes selectively impair lymphocyte responses to IL-2, skewing IL-2 responsiveness in favor of Tregs and away from effector T cells [92]. They also demonstrated that cancer-derived exosomes express CD39 and CD73 and that exosomes suppress T cell activation through adenosine production [93]. Wang et al. showed that thymus-derived exosome-like particles induce Treg development and convert thymic $CD4^{+}CD25^{-}$ T cells into Tregs [94]. Additionally, it has been shown that purified Treg exosomes prolong kidney allograft survival [95]. This result suggests an autocrine activation system of Tregs.

### 21.5.4 CD25

CD25 plays a role in the maintenance and proliferation in Tregs [96]. Denileukin diftitox (Ontak) is a recombinant protein of diphtheria toxin and IL-2 that binds the high-affinity ($\alpha-\beta-\gamma$) IL-2 receptor and, following internalization, suppresses protein synthesis [97]. A phase II study reported promising results with Ontak in patients with unresectable stage IV melanoma [98]. In contrast, Baur et al. have shown that activated but not resting Tregs were killed after internalization of Ontak and that resting Tregs showed increased survival due to Ontak-associated antiapoptotic IL-2 signaling [99].

A CD25-directed immunotoxin (LMB-2) is another candidate for selectively eliminating Tregs. LMB-2 is a fusion of a single-chain Fv fragment of the CD25-specific, anti-Tac mAb to a truncated form of the bacterial Pseudomonas exotoxin A [100]. Promising clinical trial results testing LMB-2 have been reported in patients with several hematological malignancies [101]. The capacity of LMB-2 to mediate a transient partial reduction in circulating and tumor-infiltrating Tregs in vivo has been shown [102].

### 21.5.5 *Cyclooxygenase-2 (COX-2)*

COX-2 is a membrane-bound enzyme and member of the mammalian heme-dependent peroxidase family [103] and is expressed on Foxp3$^+$CD25$^+$CD4$^+$ Tregs [104]. Studies have shown that COX-2 is involved in the immunosuppressive function of Tregs [104, 105]. Moreover, prostaglandin E2 (PGE2) produced by COX-2 mediates the suppressive function of CD4$^+$CD25$^{high}$ Tregs and induces a regulatory phenotype in CD4$^+$CD25$^-$ T cells [105]. Tumor-derived and DC-derived COX-2/PGE2 as well as Treg-derived COX-2/PGE2 increases Treg activity [103, 106]. COX-2 is also overexpressed in many human solid tumors [44]. Taken together, these results suggest that the COX-2/PGE2 pathway mediates Treg regulatory function in tumor immunity.

### 21.5.6 *Glucocorticoid-Induced Tumor Necrosis Factor Receptor (GITR)*

GITR is constitutively expressed on Tregs rather than CD4 and CD8 T cells [107, 108]. Activation of GITR signaling is thought to neutralize suppressor Tregs [107–109]. It is thought that anti-GITR antibody acting on soluble GITR ligand modulates Treg activity through the loss of Foxp3 expression [110]. David et al. have raised an important implication of the agonistic anti-GITR mAb DTA-1 in cancer immunotherapy [111].

### 21.5.7 *OX-40*

OX40 (CD134) is a co-stimulatory TNF receptor family molecule expressed constitutively on Tregs [112]. OX40 activation suppresses expression of the Foxp3 gene and inhibits suppressor Tregs [113]. Antihuman OX40 agonistic mouse mAb promotes CD4$^+$CD8$^+$ T cell proliferation and suppresses TGF-β, which induces Foxp3 expression on naive CD4$^+$ T cells and inhibits suppressor Tregs [114]. In contrast, intratumoral injection of anti-OX40 mAb decreases tumor growth dramatically [115]. These results suggest that OX40 may be a good therapeutic target candidate.

### 21.5.8 *Notch Signaling*

Notch signaling is a morphogenic signaling pathway that is reactivated in various types of cancer and has become a new potential strategy for human cancer treatment

[116]. A relationship between Notch signaling and Tregs has recently been reported. Kostianovsky et al. have shown that Tregs are generated by E3 ubiquitin ligase, a gene related to lymphocyte anergy (GRAIL) via Notch activation [117]. Notch activation augments effector T cell sensitivity to Treg-mediated suppression by regulating the Foxp3 promoter [118] and upregulating TGF-βRII expression [119]. Therefore, Notch signaling may be a potential therapeutic target for both cancer and Treg modulation.

### 21.5.9 *Drug-Induced Treg Inhibition*

Many additional agents regulate Tregs. Cyclophosphamide inhibits the production and function of $CD8^+$ and $CD4^+$ Tregs [120, 121]. Additionally, paclitaxel and fludarabine reduce the number and suppressive function of Tregs [122, 123]. Imatinib decreases the number, function, and Foxp3 expression in Tregs [124]. The humanized anti-CCR4 mAb mogamulizumab depletes Tregs, and mogamulizumab clinical trials have been conducted for advanced solid tumors [125]. These agents may provide effective therapies against cancer directly and by improving antitumor immunity.

## References

1. Berendt MJ, North RL (1980) T-cell-mediated suppression of anti-tumour immunity. An explanation for progressive growth of an immunogenic tumour. J Exp Med 151:69–80
2. Sakaguchi S, Sakaguchi N, Asano M, Itoh M, Toda M (1995) Immunologic self-tolerance maintained by activated T cells expressing IL-2 receptor alpha-chains (CD25). Breakdown of a single mechanism of self-tolerance causes various autoimmune diseases. J Immunol 155:1151–1164
3. Hori S, Nomura T, Sakaguchi S (2003) Control of regulatory T cell development by the transcription factor Foxp3. Science 299:1057–1061
4. Sakaguchi S (2004) Naturally arising $CD4^+$ regulatory T cells for immunologic self-tolerance and negative control of immune responses. Annu Rev Immunol 22:531–562
5. Sakaguchi S (2005) Naturally arising Foxp3-expressing $CD25^+$ $CD4^+$ regulatory T cells in immunological tolerance to self and non-self. Nat Immunol 6:345–352
6. Chen W, Jin W, Hardegen N, Lei KJ, Li L, Marinos N et al (2003) Conversion of peripheral $CD4^+$ $CD25^-$ naïve T cells to $CD4^+$ $CD25^+$ regulatory T cells by TGF-beta induction of transcription factor Foxp3. J Exp Med 198:1875–1886
7. Zou W (2005) Immunosuppressive networks in the tumour environment and their therapeutic relevance. Nat Rev Cancer 5:263–274
8. Olson BM, McNeel DG (2013) Monitoring regulatory immune responses in tumor immunotherapy clinical trials. Front Oncol 3:109. doi:10.3389/fonc.2013.00109
9. Huang B, Pan PY, Li Q, Sato AI, Levy DE, Bromberg J et al (2006) Gr-1+CD115+ immature myeloid suppressor cells mediate the development of tumor-induced T regulatory cells and T-cell anergy in tumor-bearing host. Cancer Res 66:1123–1131

10. Yang R, Cai Z, Zhang Y, Yutzy WH 4th, Roby KF, Roden RB (2006) CD80 in immune suppression by mouse ovarian carcinoma-associated Gr-1+CD11b+ myeloid cells. Cancer Res 66:6807–6815
11. Serafini P, Mgebroff S, Noonan K, Borrello I (2008) Myeloid-derived suppressor cells promote cross-tolerance in B-cell lymphoma by expanding regulatory T cells. Cancer Res 68:5439–5449
12. Groux H, O'Garra A, Bigler M, Rouleau M, Antonenko S, De Vries JE et al (1997) A CD4+ T-cell subset inhibits antigen-specific T-cell responses and prevents colitis. Nature 389:737–742
13. Roncarolo MG, Bacchetta R, Bordignon C, Narula S, Levings MK (2001) Type 1 T regulatory cells. Immunol Rev 182:68–79
14. Levings MK, Gregori S, Tresoldi E, Cazzaniga S, Bonini C, Roncarolo MG (2005) Differentiation of Tr1 cells by immature dendritic cells requires IL-10 but not $CD25^{+}CD4^{+}$ Tr cells. Blood 105:1162–1169
15. Chen Y, Kuchroo VK, Inobe J, Hafler DA, Weiner HL (1994) Regulatory T cell clones induced by oral tolerance suppression of autoimmune encephalomyelitis. Science 265:1237–1240
16. Weiner HL (2001) Induction and mechanism of action of transforming growth factor-beta-secreting Th3 regulatory cells. Immunol Rev 182:207–214
17. Collison LW, Chaturvedi V, Henderson AL, Giacomin PR, Guy C, Bankoti J et al (2010) IL-35-mediated induction of a potent regulatory T cell population. Nat Immunol 11:1093–1101
18. Tsai S, Clemente-Casares X, Santamaria P (2011) CD8+ Tregs in autoimmunity: learning "self"-control from experience. Cell Mol Life Sci 68:3781–3795
19. Hayday A, Geng L (1997) γδ-T-cells regulate autoimmunity. Curr Opin Immunol 9:884–889
20. Ye J, Ma C, Hsueh EC, Eickhoff CS, Zhang Y, Varvares MA et al (2013) Tumor-derived γδ regulatory T cells suppress innate and adaptive immunity through the induction of immunosenescence. J Immunol 190:2403–2414
21. Landskron J, Taskén K (2013) CD147 in regulatory T cells. Cell Immunol 282:17–20
22. Miyara M, Yoshioka Y, Kitoh A, Shima T, Wing K, Niwa A et al (2009) Functional delineation and differentiation dynamics of human CD4+ T cells expressing the FoxP3 transcription factor. Immunity 30:899–911
23. Miyauchi T, Masuzawa Y, Muramatsu T (1991) The basigin group of the immunoglobulin superfamily: complete conservation of a segment in and around transmembrane domains of human and mouse basigin and chicken HT7 antigen. J Biochem 110:770–774
24. Ross EM, Bourges D, Hogan TV, Gleeson PA, van Driel IR (2014) Helios defines T cells being driven to tolerance in the periphery and thymus. Eur J Immunol. doi:10.1002/eji.201343999
25. Getnet D, Grosso JF, Goldberg MV, Harris TJ, Yen HR, Bruno TC et al (2010) A role for the transcription factor Helios in human CD4(+)CD25(+) regulatory T cells. Mol Immunol 47:1595–1600
26. Thornton AM, Korty PE, Tran DQ, Wohlfert EA, Murray PE, Belkaid Y et al (2010) Expression of Helios, an Ikaros transcription factor family member, differentiates thymic-derived from peripherally induced Foxp3+ T regulatory cells. J Immunol 184:3433–3441
27. Gottschalk RA, Corse E, Allison JP (2012) Expression of Helios in peripherally induced Foxp3+ regulatory T cells. J Immunol 188:976–980
28. Himmel ME, MacDonald KG, Garcia RV, Steiner TS, Vevings M (2013) Helios+ and Helios- cells coexist within the natural FOXP3+ T regulatory cell subset in humans. J Immunol 190:2001–2008
29. Bilate AM, Lafaille JJ (2012) Induced $CD4^{+}Foxp3^{+}$ regulatory T cells in immune tolerance. Annu Rev Immunol 30:733–758
30. Horwitz DA, Zheng SG, Gray JD (2008) Natural and TGF-β-induced $Foxp3^{+}CD4^{+}$ $CD25^{+}$ regulatory T cells are not mirror images of each other. Trends Immunol 29:429–435

31. Mucida D, Park Y, Kim G, Turovskaya O, Scott I, Kronenberg M et al (2007) Reciprocal TH17 and regulatory T cell differentiation mediated by retinoic acid. Science 317:256–260
32. Kim HP, Leonard WJ (2007) CREB/ATF-dependent T cell receptor-induced FoxP3 gene expression: a role for DNA methylation. J Exp Med 204:1543–1551
33. Baron U, Floess S, Wieczorek G, Baumann K, Grützkau A, Dong J et al (2007) DNA demethylation in the human FOXP3 locus discriminates regulatory T cells from activated FOXP3(+) conventional T cells. Eur J Immunol 37:2378–2389
34. Stockis J, Fink W, Francois V, Connerotte T, de Smet C, Knoops L et al (2009) Comparison of stable human Treg and Th clones by transcriptional profiling. Eur J Immunol 39:869–882
35. Lal G, Zhang N, van der Touw W, Ding Y, Ju W, Bottinger EP et al (2009) Epigenetic regulation of Foxp3 expression in regulatory T cells by DNA methylation. J Immunol 182:259–273
36. Campbell DJ, Koch MA (2011) Phenotypical and functional specialization of FOXP3+ regulatory T cells. Nat Rev Immunol 11:119–130
37. Pandiyan P, Zheng L, Ishihara S, Reed J, Lenardo MJ (2007) CD4+CD25+Foxp3+ regulatory T cells induce cytokine deprivation-mediated apoptosis of effector CD4+ cells. Nat Immunol 8:1353–1362
38. Onizuka S, Tawara I, Shimizu J, Sakaguchi S, Fujita T, Nakayama E et al (1999) Tumor rejection by in vivo administration of anti-CD25 (interleukin-2 receptor alpha) monoclonal antibody. Cancer Res 59:3128–3133
39. Sakaguchi S, Wing K, Onishi Y, Prieto-Martin P, Yamaguchi T (2009) Regulatory T cells: how do they suppress immune responses? Int Immunol 21:1105–1111
40. Vercoulen Y, Wehrens EJ, van Teijlingen NH, de Jager W, Beekman JM, Prakken BJ (2009) Human regulatory T cell suppressive function is independent of apoptosis induction in activated effector T cells. PLoS One 4:e7183. doi:10.1371/journal.pone.0007183
41. Wing K, Onishi Y, Prieto-Martin P, Yamaguchi T, Miyara M, Fehervari Z et al (2008) CTLA-4 control over Foxp3+ regulatory T cell function. Science 322:271–275
42. Mellor AL, Munn DH (2004) IDO expression by dendritic cells: tolerance and tryptophan catabolism. Nat Rev Immunol 4:762–774
43. Qureshi OS, Zheng Y, Nakamura K, Attridge K, Manzotti C, Schmidt EM et al (2011) Trans-endocytosis of CD80 and CD86: a molecular basis for the cell-extrinsic function of CTLA-4. Science 332:600–603
44. Whiteside TL (2014) Regulatory T cell subsets in human cancer: are they regulating for or against tumor progression? Cancer Immunol Immunother 63:67–72
45. Bopp T, Becker C, Klein M, Klein-Hessling S, Palmetshofer A, Serfling E et al (2007) Cyclic adenosine monophosphate is a key component of regulatory T cell-mediated suppression. J Exp Med 204:1303–1310
46. Bashyam H (2007) cAMP crosses junctions. J Exp Med 204:1240b
47. Peng G, Guo Z, Kiniwa Y, Voo KS, Peng W, Fu T et al (2005) Toll-like receptor 8-mediated reversal of CD4+ regulatory T cell function. Science 309:1380–1384
48. Huber S, Schrader J, Fritz G, Presser K, Schmitt S, Waisman A et al (2008) P38 MAP kinase signaling is required for the conversion of $CD4^{+}CD25^{-}$ T cells into iTreg. PLoS One 3:e3302. doi:10.1371/journal.pone.0003302
49. Wang HY, Lee DA, Peng G, Guo Z, Li Y, Kiniwa Y et al (2004) Tumor-specific human $CD4^{+}$ regulatory T cells and their ligands: implications for immunotherapy. Immunity 20:107–118
50. van der Burg SH, Piersma SJ, de Jong A, van der Hulst JM, Kwappenberg KM, van den Hende M et al (2007) Association of cervical cancer with the presence of $CD4^{+}$ regulatory T cells specific for human papillomavirus antigens. Proc Natl Acad Sci U S A 104:12087–12092
51. Bonertz A, Weitz J, Pietsch DH, Rahbari NN, Schlude C, Ge Y et al (2009) Antigen-specific Tregs control T cell responses against a limited repertoire of tumor antigens in patients with colorectal carcinoma. J Clin Invest 119:3311–3321

52. Wada J, Yamasaki A, Nagai S, Yanai K, Fuchino K, Kameda C et al (2008) Regulatory T-cells are possible effect prediction markers of immunotherapy for cancer patients. Anticancer Res 28:2401–2408
53. Curiel TJ, Coukos G, Zou L, Alvarez X, Cheng P, Mottram P et al (2004) Specific recruitment of regulatory T cells in ovarian carcinoma fosters immune privilege and predicts reduced survival. Nat Med 10:942–949
54. Ormandy LA, Hillemann T, Wedemeyer H, Manns MP, Greten TF, Korangy F (2005) Increased populations of regulatory T cells in peripheral blood of patients with hepatocellular carcinoma. Cancer Res 65:2457–2464
55. Kono K, Kawaida H, Takahashi A, Sugai H, Mimura K, Miyagawa N et al (2006) CD4(+) CD25high regulatory T cells increase with tumor stage in patients with gastric and esophageal cancers. Cancer Immunol Immunother 55:1064–1071
56. Miller AM, Lundberg K, Ozenci V, Banham AH, Hellstrom M, Egevad L et al (2006) $CD4^{+}CD25^{high}$ T cells are enriched in the tumor and peripheral blood of prostate cancer patients. J Immunol 177:7398–7405
57. Ling KL, Pratap SE, Bates GJ, Singh B, Mortensen NJ, George BD et al (2007) Increased frequency of regulatory T cells in peripheral blood and tumour infiltrating lymphocytes in colorectal cancer patients. Cancer Immun 7:7
58. Gao Q, Qiu SJ, Fan J, Zhou J, Wang XY, Xiao YS et al (2007) Intratumoral balance of regulatory and cytotoxic T cells is associated with prognosis of hepatocellular carcinoma after resection. J Clin Oncol 25:2586–2593
59. Hiraoka N, Onozato K, Kosuge T, Hirohashi S (2006) Prevalence of FOXP3+ regulatory T cells increases during the progression of pancreatic ductal adenocarcinoma and its premalignant lesions. Clin Cancer Res 12:5423–5434
60. Bates GJ, Fox SB, Han C, Leek RD, Garcia JF, Harris AL et al (2006) Quantification of regulatory T cells enables the identification of high-risk breast cancer patients and those at risk of late relapse. J Clin Oncol 24:5373–5380
61. Suzuki H, Chikazawa N, Tasaka T, Wada J, Yamasaki A, Kitaura Y et al (2010) Intratumoral CD8(+) T/FOXP3 (+) cell ratio is a predictive marker for survival in patients with colorectal cancer. Cancer Immunol Immunother 59:653–661
62. Sasada T, Kimura M, Yoshida Y, Kanai M, Takabayashi A (2003) CD4+CD25+ regulatory T cells in patients with gastrointestinal malignancies: possible involvement of regulatory T cells in disease progression. Cancer 98:1089–1099
63. Tzankov A, Meier C, Hirschmann P, Went P, Pileri SA, Dirnhofer S (2008) Correlation of high numbers of intratumoral FOXP3+ regulatory T cells with improved survival in germinal center-like diffuse large B-cell lymphoma, follicular lymphoma and classical Hodgkin's lymphoma. Haematologica 93:193–200
64. Nishikawa H, Sakaguchi S (2014) Regulatory T cells in cancer immunotherapy. Curr Opin Immunol 27:1–7
65. Tanchot C, Terme M, Pere H, Tran T, Benhamouda N, Strioga M et al (2013) Tumor-infiltrating regulatory T cells: phenotype, role, mechanism of expansion in situ and clinical significance. Cancer Microenviron 6:147–157
66. Mougiakakos D, Choudhurt A, Lladser A, Kiessling R, Johansson CC (2010) Regulatory T cells in cancer. Adv Cancer Res 107:57–117
67. Peggs KS, Quezada SA, Chambers CA, Korman AJ, Allison JP (2009) Blockade of CTLA-4 on both effector and regulatory T cell compartments contributes to the antitumor activity of anti-CTLA-4 antibodies. J Exp Med 206:1717–1725
68. Wang W, Lau R, Yu D, Zhu W, Korman A, Weber J (2009) PD1 blockade reverses the suppression of melanoma antigen-specific CTL by CD4+ CD25(Hi) regulatory T cells. Int Immunol 21:1065–1077
69. Walunas TL, Lenschow DJ, Bakker CY, Linsley PS, Freeman GJ, Green JM et al (1994) CTLA-4 can function as a negative regulator of T cell activation. Immunity 1:405–413

70. Waterhouse P, Penninger JM, Timms E, Wakeham A, Shahinian A, Lee KP et al (1995) Lymphoproliferative disorders with early lethality in mice deficient in Ctla-4. Science 270:985–988
71. Torino F, Barnabei A, De Vecchis L, Sini V, Schittulli F, Marchetti P et al (2014) Chemotherapy-induced ovarian toxicity in patients affected by endocrine-responsive early breast cancer. Crit Rev Oncol Hematol 89:27–42
72. Reichert JM, Reichert JM (2012) Marketed therapeutic antibodies compendium. MAbs 4:413–415
73. Hodi FS, O'Day SJ, McDermott DF, Weber RW, Sosman JA, Haanen JB et al (2010) Improved survival with ipilimumab in patients with metastatic melanoma. N Engl J Med 363:711–723
74. Robert C, Thomas L, Bondarenko I, O'Day S, Weber J, Garbe C et al (2011) Ipilimumab plus dacarbazine for previously untreated metastatic melanoma. N Engl J Med 364:2517–2526
75. Topalian SL, Hodi FS, Brahmer JR, Gettinger SN, Smith DC, McDermott DF et al (2012) Safety, activity, and immune correlates of anti-PD-1 antibody in cancer. N Engl J Med 366:2443–2454
76. O'Sullivan Coyne G, Madan RA, Gulley JL (2014) Nivolumab: promising survival signal coupled with limited toxicity raises expectations. J Clin Oncol 32:986–988
77. Wolchok JD, Kluger H, Callahan MK, Postow MA, Rizvi NA, Lesokhin AM et al (2013) Nivolumab plus ipilimumab in advanced melanoma. N Engl J Med 369:122–133
78. Suzuki H, Onishi H, Wada J, Yamasaki A, Tanaka H, Nakano K et al (2010) VEGFR2 is selectively expressed by FOXP3high CD4+ Treg. Eur J Immunol 40:197–203
79. Suzuki H, Onishi H, Morisaki T, Tanaka M, Katano M (2013) Intratumoral FOXP3+VEGFR2+ regulatory T cells are predictive markers for recurrence and survival in patients with colorectal cancer. Clin Immunol 146:26–33
80. Terme M, Pernot S, Marcheteau E, Sandoval F, Benhamouda N, Colussi O et al (2013) VEGFA-VEGFR pathway blockade inhibits tumor-induced regulatory T-cell proliferation in colorectal cancer. Cancer Res 73:539–549
81. Terme M, Tartour E, Taieb J (2013) VEGFA/VEGFR2-targeted therapies prevent the VEGFA-induced proliferation of regulatory T cells in cancer. Oncoimmunology 2:e25156
82. Finke JH, Rini B, Ireland J, Rayman P, Richmond A, Golshayan A et al (2008) Sunitinib reverses type-1 immune suppression and decreases T-regulatory cells in renal cell carcinoma patients. Clin Cancer Res 14:6674–6682
83. Cabrera R, Ararat M, Xu Y, Brusko T, Wasserfall C, Atkinson MA et al (2013) Immune modulation of effector CD4+ and regulatory T cell function by sorafenib in patients with hepatocellular carcinoma. Cancer Immunol Immunother 62:737–746
84. Ben-Shoshan J, Maysel-Auslender S, Mor A, Keren G, George J (2008) Hypoxia controls $CD4^+CD25^+$ regulatory T-cell homeostasis via hypoxia-inducible factor-1alpha. Eur J Immunol 38:2412–2418
85. Ogino T, Onishi H, Suzuki H, Morisaki T, Tanaka M, Katano M (2012) Inclusive estimation of complex antigen presentation functions of monocyte-derived dendritic cells differentiated under normoxia and hypoxia conditions. Cancer Immunol Immunother 61:409–424
86. Trams EG, Lauter CJ, Salem N Jr, Heine U (1981) Exfoliation of membrane ecto-enzymes in the form of micro-vesicles. Biochim Biophys Acta 645:63–70
87. Johnstone RM, Adam M, Hammond JR, Orr L, Turbide C (1987) Vesicle formation during reticulocyte maturation. Association of plasma membrane activities with released vesicles (exosomes). J Biol Chem 262:9412–9420
88. Raposo G, Nijman HW, Stoorvogel W, Liejendekker R, Harding CV, Melief CJ et al (1996) B lymphocytes secrete antigen-presenting vesicles. J Exp Med 183:1161–1172
89. Mignot G, Roux S, Thery C, Ségura E, Zitvogel L (2006) Prospects for exosomes in immunotherapy of cancer. J Cell Mol Med 10:376–388

90. Laulagnier K, Motta C, Hamdi S, Roy S, Fauvelle F, Pageaux JF et al (2004) Mast cell- and dendritic cell-derived exosomes display a specific lipid composition and an unusual membrane organization. Biochem J 380:161–171
91. Wada J, Onishi H, Suzuki H, Yamasaki A, Nagai S, Morisaki T et al (2010) Surface-bound TGF-beta1 on effusion-derived exosomes participates in maintenance of number and suppressive function of regulatory T-cells in malignant effusions. Anticancer Res 30:3747–3757
92. Clayton A, Mitchell JP, Court J, Mason MD, Tabi Z (2007) Human tumor-derived exosomes selectively impair lymphocyte responses to interleukin-2. Cancer Res 67:7458–7466
93. Clayton A, Al-Taei S, Webber J, Mason MD, Tabi Z (2011) Cancer exosomes express CD39 and CD73, which suppress T cells through adenosine production. J Immunol 187:676–683
94. Wang GJ, Liu Y, Qin A, Shah SV, Deng ZB, Xiang X et al (2008) Thymus exosomes-like particles induce regulatory T cells. J Immunol 181:5242–5248
95. Yu X, Huang C, Song B, Xiao Y, Fang M, Feng J et al (2013) CD4+CD25+ regulatory T cells-derived exosomes prolonged kidney allograft survival in a rat model. Cell Immunol 285:62–68
96. Sharma R, Zheng L, Deshmukh US, Jarjour WN, Sung SS, Fu SM et al (2007) A regulatory T cell-dependent novel function of CD25 (IL-2Ralpha) controlling memory CD8(+) T cell homeostasis. J Immunol 178:1251–1255
97. Foss FM (2000) DAB(389)IL-2 (denileukin diftitox, ONTAK): a new fusion protein technology. Clin Lymphoma 1:S27–S31
98. Telang S, Rasku MA, Clem AL, Carter K, Klarer AC, Badger WR et al (2011) Phase II trial of the regulatory T cell-depleting agent, denileukin diftitox, in patients with unresectable stage IV melanoma. BMC Cancer 11:515. doi:10.1186/1471-2407-11-515
99. Baur AS, Lutz MB, Schierer S, Beltrame L, Theiner G, Zinser E et al (2013) Denileukin diftitox (ONTAK) induces a tolerogenic phenotype in dendritic cells and stimulates survival of resting Treg. Blood 122:2185–2194
100. Kreitman RJ, Batra JK, Seetharam S, Chaudhary VK, FitzGerald DJ, Pastan I (1993) Single-chain immunotoxin fusions between anti-Tac and Pseudomonas exotoxin: relative importance of the two toxin disulfide bonds. Bioconjug Chem 4:112–120
101. Kreitman RJ (2009) Recombinant immunotoxins for the treatment of chemoresistant hematologic malignancies. Curr Pharm Des 15:2652–2664
102. Powell DJ Jr, Felipe-Silva A, Merino MJ, Ahmadzadeh M, Allen T, Levy C et al (2007) Administration of a CD25-directed immunotoxin, LMB-2, to patients with metastatic melanoma induces a selective partial reduction in regulatory T cells in vivo. J Immunol 179:4919–4928
103. Sahin M, Sahin E, Koksoy S (2013) Regulatory T cells in cancer: an overview and perspectives on cyclooxygenase-2 and Foxp3 DNA methylation. Hum Immunol 74:1061–1068
104. Mahic M, Yaqub S, Johansson CC, Tasken K, Aandahl EM (2006) FOXP3$^{+}$CD4$^{+}$CD25$^{+}$ adaptive regulatory T cells express cyclooxygenase-2 and suppress effector T cells by a prostaglandin E2-dependent mechanism. J Immunol 177:246–254
105. Baratelli F, Lin Y, Zhu L, Yang SC, Heuzé-Vourc'h N, Zeng G et al (2005) Prostaglandin E2 induces FOXP3 gene expression and T regulatory cell function in human CD4+ T cells. J Immunol 175:1483–1490
106. Trinath J, Hegde P, Sharma M, Maddur MS, Rabin M, Vallat JM et al (2013) Intravenous immunoglobulin expands regulatory T cells via induction of cyclooxygenase-2-dependent prostaglandin E2 in human dendritic cells. Blood 122:1419–1427
107. Shimizu J, Yamazaki S, Takahashi T, Ishida Y, Sakaguchi S (2002) Stimulation of CD25(+) CD4(+) regulatory T cells through GITR breaks immunological self-tolerance. Nat Immunol 3:135–142
108. McHugh RS, Whitters MJ, Piccirillo CA, Young DA, Shevach EM, Collins M et al (2002) CD4(+)CD25(+) immunoregulatory T cells: gene expression analysis reveals a functional role for the glucocorticoid-induced TNF receptor. Immunity 16:311–323

109. Ji HB, Liao G, Faubion WA, Abadía-Molina AC, Cozzo C, Laroux FS et al (2004) Cutting edge: the natural ligand for glucocorticoid-induced TNF receptor-related protein abrogates regulatory T cell suppression. J Immunol 172:5823–5827
110. Schaer DA, Murphy JT, Wolchok JD (2012) Modulation of GITR for cancer immunotherapy. Curr Opin Immunol 24:217–224
111. Coe D, Begom S, Addey C, White M, Dyson J, Chai JG (2010) Depletion of regulatory T cells by anti-GITR mAb as a novel mechanism for cancer immunotherapy. Cancer Immunol Immunother 59:1367–1377
112. Sagamura K, Ishii N, Weinberg AD (2004) Therapeutic targeting of the effector T-cell co-stimulatory molecule OX40. Nat Rev Immunol 4:420–431
113. Vu MD, Xiao X, Gao W, Degauque N, Chen M, Kroemer A et al (2007) OX40 costimulation turns off Foxp3+ Tregs. Blood 110:2501–2510
114. Voo KS, Bover L, Harline ML, Vien LT, Facchinetti V, Arima K et al (2013) Antibodies targeting human OX40 expand effector T cells and block inducible and natural regulatory T cell function. J Immunol 191:3641–3650
115. Piconese S, Valzasina B, Colombo MP (2008) OX40 triggering blocks suppression by regulatory T cells and facilitates tumor rejection. J Exp Med 205:825–839
116. Takebe N, Nguyen D, Yang SX (2014) Targeting notch signaling pathway in cancer: clinical development advances and challenges. Pharmacol Ther 141:140–149
117. Kostianovsky AM, Maier LM, Baecher-Allan C, Anderson AC, Anderson DE (2007) Up-regulation of gene related to anergy in lymphocytes is associated with Notch-mediated human T cell suppression. J Immunol 178:6158–6163
118. Qu-Yang HF, Zhang HW, Wu CG, Zhang P, Zhang J, Li JC et al (2009) Notch signaling regulates the FOXP3 promoter through RBP-J- and Hes1-dependent mechanisms. Mol Cell Biochem 320:109–114
119. Hue S, Kared H, Mehwish Y, Mouhamad S, Balbo M, Levy Y (2012) Notch activation on effector T cells increases their sensitivity to Treg cell-mediated suppression through upregulation of TGF-βRII expression. Eur J Immunol 42:1796–1803
120. Lutsiak ME, Semnani RT, De Pascalis R, Kashmiri SV, Schlom J, Sabzevari H (2005) Inhibition of CD4(+)25+ T regulatory cell function implicated in enhanced immune response by low-dose cyclophosphamide. Blood 105:2862–2868
121. Traverso I, Fenoglio D, Negrini S, Parodi A, Battaglia F, Kalli F et al (2012) Cyclophosphamide inhibits the generation and function of CD8(+) regulatory T cells. Hum Immunol 73:207–213
122. Zhang L, Dermawan K, Jin M, Liu R, Zheng H, Xu L et al (2008) Differential impairment of regulatory T cells rather than effector T cells by paclitaxel-based chemotherapy. Clin Immunol 129:219–229
123. Beyer M, Kochanek M, Darabi K, Popov A, Jensen M, Engl E et al (2005) Reduced frequencies and suppressive function of CD4+CD25hi regulatory T cells in patients with chronic lymphocytic leukemia after therapy with fludarabine. Blood 106:2018–2025
124. Chen J, Schmitt A, Giannopoulos K, Chen B, Rojewski M, Döhner H et al (2007) Imatinib impairs the proliferation and function of CD4+CD25+ regulatory T cells in a dose-dependent manner. Int J Oncol 31:1133–1139
125. Kurose K, Ohue Y, Oka M (2013) Anti-CCR4 mAb and regulatory T cells. Gan To Kagaku Ryoho (Japanese) 40:1150–1155

# Chapter 22
# MDSC: Myeloid-Derived Suppressor Cells

**Masahiko Shibata, Kenji Gonda, and Seiichi Takenoshita**

**Abstract** Myeloid-derived suppressor cells (MDSC) are a heterogeneous population of immature myeloid cells whose numbers are increased in states of cancer, inflammation, or infection. MDSC are reported to be induced by tumor-produced growth factors in cancer-bearing hosts. Mechanisms of immune suppression by MDSC include production of arginase-1, reactive oxygen species, and nitric oxide and secretion of immunosuppressive cytokines including IL-10. MDSC have been reported to be one of the strongest barriers to cancer immunotherapy because of their extensive suppression of immune functions. Inhibition of MDSC is thus essential for improving anticancer immunotherapy. Several compounds and agents that were reported to inhibit MDSC in mice are now being proven effective for inhibition of MDSC in patients with cancer. In this chapter, mechanisms of MDSC production and MDSC suppression of immune responses are described, and strategies to inhibit MDSC are addressed.

**Keywords** Immune suppression • Inflammation • MDSC

## 22.1 Introduction

Much progress and significant therapeutic advances have been made in the field of anticancer treatment in recent decades. Immunotherapy is a promising treatment modality for many types of cancer [1]. Several tumor-associated antigens that are recognized by specific monoclonal antibodies and T cells have been identified, providing essential tools for the development of immunotherapies, including

M. Shibata (✉)
Saitama Medical University International Medical Center, 1397-1 Yamane, Hidaka, Saitama 350-1298, Japan

Fukushima Medical University, Fukushima, Japan
e-mail: mshibata@saitama-med.ac.jpc

K. Gonda
Saitama Medical University International Medical Center, 1397-1 Yamane, Hidaka, Saitama 350-1298, Japan

S. Takenoshita
Fukushima Medical University, Fukushima, Japan



Y. Yamaguchi (ed.), *Immunotherapy of Cancer*,
DOI 10.1007/978-4-431-55031-0_22

dendritic cell (DC)-based vaccination and adoptive cell transfer [2]. However, even if vaccine-induced immune effector cells with antitumor reactivity are present, there are not always good clinical outcomes of immunotherapy [3]. This is because many different local and systemic mechanisms and regulatory pathways exist that can suppress antitumor immune responses [4]. A major paradigm shift in the field of tumor immunotherapy occurred following the recognition of tumor escape from immune elimination as an emerging additional hallmark of cancer. Myeloid-derived suppressor cells (MDSC) are a population of immature myeloid cells that are expanded in various conditions including cancer and inflammation and are capable of immune suppression [5]. The myeloid marker Gr1 is expressed on mouse MDSC, but CD11b and CD33 are expressed on human MDSC, which are also usually negative for HLA-DR, CD3, CD19, and CD57 [6, 7]. The MDSC of almost all patients with cancer, and of almost all tumor-bearing mice, are present in the proportion of approximately 75 % granulocytic MDSC (G-MDSC) and approximately 25 % monocytic MDSC (M-MDSC) [8, 9]. Increased production of intratumoral granulocyte (GCSF) or granulocyte-macrophage colony-stimulating factors (GM-CSF) may account for the differences seen in G-MDSC and M-MDSC levels. In addition to their generation by GCSF and GM-CSF, MDSC can also be generated in the bone marrow in response to cancer-derived factors such as interleukin (IL)-6, IL-1β, prostaglandin E2 (PGE2), tumor necrosis factor-α (TNFα), and vascular endothelial growth factor (VEGF). Chemokines such as CCL2, CXCL12, and CXCL5 have been reported to recruit MDSC to tumor sites [10–12].

## 22.2 Origin and Markers of MDSC

A number of studies of tumor-bearing mice have established that a group of bone marrow-derived cells, the MDSC, are directly involved in the suppression of immune responses in cancer [11]. These cells express both Gr1 (Ly6G and Ly6C: myeloid lineage differentiation antigens) and CD11b (αM integrin). Inoculation with tumor cells or development of spontaneous tumors results in a marked systemic expansion of these cells [13, 14]. Under these conditions the number of MDSC in the spleen increases by 5- to 20-fold. In humans, MDSC are generally defined as CD14-CD11b+ cells, or, more narrowly, as the cells that express the common myeloid marker CD33 but lack the expression of markers of mature myeloid and lymphoid cells. Many different phenotypes have been utilized to define MDSC in humans, but they are usually defined as CD33+CD11b+HLA-DR$^{neg/low}$ or CD33+CD11b+CD14- [15, 16]. Two main MDSC subtypes have been reported in tumor-bearing mice, granulocytic (G-MDSC). MDSC populations are even more complex in humans; however, in humans M-MDSC are predominantly CD14+, whereas G-MDSC are CD15+, and both populations are CD33+HLA-DR-.

MDSC that are expanded under pathological conditions are not a defined subset of myeloid cells but are rather a heterogeneous population of activated immature myeloid cells that have been prevented from fully differentiating into mature cells. These MDSC lack the expression of cell surface markers that are specifically expressed by monocytes, macrophages, or DC and comprise a mixture of myeloid cells that have the morphology of granulocytes or monocytes. These two subsets of MDSC, termed G-MDSC and M-MDSC, respectively, may have different functions in cancer and infectious and autoimmune diseases. Both of these subsets of MDSC are expanded in mouse tumor models, but in most cases the expansion of G-MDSC is much greater than that of M-MDSC. These two MDSC subsets appear to have different mechanism of immune suppression. In addition, the ability to differentiate into mature DC and macrophages in vitro has been shown to be restricted to M-MDSC.

In recent years, attempts have been made to identify additional subsets of MDSC by using several other surface molecules including CD80 (known as B7.1), CD115 (macrophage colony-stimulating factor receptor), and CD124.

## 22.3 Immunosuppressive Mechanisms of MDSC (Fig. 22.1)

Many tumor models and clinical trials have demonstrated that immunotherapy of advanced tumors in both animal models and human patients failed to achieve a therapeutic response as a result of loss of T-cell responses [1, 2]. In some cases these poor outcomes were associated with tumor progression despite a robust T-cell response. The development of mechanisms that cause T-cell anergy provided important data regarding the pathway by which cancer (or chronic inflammation) can induce T cell dysfunction. It has been reported that MDSC play an important role in these mechanisms [17–19].

The most important function of MDSC is to inhibit the cytotoxic response mediated by T lymphocytes and NK cells. M-MDSC have been reported to inhibit T-cell responses through depletion of L-arginine, via both arginase I and iNOS [20–22]. On the other hand, it has been reported that G-MDSC inhibit T-cell responses through reactive oxygen species (ROS) [14, 23]. Both M-MDSC and G-MDSC use antigen-specific and nonspecific mechanisms to regulate immune responses. In addition to directly suppressing immune responses, MDSC inhibit T-cell-mediated cytotoxicity through indirect mechanisms. Thus, MDSC also produce indoleamine 2,3-dioxygenase (IDO) [24], NADPH oxidase, and immunosuppressive cytokines that have the potential to inhibit cytotoxic T lymphocytes (CTL), dendritic cells (DC), and natural killer (NK) cells as well as to expand regulatory T cells (Treg) [11, 17, 25, 26].

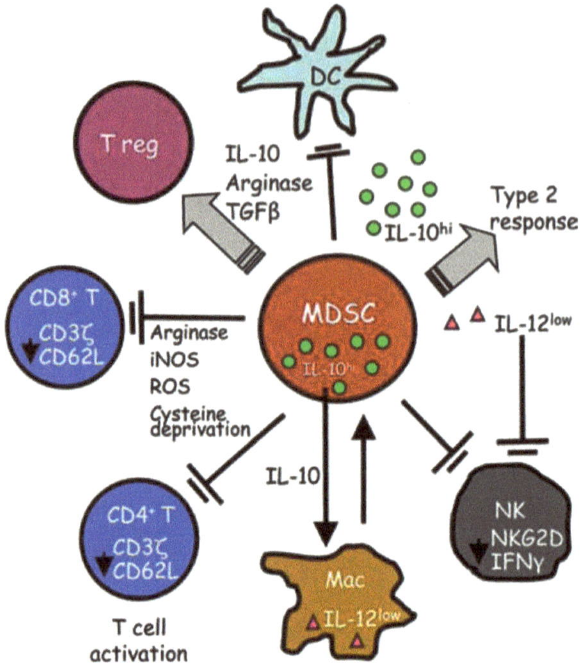


**Fig. 22.1** Immunosuppressive mechanisms of MDSC (Ostrand-Rosenberg and Sinha [25]). MDSC suppress antitumor immunity through a variety of diverse mechanisms. T-cell activation is suppressed by the production of arginase and ROS, the nitration of the TCR, the nitration of the TCR, cysteine deprivation, and the induction of Tregs. Innate immunity is impaired by the downregulation of macrophage-produced IL-12, the increase in MDSC production of IL-10, and the suppression of NK cell cytotoxicity. Ag presentation is limited by the expansion of MDSC at the expense of DC

## 22.4 MDSC in Cancer Patients

MDSC were first characterized in tumor-bearing mice and in patients with cancer. These cells have been shown to display marked systemic expansion when mice were inoculated with transplantable tumor cells. In addition, up to a tenfold increase in MDSC numbers was detected in the circulating blood of patients with cancer. Furthermore, MDSC are found in tumor tissues and in the lymph nodes of tumor -bearing mice [10, 11, 17, 26].

A dysfunctional immune response in cancer patients that was manifested by the loss of delayed type hypersensitivity was demonstrated several decades ago [27–30]. However, although cancer patients do not develop the characteristic opportunistic infections seen in patients that have received high-dose chemotherapy, they do show impaired T-cell responses against bacterial antigens [27–30]. This development of specific immune suppression in cancer patients has been investigated for many years, and the impact of MDSC on these phenomena is becoming increasingly better understood. MDSC can synergize with Tregs to prevent antitumor immunity, whereas reciprocal communications with many types of immunocompetent cells can be either antitumorigenic or pro-tumorigenic [31, 32]. These important findings were derived from animal studies, and it will be essential to determine whether they can be extrapolated to a human setting. MDSC have been reported to be present in many types of human cancers [33–36]. We recently reported that circulating levels of MDSC were significantly increased in patients with gastrointestinal, breast, pulmonary, ovarian, and thyroid cancer. Moreover, the levels of MDSC significantly correlated with immunosuppression, malnutrition, and inflammation. MDSC have also been reported to correlate with clinical stages of several types of cancer and with increased levels of IL-6 or IL-10. Our laboratory has found that increased levels of MDSC were significantly correlated with the plasma levels of VEGF, which is an important factor for the induction and proliferation of MDSC [37]. In a recent human setting of immunotherapy, clinical responders to therapy with the anti-CTLA-4 antibody, ipilimumab, had significantly fewer M-MDSC as compared to nonresponders [18].

MDSC expansion is also associated with autoimmunity and inflammation. A large increase in the number of MDSC was found in experimental mouse models of multiple sclerosis, inflammatory bowel diseases, or intraocular autoimmune inflammatory disease [38–41].

## 22.5 Strategies of MDSC Inhibition (Fig. 22.2)

Multiple mechanisms of cancer immune evasion and immunoinhibitory pathways have been identified. It has been well established that tumors can promote immunosuppressive cells including Tregs, MDSC, immature DCs, and type 2 macrophages [42]. These cells inhibit anticancer immunity and compromise the efficacy of anticancer immunotherapy. Inhibition or depletion of MDSC enhances the activities of cancer vaccines in animal models. It has been demonstrated that MDSC elimination, inhibition, or the induction of their differentiation into proinflammatory cells using anticancer agents, in patients with different types of cancer, enhances anticancer immunity and fosters the response to immunotherapy [43].

Phosphodiesterase-5 (PDE-5) inhibitors may reduce expression of the arginase-1 gene *ARG 1* and the nitric oxide synthase 2 gene NOS2 [44, 45]. Arginase-1-mediated depletion of L-arginine from the tumor microenvironment may be one of the mechanisms of MDSC-induced T-cell suppression. The production of nitric oxide may be a direct cause of MDSC-induced suppression of T-cell responses [46]. The nitro (NO)-aspirin inhibits inducible NOS via various mechanisms and may inhibit MDSC action [47]. MDSC display increased expression of prostaglandin E receptors, and cyclooxygenase 2 (COX-2) is involved in the synthesis of prostaglandin E. Administration of the widely used COX-2 inhibitor, celecoxib, to mice was associated with lower levels of MDSC and a higher number of tumor-

**Strategies of MDSC Inhibition Under Investigation**

| Deactivation of MDSC | Differentiation of MDSC into mature cells | Blocking Development of MDSC | Depletion of MDSC |
|---|---|---|---|
| **NO Inhibitors**<br>•PDE-5 inhibitors*<br>• NO-aspirins*<br>•L-NAME<br>**Arginase Inhibitors**<br>•PDE-5 Inhibitors*<br>•COX2 inhibitors<br>•NOHA<br>•L-NAME<br>**ROS Inhibitors**<br>•Synthetic Triterpenoids*<br>**MDSC Migration Inhibitors**<br>•Anti-glycan antibodies<br>•CSF-1R inhibitors*<br>**Others**<br>•Histamine inhibitors<br>•Anti-IL-17 Antibodies | **Vitamins**<br>•ATRA*<br>•Vitamin A<br>•Vitamin D3*<br>**Cytokines**<br>•IL-12<br>**Others:**<br>•CpG | **Bisphosphonates**<br>•Zoledronic Acid*<br>**Modulators of Cell Signaling**<br>•JAK2/STAT3 inhibitors*<br>•Multi-Kinase Inhibitors*<br>•VEGF Inhibitors* | **Cytotoxic Agents**<br>•Gemcitabine<br>•Cisplatin<br>•Paclitaxel<br>•5-Fluorouracil<br>**HSP 90 Inhibitors**<br>•17-DMAG<br>**•Others**<br>•IL-6R blockers<br>•Antibody Drug Conjugates (ex IL-13-PE) |

**Fig. 22.2** Graphical presentation of MDSC inhibition strategies (Wesolowski et al. [26])

infiltrating lymphocytes [48]. Therefore, the COX-2 inhibitor may be effective in reducing MDSC activity [49–51]. N-hydroxy-L-arginine (NOHA) and N-nitro-L-arginine methyl ester (L-NAME) are compounds that inhibit arginase-1, and these drugs were shown to decrease immunosuppressive MDSC activity [52, 53]. Histamine H2 blockers such as cimetidine appear to induce apoptosis of MDSC through induction of Fas and FasL [54]. IL-17 is also an important cytokine for recruitment of MDSC to tumor sites in murine models, and anti-IL-17 antibody administration may lead to a decrease in MDSC at tumor sites [55]. As for MDSC differentiating agents, all-trans retinoic acid (ATRA) is a metabolite of vitamin A and can differentiate MDSC into DC, granulocytes, and monocytes, which is associated with improvements in CTL (cytotoxic T-lymphocyte)-mediated immune response. Vitamins such as vitamin D3 or vitamin A may also enhance the maturation of myeloid cells [56–59].

Tyrosine kinase signaling has been implicated in the stimulation of early myeloid cell differentiation into MDSC [60]. Sunitinib is a multi-kinase inhibitor that has multiple targets including the VEGFR and c-kit. Treatment of patients with renal cell carcinoma with sunitinib led to a reduction in circulating MDSC levels with improved Th1 functions [61]. We have reported that plasma levels of VEGF are increased in patients with gastrointestinal cancers and are correlated with immune suppression, MDSC levels, and low production of IL-12 [62]. Anti-VEGF antibody treatment of patients with renal cell carcinoma did not result in a decrease in circulating MDSC levels, but the circulating levels of mature DC were increased [63].

Some cytotoxic chemotherapeutic agents have been found to cause MDSC depletion through as yet incompletely understood mechanisms. Administration of gemcitabine, an antimetabolite drug that is used for the treatment of pancreatic, breast, ovarian, and lung carcinomas and of malignant lymphoma, to tumor-bearing mice has been reported to deplete MDSC, resulting in improvement of antitumoral immune responses [64, 65]. 5-Fluorouracil, another antimetabolite, has also been reported to induce apoptosis of MDSC [66, 67]. Docetaxel, a mitotic inhibitor, was shown to impair MDSC-immunosuppressive function by blocking STAT3 (signal transduction and activator of transcription) phosphorylation and by promoting MDSC differentiation into M1 macrophages [43]. Immunomodulatory effects of the chemotherapeutic anthracycline agent, doxorubicin, have been reported. It is noteworthy that MDSC number remained low following immunotherapy in combination with chemotherapy that included doxorubicin, whereas MDSC number significantly increased after treatment with immunotherapy alone. Cisplatin-treated tumor-bearing mice displayed reduced numbers of MDSC and Tregs compared to untreated mice [66]. Other cytotoxic agents may also inhibit MDSC. 5-Fluorouracil has been widely used in clinical practice for many years. Circulating numbers of MDSC in patients with gastrointestinal cancers have been reported to decrease after treatment with 5-fluorouracil-including regimens [67, 68]. We have measured circulating MDSC levels before and after treatments including gemcitabine as well as other regimens that included 5-fluorouracil, paclitaxel, and cisplatin and reported that it decreased mainly in patients with clinical effects [69]. This observation means that not only is there a direct decrease of MDSC uniformly induced by chemotherapeutic agents but that this decrease is secondary to immunomodulatory effects that result from tumor unloading such as tumor shrinkage, which may be also be important in clinical practice.

Antitumor immunotherapy has been reported to be more effective in patients with lower levels of MDSC than in patients with higher MDSC levels. Also, preclinical evidence suggests that cancer vaccines are more effective in tumor-bearing mice that have been depleted of MDSC [70–73]. MDSC may be inhibited by numerous molecules including the molecules described in this chapter. The ability of agents such as ATRA, PDE-5 inhibitors, NO-aspirins, and tyrosine kinase inhibitors to inhibit MDSC and to enhance antitumor immunity in humans is already being tested in clinical trials. Other compounds are still undergoing testing as MDSC inhibitors in preclinical models.

## 22.6 Conclusion

It has been established that tumor progression can be associated with a progressive accumulation of immature myeloid cells in the circulating blood, lymph nodes, spleen, and primary tumor site, due to tumor-derived factors. This aberrant balance between immature and mature myeloid cells is a hallmark of cancer and may be one of the central mechanisms of tumor evasion of the immune system and subsequent tumor progression.

The advent of immunotherapy of cancer made it apparent that, despite powerful biological agents that can prime tumor-specific T cells, tumors have sophisticated mechanisms including MDSC for escape from immune responses. However, MDSC are not unique to cancer. Trauma patients and patients with chronic infections also have increased numbers of MDSC, which express arginase I that inhibits T-cell responses. Our understanding of the role that MDSC play in tumor progression has greatly increased over the last 10 years. Multiple approaches have been taken to suppress MDSC including the use of ATRA, inhibition of nitric oxide function using NO-aspirin, inhibition of PDE-5, blockage of arginase activity with specific arginase inhibitors, or blockage of MDSC accumulation using antibodies against specific markers expressed on MDSC. As previously mentioned, MDSC accumulation can be inhibited by using the chemotherapeutic agents sunitinib, gemcitabine, or 5-fluorouracil. It is likely that appropriate combinations of inhibitors that inhibit the functions of MDSC with stimuli that protect T cells may overcome these powerful tumor-derived mechanisms that impair the promise of cancer immunotherapy. Further research is needed to identify the most promising compound for clinical development.

## References


1. Dougan M, Granoff G (2009) Immune therapy for cancer. Annu Rev Immunol 27:83–117
2. Kantoff PW, Higano CD, Shore ND, Berger ER, Small EJ, Penson DF et al (2010) Sipuleucel-T immunotherapy for castration-resistant prostate cancer. N Engl J Med 363:411–422
3. Hanahan D, Weinberg RA (2011) Hallmarks of cancer: the next generation. Cell 144:646–674
4. Vesely MD, Kenshaw MH, Schreiber RD, Smyth MJ (2011) Natural innate and adaptive immunity to cancer. Annu Rev Immunol 29:235–271
5. Kamo I, Friedman H (1977) Immunosuppression and the role of suppressive factors in cancer. Adv Cancer Res 25:271–321
6. Gabrilovich DI, Bronte V, Chen SH, Colombo MP, Ochoa A, Ostrand-Rosenberg S, Schreiber H (2007) The terminology issue for myeloid-derived suppressor cells. Cancer Res 67:425–426
7. Bronte V, Appoloni A, Cabrelle A, Ronca R, Serafini P, Zamboni P, Restifo NP, Zanovello P (2000) Identification of a CD11b(+)/Gr-1(+)/CD31(+)myeloid progenitor capable of activating or suppressing CD8(+) T cells. Blood 96:3838–3846
8. Schmielau J, Finn OJ (2011) Activated granulocytes and granulocyte-derived hydrogen peroxide are the underlying mechanism of suppression of T-cell function in advanced cancer patients. Cancer Res 61:4756–4760
9. Kusmartsev S, Nefedova Y, Yoder D, Gabrilovich DI (2004) Antigen-specific inhibition of CD8+ T cell response by immature myeloid cells in cancer is mediated by reactive oxygen species. J Immunol 172:989–999
10. Lindau I, Gielen P, Kroesen M, Wesseling P, Adena GJ (2012) The immunosuppressive tumour network: myeloid-derived suppressor cells, regulatory T cells and natural killer T cells. Immunology 138:105–115
11. Gabrilovich DI, Nagaraj S (2009) Myeloid-derived suppressor cells as regulators of the immune system. Nat Rev Immunol 9:162–174
12. Sawanobori Y, Ueha S, Kurachi M, Shimaoka T, Talmadge JE, Abe J et al (2008) Chemokine-mediated rapid turnover of myeloid-derived suppressor cells in tumor-bearing mice. Blood 118:5457–5466

13. Huang B, Pan PY, Li Q, Sato AI, Levy DE, Bromberg J, Divino CM, Chen SH (2006) Gr-1′CD115′ immature myeloid suppressor cells mediate the development of tumor-induced T regulatory and T-cell anergy in tumor-bearing host. Cancer Res 66:1123–1131
14. Youn JI, Nagarj S, Collazo M, Gabrilovich DI (2008) Subsets of myeloid-derived suppressor cells in tumor-bearing mice. J Immunol 181:5791–5802
15. Ochoa AC, Zea AH, Hernandez C, Rodriguez PC (2007) Arginase, prostaglandins, and myeloid-derived suppressor cells in renal cell carcinoma. Clin Cancer Res 13:721s–726s
16. Almand B, Clark JI, Nikitina E, van Beynen J, English NR, Knight SC et al (2001) Increased production of immature myeloid cells in cancer patients. A mechanism of immunosuppression in cancer. J Immunol 166:678–689
17. Nagaraj S, Gabrilovich DI (2008) Tumor escape mechanism governed by myeloid-derived suppressor cells. Cancer Res 68:2561–2563
18. Laborde RR, Lin Y, Gustafson MP, Bulur PA, Diets AB (2014) Cancer vaccines in the world of immune suppressive monocytes (CD14+HLA-DRlo/neg Cells): the gateway to improved responses. Front Immunol 5:1–5
19. Serafini P, Carbley R, Noonan KA, Tan G, Bronte V, Borello I (2004) High-dose GM-CSF producing vaccines impair the immune response through the recruitment of myeloid suppressor cells. Cancer Res 64:6337–6343
20. Rodriguez PC, Zea AH, Culotta KS, Zabaleta J, Ochoa JB, Ochoa AC (2002) Regulation of T cell receptor CD3zeta chain expression by L-arginine. J Biol Chem 2777:21123–21129
21. Bronte V, Zanovello P (2005) Regulation of immune responses by L-arginine metabolism. Nat Rev Immunol 5:641–654
22. Rodriguez PC, Ochoa AC (2008) Arginine regulation by myeloid-derived suppressor cells and tolerance in cancer: mechanisms and therapeutic perspectives. Immunol Rev 222:180–191
23. Dolcetti L, Peranzoni E, Ugel S, Marigo I, Fernandez Gomez A, Mesa C et al (2010) Hierarchy of immunosuppressive strength among myeloid-derived suppressor cell subsets is determined by GM-CSF. Eur J Immunol 40:22–35
24. Mao Y, Poschke I, Kiessling R (2014) Tumor-induced immune-suppression: role of inflammatory mediators released by myelomonocytic cells. J Int Med 276:154–179
25. Ostrand-Rosenberg S, Sinha P (2009) Myeloid-derived suppressor cells: linking inflammation and cancer. J Immunol 182:4499–4506
26. Wesolowski R, Markowitz J, Carson WE III (2013) Myeloid derived suppressor cells-a new therapeutic target in the treatment of cancer. J Immunother Cancer 1:10
27. Miescher S, Stoeck M, Qiao L, Barras C, Barrelet L, von Fliedner V (1988) Preferential clonogenic deficit of CD8-positive T-lymphocytes infiltrating human solid tumors. Cancer Res 48:2094–2103
28. Miescher S, Whiteside TL, Carrel S, von Fliedner V (1986) Functional properties of tumor-infiltrating and blood lymphocytes in patients with solid tumors: effects of tumor cells and their supernatants on proliferative responses of lymphocytes. J Immunol 136:1899–1907
29. Whiteside TL, Miescher S, Moretta L, von Fliedner V (1988) Cloning and proliferating precursor frequencies of tumor-infiltrating lymphocytes from human solid tumors. Transplant Proc 20:342–343
30. Whiteside TL, Rabinowich H (1988) The role of Fas/FasL in immunosuppression induced by human tumors. Cancer Immunol Immunother 46:175–184
31. Yang R, Cai Z, Zhang Y, Yutzy WH 4th, Roby KF, Roden RB (2006) CD80 in immune suppression by mouse ovarian carcinoma-associated Gr-1′CD11b’ myeloid cells. Cancer Res 66:6807–6815
32. Huang B, Pan PY, Li Q, Sato AI, Levy DE, Bromberg J et al (2006) Gr-1+CD115+ immature myeloid suppressor cells mediate the development of tumor-induced T regulatory cells and T-cell anergy in tumor bearing host. Cancer Res 66:1125–1131
33. Ohki S, Shibata M, Gonda K, Machida T, Shimura T, Nakamura I et al (2012) Circulating myeloid-derived suppressor cells are increased and correlate to immune suppression, inflammation and hypoalbuminemia in patients with cancer. Oncol Rep 28:453–458

34. Gonda K, Shibata M, Shimura T, Machida T, Suzuki S, Nakamura I et al (2012) Serum soluble interleukin-2 receptor is increased in malnourished and immunosuppressed patients with gastric and colorectal cancer: possible influence of myeloid-derived suppressor cells. World J Oncol 3:158–164
35. Yazawa T, Shibata M, Gonda K, Machida T, Suzuki S, Kenjo A et al (2013) Increased IL-17 production correlates with immunosuppression involving myeloid-derived suppressor cells and nutritional impairment in patients with various gastrointestinal cancers. Mol Clin Oncol 1:675–679
36. Suzuki S, Shibata M, Gonda K, Kanke Y, Ashizawa M, Ujiie D et al (2013) Immunosuppression involving increased myeloid-derived suppressor cells, systemic inflammation and hypoalbuminemia are present in patients with anaplastic thyroid cancer. Mol Clin Oncol 1:959–964
37. Watanabe T, Shibata M, Nishiyama H, Soeda S, Furukawa S, Gonda K, Takenoshita S, Fujimori K (2013) Elevated serum levels of vascular endothelial growth factor is effective as a marker for malnutrition and inflammation in patients with ovarian cancer. Biomed Rep 1:197–201
38. Zhu B, Bando Y, Xiao S, Yang K, Anderson AC, Kuchroo VK, Khoury SJ (2007) $CD11b^{+}$ $Ly\text{-}6C^{DM}$ suppressive monocytes in experimental autoimmune encephalomyelitis. J Immunol 179:5228–5237
39. Kerr EC, Raveney BJ, Copland DA, Dick AD, Nicholson LB (2008) Analysis of retinal cellular infiltrate in experimental autoimmune uveoretinitis reveals multiple regulatory cell populations. J Autoimmun 31:354–361
40. Marhaba R, Vitacolonna M, Hildebrand D, Baniyask M, Freyschmidt-Paul P, Zoller M (2007) The importance of myeloid-derived suppressor cells in the regulation of autoimmune effector cells by a chronic contact eczema. J Immunol 179:5071–5081
41. Haile LA, von Wasielewski R, Gamrekelashvili J, Kruger C, Bachman O, Westendorf AM et al (2008) Myeloid-derived suppressor cells in inflammatory bowel disease: a new immunoregulatory pathway. Gastroenterology 135:871–881
42. Ostrand-Rosenberg S, Sinha P, Beury DW, Clements VK (2012) Cross-talk between myeloid-derived suppressor cells (MDSC), macrophages, and dendritic cells enhances tumor-induced immune suppression. Semin Cancer Biol 22:275–281
43. Kao J, Ko EC, Sikora AT, Fu S, S-h C (2011) Targeting immune suppressing myeloid-derived suppressor cells in oncology. Crit Rev Oncol Hematol 77:12–19
44. Serafini P, Meckel K, Kelso M, Noonan K, Califano J, Koch W et al (2006) Phosphodiesterase-5 inhibition augments endogenous antitumor immunity by reducing myeloid-derived suppressor cell function. J Exp Med 203:2691–2702
45. Nagaraj S, Schrum AG, Cho HI, Celis E, Gabrilovich DI (2010) Mechanism of T cell tolerance induced by myeloid-derived suppressor cells. J Immunol 184:3106–3116
46. Molon B, Ugel S, Del Pozo F, Sondani C, Zilio S, Avella D et al (2011) Chemokine nitration prevent intratumoral infiltration of antigen-specific T cells. J Exp Med 208:1949–1962
47. Fiorucci S, Santucci S, Cirino G, Mencarelli A, Familiari L, Soldano PD, Morelli A (2000) IL-1 beta converting enzyme is a target for nitric oxide-releasing aspirin: new insight in the anti-inflammatory mechanism of nitric oxide-releasing nonsteroidal anti-inflammatory drugs. J Immunol 165:5245–5254
48. Veltman JD, Lambers ME, van Nimwegen M, Hendriks RW, Hoogsteden HC, Aerts JG, Hegmans JP (2010) COX-2 inhibition improves immunotherapy and is associated with decreased numbers of myeloid-derived suppressor cells in mesothelioma. Celecoxib influences MDSC function. BMC Cancer 10:464
49. Sinha P, Clements VK, Fulton AM, Ostrand-Rosenberg S (2007) Prostaglandin E2 promotes tumor progression by inducing myeloid-derived suppressor cells. Cancer Res 67:4507–4513
50. Rodriguez PC, Hernadez CP, Quiceno D, Rubinett SM, Zabaleta J, Ochoa JB, Ochoa AC (2005) Arginase 1 in myeloid suppressor cells in induced by COX-2 in lung carcinoma. J Exp Med 202:931–939

51. Talmadge JE, Hood KC, Zobel LC, Shafer LR, Coles M, Toth B (2007) Chemoprevention by cyclooxygenase-2 inhibition reduces immature myeloid suppressor cell expansion. Int Immunopharmacol 7:140–151
52. Stuehr DJ, Kwon NS, Nathan CF, Griffith OW, Feldman PL, Wiseman J (1991) N omega-hydoxy-l-arginine is an intermediate in the biosynthesis of nitric oxide from l-arginine. J Biol Chem 266:6259–6263
53. Reisser D, Onier-Cherix N, Jennin JF (2002) Arginase activity is inhibited by L-NAME, both in vitro and in vivo. J Enzyme Inhibit Med Chem 17:267–270
54. Zheng Y, Xu M, Li X, Jia J, Fan K, Lai G (2012) Cimetidine suppresses lung tumor growth in mice trough proapoptosis of myeloid-derived suppressor cells. Mol Immunol 54:74–83
55. He D, Li H, Yasuf N, Elmets CA, Li J, Mounts JD, Xu H (2010) IL-17 promotes tumor development through the induction of promoting microenvironments at tumor sites and myeloid-derived suppressor cells. J Immunol 184:2281–2288
56. Bastien J, Richette-Egly C (2004) Nuclear retinoid receptors and the transcription of retinoid-target genes. Gene 328:1–16
57. Hengesbach LM, Hoag KA (2004) Physiological concentrations of retinoic acid favor myeloid dendritic cells development over granulocyte development in cultures of bone marrow cells from mice. J Nutr 134:2653–2659
58. Kusmartsev S, Su Z, Heiser A, Dannul J, Erushanov E, Kubler H et al (2008) Reversal of myeloid cell-mediated immunosuppression in patients with metastatic renal cell carcinoma. Clin Cancer Res 14:8270–8278
59. Mirza N, Fishman M, Fricke I, Dunn M, Neuger AM, Frost TJ et al (2006) All-trans retinoic acid improves differentiation of myeloid cells and immune response in cancer patients. Cancer Res 66:9299–9307
60. Ugel S, Delpozzo F, Desantis G, Papalini F, Simonato F, Sonda N, Zilio S, Bronte V (2009) Cur Opin Pharmacol 9:470–481
61. Ko JS, Zea AH, Rini BI, Irelan JL, Elon P, Cohen P et al (2009) Sunitinib mediates reversal of myeloid-derived suppressor cell accumulation in renal cell carcinoma patients. Clin Cancer Res 15:2148–2157
62. Nakamura I, Shibata M, Gonda K, Yazawa T, Shimura T, Anazawa T et al (2013) Serum levels of vascular endothelial growth factor are increased and correlate with malnutrition, immuno-suppression involving MDSCs and systemic inflammation in patients with cancer of the digestive system. Oncol Let 5:1682–1686
63. Rodriguez PC, Emstoff MS, Hernandez C, Atkins M, Zabaleta J, Sierra R, Ochoa AC (2009) Arginase I-producing myeloid-derived suppressor cells in renal cell carcinoma are a subpopulation of activated granulocytes. Cancer Res 69:1553–1560
64. Suzuki E, Kapoor V, Jassar AS, Kaiser LR, Albelda SM (2005) Gemcitabine selectively eliminates splenic Gr-1+?CD11b+ myeloid suppressor cells I tumor-bearing animals and enhances antitumor immune activity. Clin Cancer Res 11:6713–6721
65. Le HK, Graham L, Cha E, Morales JK, Manjili MH, Bear HD (2009) Gemcitabine directly inhibits myeloid derived suppressor cells in BALB/c mice bearing 4T1 mammary carcinoma and augments expansion of T cells from tumor-bearing mice. Int Immunopharmacol 9:900–909
66. Tseng CW, Hung CF, Alvarez RD, Trimble C, Huh WK, Kim D et al (2008) Pretreatment with cisplatin enhances E7-specific CD8; T-cell-mediated antitumor immunity induced by DNA vaccination. Clin Cancer Res 14:3185–3192
67. Naiditch H, Shurin MR, Shurin GV (2011) Targeting myeloid regulatory cells in cancer by chemotherapeutic agents. Immunol Res 50:276–285
68. Vincent J, Mignot G, Chalmin F, Ladoire S, Bruchard M, Chebriaux A et al (2010) 5-fluorouracil selectively kills tumor-associated myeloid-derived suppressor cells resulting in enhanced T cell-dependent antitumor immunity. Cancer Res 70:3052–3061
69. Shibata M, Gonda K, Nakamura I, Shimura T, Ohki S, Ohtake T et al (2013) Increased myeloid-derived suppressor cells (MDSC) correlated to immune suppression and chronic

inflammation in patients with cancer. In: Cancer immunology and immunotherapy Keystone Symposium, Vancouver
70. Kusmartsev S, Cheng F, Yu B, Nefedova Y, Sotomayor E, Lush R, Gabrilovich DI (2003) All-trans-retinoic-acid eliminates immature myeloid cells from tumor bearing mice and improves the effect of vaccination. Cancer Res 63:4441–4449
71. De Santo C, Serafini P, Marigo I, Dolcetti L, Bolla M, Del Soldato P et al (2005) Nitroaspirin corrects immune dysfunction in tumor-bearing hosts and promotes tumor eradication by cancer vaccination. Proc Natl Acad Sci U S A 102:4185–4190
72. Nagaraj S, Youn JI, Weber H, Iclozan C, Lu L, Cotter MJ et al (2010) Anti-inflammatory triterpenoid blocks immune suppressive function of MDSC and improves immune response in cancer. Clin Cancer Res 16:1812–1823
73. Melani C, Sangaletti S, Barazzetta FM, Werb Z, Colombo MP (2007) Amino-biphosphonate-mediated MMP-9 inhibition breaks the tumor-bone marrow axis responsible for myeloid-derived suppressor cell expansion and macrophage infiltration in tumor stroma. Cancer Res 67:11438–11446

# Part VIII
# Immune-Related Response Criteria and Guidance for Clinical Trials

# Chapter 23
# Immune-Related Response Criteria and Guidance for Clinical Trials

**Hiroyuki Suzuki**

**Abstract** Recent progression in the field of tumor immunology has enabled the contribution of cancer immunotherapy to standard cancer treatments. However, to date, most clinical trials investigating novel treatments such as therapeutic peptide vaccines have failed possibly because of the lack of correct evaluation and/or trial setting. According to this context, immunotherapy-specific novel concepts were devised. Immune-related response criteria (irRC) are used in an immunotherapy-specific evaluation protocol. In addition, publication of the "Guidance of clinical trials" for immunotherapy has helped develop cancer immunotherapeutic agents established by the US Food and Drug Administration. Furthermore, The Japanese Society has also created "Guidance for peptide vaccines for the treatment of cancer" by biological therapy. This unique and specific guidance has aided the development of peptide vaccines. These evolutions have clearly contributed to this field, and novel drugs such as ipilimumab have recently been approved by using these concepts.

**Keywords** Immune-related response criteria (irRC) • Guidance for clinical trials • Guidance for peptide vaccines for the treatment of cancer

## 23.1 Introduction

Recent remarkable progress in the field of cancer immunotherapy is based on a defined understanding of the molecular basis of immune responses against cancer including the identification of tumor antigens, dendritic cells, and immunosuppressive mechanisms. Encouraged by this progress, many small studies have been accomplished. Rosenberg et al. [1] summarized these results in 2004 and reported that the clinical effectiveness of cancer immunotherapy including cancer vaccines and dendritic cell-based immunotherapy was limited when evaluations used the conventional World Health Organization (WHO) response criteria [2] or Response

H. Suzuki, M.D., Ph.D. (✉)
Department of Regenerative Surgery, Fukushima Medical University, 1 Hikarigaoka, Fukushima 960-1295, Japan
e-mail: hiro@fmu.ac.jp



Y. Yamaguchi (ed.), *Immunotherapy of Cancer*,
DOI 10.1007/978-4-431-55031-0_23

Evaluation Criteria in Solid Tumors (RECIST) [3]. However, many physicians and experts have experienced the effectiveness of immunotherapy in the clinic. In 2004 and 2005, approximately 200 oncologists, immunotherapists, and regulatory experts in the USA convened to discuss the evaluation of immunotherapy and subsequently established novel and specific criteria for immunotherapy evaluation termed the immune-related response criteria (irRC), as reported by Wolchock et al. [4].

During the establishment of the irRC, the US Food and Drug Administration (FDA) released a draft of Guidance of Industry in September 2009 [5], which contained clinical considerations for cancer vaccines and which was finalized in 2011. This guidance described the basic concept and considerations of developing novel cancer vaccines throughout the preclinical and clinical phases. Similar guidance has been developed in Japan by The Japanese Society for Biological Therapy, a group of researchers focused on biological therapies for cancer, mainly in the field of immunotherapy, which has published "Guidance for peptides vaccines for the treatment of cancer" [6].

These important revolutions have contributed and accelerated the development of cancer immunotherapeutic drugs not only as vaccines but also as antibody-based immunotherapeutic drugs.

In this chapter, the details of irRC and guidance of clinical trials will be summarized.

## 23.2 irRC

It was widely known that there is a difference in the pattern of effects between conventional cytotoxic chemotherapy and immunotherapy. In chemotherapy, we define a complete response (CR) and partial response (PR) as effective and stable disease (SD), but this does not define drug efficacy, because SD often rapidly develops into progressive disease (PD). However, recently established targeted therapies including immunotherapy have sometimes induced a long SD. Wolchok et al. reported that several distinct patterns of responses were observed in an ipilimumab trial for patients with melanoma [7]. Interestingly, some patients showed an initial increase in tumor volume followed by a decrease. A similar phenomenon was also observed in our peptide vaccine trial where metastatic cervical lymph nodes in patients with lung cancer were initially increased and highly accumulated by fludeoxyglucose-positron emission tomography (FDG-PET) scan followed by a remarkable response (Fig. 23.1) [8]. These responses were thought to be distinctive to immunotherapy. Thus, when considering immunotherapy, novel and specific evaluation protocols are required and were established in 2004 and 2005, with irRC in 2009. The major points of the irRC are summarized: (a) the appearance of measurable antitumor activity may take longer for immune therapies than for cytotoxic therapies; (b) responses to immune therapies may occur after conventional PD; (c) discontinuation of immune therapy may

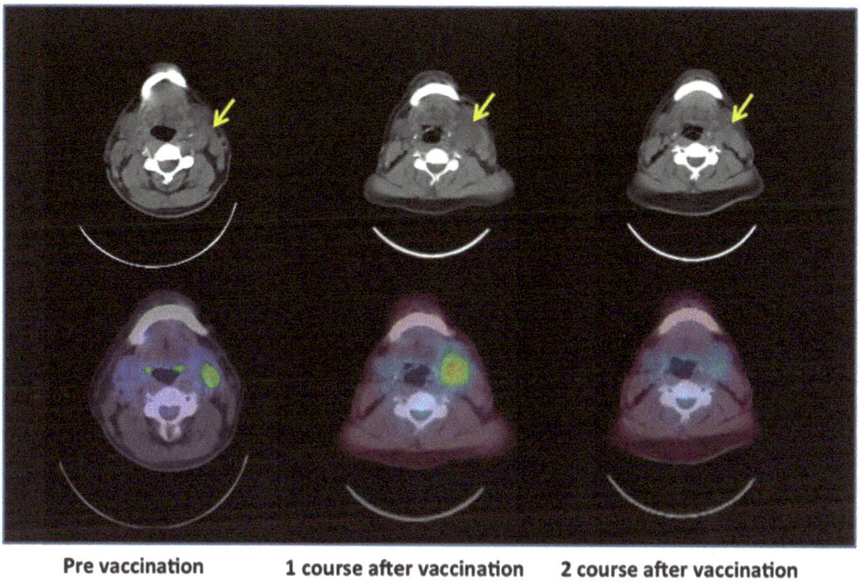


**Fig. 23.1** Metastatic lymph node detected by FDG-PET scan in patients with lung cancer treated by peptide vaccine. A metastatic lesion was enlarged after one course (four times) of vaccination but then decreased after the two course (eight times) of vaccination

not be appropriate in some cases, unless PD is confirmed (as is usually done for responses); (d) allowance for "clinically insignificant" PD (e.g., small new lesions in the presence of other responsive lesions) is recommended; and (e) durable SD may represent antitumor activity [4]. Thus, the irRC was created based on WHO response criteria and considering these essential points above [4, 9, 10].

The details of irRC and a comparison with WHO criteria are shown in Tables 23.1 and 23.2 [4]. The essential points were cited from Wolchok et al. and described as follows. By irRC, only index and measurable new lesions are taken into account (in contrast to conventional WHO criteria that do not require the measurement of new lesions or new lesion measurements for the characterization of evolving tumor burden). At baseline tumor assessment, the sum of the products of the two largest perpendicular diameters (SPD) of all index lesions (five lesions per organ, up to ten visceral lesions, and five cutaneous index lesions) is calculated. At each subsequent tumor assessment, the SPD of the index lesions and of new, measurable lesions ($\geq 5 \times 5$ mm; up to five new lesions per organ, five new cutaneous lesions, and ten visceral lesions) is added together to provide the total tumor burden.

The overall response according to the irRC is derived from time-point response assessments (based on tumor burden) as follows: irCR, complete disappearance of all lesions (whether measurable or not and no new lesions) confirmation by a repeat, consecutive assessment no less than 4 weeks from the date first documented; irPR, decrease in tumor burden $\geq 50$ % relative to baseline confirmed by a consecutive

**Table 23.1** Comparison between WHO criteria and irRC

| | WHO | irRC |
|---|---|---|
| New, measurable lesions (≥5 × 5 mm) | Always represent PD | Incorporated into tumor burden |
| New, nonmeasurable lesions (≥5 × 5 mm) | Always represent PD | Do not define progression (but preclude irRC) |
| Non-index lesions | Changes contribute to defining BOR of CR, PR, SD, and PD | Contribute to defining irRC (complete disappearance required) |
| CR | Disappearance of all lesions in two consecutive observations not less than 4 weeks apart | Disappearance of all lesions in two consecutive observations not less than 4 weeks apart |
| PR | ≥50 % decrease in SPD of all index lesions compared with baseline in two consecutive observations at least 4 weeks apart, in the absence of new lesions or unequivocal progression of non-index lesions | ≥50 % decrease in tumor burden compared with baseline in two consecutive observations at least 4 weeks apart |
| SD | 50 % decrease in SPD compared with baseline cannot be established nor 25 % increase compared with nadir, in the absence of new lesions or unequivocal progression of non-index lesions | 50 % decrease in tumor burden compared with baseline cannot be established, nor 25 % increase compared with nadir |
| PD | At least 25 % increase in SPD compared with nadir and/or unequivocal progression of non-index lesions and/or appearance of new lesions (at any single time point) | At least 25 % increase in tumor burden compared with nadir (at any single time point) in two consecutive observations at least 4 weeks apart |

*WHO* World Health Organization, *irRC* immune-related response criteria, *BOR* best overall response, *SPD* sum of the products of the two largest perpendicular diameters, *CR* complete response, *PR* partial response, *SD* stable disease, *PD* progressive disease, *wk* week (Reprinted from Wolchok et al. (American Association for Cancer Research))

assessment at least 4 weeks after first documentation; irSD, not meeting criteria for irCR or irPR in the absence of irPD; irPD, increase in tumor burden ≥25 % relative to nadir (minimum recorded tumor burden) confirmation by a repeat, consecutive assessment no less than 4 weeks from the date first documented.

By using irRC, two major ipilimumab trials for patients with melanoma and non-small cell lung cancer were completed and indicated irRC was useful [4, 11]. However, several problems were also observed when using irRC. One of the most important issues is the comparison irRC with RECIST. There are major differences between irRC and RECIST in the procedure of measuring tumor size. By irRC, bidimensional measurements were applied because it was based on WHO criteria. However, RECIST guidelines use a unidimensional measurement that is simpler than the WHO criteria. Furthermore, RECIST guidelines have been more

**Table 23.2** Deviation of irRC overall responses

| Measurable response | Nonmeasurable response | | Overall response |
|---|---|---|---|
| Index and new, measurable lesions (tumor burden)[a], % | Non-index lesions | New, nonmeasurable lesions | Using irRC |
| ↓100 | Absent | Absent | irCR[b] |
| ↓100 | Stable | Any | irPR[b] |
| ↓100 | Unequivocal progression | Any | irPR[b] |
| ↓≥50 | Absent/stable | Any | irPR[b] |
| ↓≥50 | Unequivocal progression | Any | irPR[b] |
| ↓<50 to <25↑ | Absent/stable | Any | irSD |
| ↓<50 to <25↑ | Unequivocal progression | Any | irSD |
| ≥25? | Any | Any | irPD[b] |

*irRC* immune-related response criteria, *irCR* immune-related complete response, *irPR* immune-related partial response, *irSD* immune-related stable disease, *irPD* immune-related progressive disease

[a]Decreases assessed relative to baseline including measurable lesions only (>5 × 5 mm)

[b]Assuming response (irCR) and progression (irPD) are confirmed by a second, consecutive assessment at least 4 weeks apart

widely used in cancer drug trials. More recently, Nishino et al. reported the usefulness of unidimensional irRC based on RECIST guidelines [12]. They analyzed data from an ipilimumab study and demonstrated concordance between these two measurement protocols. Interestingly, they showed that unidimensional measurements were more reproducible than bidimensional measurements. Thus, unidimensional measurements by irRC could be a more useful procedure in the future.

## 23.3 Guidance for Clinical Trials

### *23.3.1 Background*

To date, large numbers of clinical trials have been conducted in the field of cancer immunotherapy and most have failed [13, 14]. The major reason for these failures is thought to be a misunderstanding of the specific effects and/or distinguishing types of responses (delayed response to tumor with minimum effect in tumor reduction and elongation of survival time) of immunotherapy on cancer. In 2007, the Cancer Vaccine Clinical Trial Working Group reported on the development of cancer immunotherapy using these concepts [15]. They proposed two types of clinical trials, efficacy trials and exploratory proof-of-principle trials, which could be performed during conventional phase I and II trials.

## 23.3.2 Basic Concept for Clinical Trials by Cancer Vaccine Clinical Trial Working Group

### 23.3.2.1 Proof-of-Principle Trials

There are four essential points in proof-of-principle trials: safety, dose, schedule of administration, and biologic activity of drug. It was recommended that more than 20 patients should be investigated to understand the safety aspects. Optimal dose and schedule should also be analyzed in these exploratory trials. An important difference between conventional phase I trials and proof-of-principle trials using immunotherapy is in determining the maximum tolerated dose. Because most immunotherapies, including vaccines, are relatively less harmful than other cancer treatments, exploratory trials should carefully consider the relationship between drug dose or schedule of administration and biological responses, while observing toxicity. To acquire the proof of principle, immunological evaluation is also important. Immunological monitoring is a quick and effective way to understand the biological activity of a drug. Thus far, several methods have been used for immune monitoring of cancer immunotherapy including cytotoxicity assays, intracellular cytokine assays, tetramer assays, and (enzyme-linked immunospot) ELISPOT assay. However, one problem of immune monitoring is that these techniques are not well validated. Therefore, to apply these techniques for monitoring, the following points should be determined: (1) the maximum justifiable amount of sample material per patient should be collected to perform the assay and permit for repeat testing; (2) samples should be taken sequentially; (3) a minimum of three assay time points should be investigated – baseline and at least two follow-up time points; (4) assays should be established, reproducible, and technically validated in the respective laboratory (no proved correlation with clinical outcomes should be required); (5) a minimum of two such assays should be applied; and (6) the frequency and magnitude of an immune response should be prospectively defined for the population under study. Only the ELISPOT assay has been well validated by the interlaboratory large-scale harmonization program. In a proof-of-principle trial, if safety of a drug has been indicated with clinical efficacy including immune responses using the above-mentioned techniques, we can consider moving forward to advanced stage clinical trials such as efficacy trials.

## *23.3.3 Basic Concept of Efficacy Trials*

### 23.3.3.1 Phase II Trials

The main purpose of an efficacy trial is to understand clinical efficacy of a drug, and therefore randomized phase II and III trials are often performed. Several types of randomized phase II trial have been described including non-comparative randomized trials, comparative randomized trials, and comparative randomized trials with an adaptive component. Non-comparative randomized phase II trials are single-group historically controlled trials where patients are allocated randomly to the trials. Comparative randomized phase II trials aim to detect significant differences in efficacy using two individual intervention arms. Comparative randomized phase II trials with an adaptive component are a specific phase II component within phase II/III trials. When clinical efficacy is observed in the phase II study, then the trial usually progresses to a phase III trial. If efficacy is not determined, the trial is usually terminated.

### 23.3.3.2 Phase III Trials

Phase III trials are definitive, confirmative, and the final stage of a clinical trial to determine the clinical benefits of a novel drug. These are usually large-scale randomized studies. For conventional cancer drugs such as cytotoxic agents, end points are usually defined by both progression-free survival and overall survival. However, in cancer immunotherapy, it is recommended to use overall survival only as an end point because of the specific features of biological responses.

## *23.3.4 Guidance for Industry: Clinical Considerations for Therapeutic Cancer Vaccines by the US Department of Health and Human Services*

These ideas led to the publication of "Guidance for industry [5]: clinical considerations for therapeutic cancer vaccines" established by the FDA [15], which states "The course of antigen presentation and processing, activation of lymphocytes, and tumor cell killing, is expected to require a substantial time in vivo. Thus, development of a cancer vaccine can present different considerations for clinical trial design than development of a more traditional biological product or cytotoxic drug for the treatment of cancer."

The essential points of this guidance are summarized in Tables 23.3 and 23.4. The basic concepts of this guidance were used by the Cancer Vaccine Clinical Trial Working Group, which also described statistical issues. Importantly, the FDA recommends the use of a superiority trial design to determine the efficacy of

**Table 23.3** Major points in early-phase clinical trial from guidance for industry

| Factors | Comment |
|---|---|
| Purpose | Assess safety |
| | Determine optimal dose and dosing schedule |
| | Identify and study potential biological activities |
| Dose escalation | "3 + 3 design" may not be the most suitable approach to gathering information |
| MTD | MTD for an cancer vaccine may not be identified |
| Dose findings | If no DLT is expected or achieved, optimization of other outcomes, such as the immune response, can be useful to identify doses for subsequent studies |

*MTD* maximum tolerated doses, *DLT* dose-limiting toxicity

**Table 23.4** Major points in late-phase clinical trials from guidance for industry

| Factors | Comment |
|---|---|
| Purpose | Gather additional information about effectiveness and safety |
| Study design | Recommend use of a superiority trial design to demonstrate a cancer vaccine treatment effect |
| | Non-inferiority design may be considered but should be carefully assessed |
| End points | Choose clinically meaningful end points |
| | Increased survival and symptomatic improvement should be considered |
| Other issues | Should have appropriate controls such as placebo |
| | Should monitor delayed vaccine effects |

therapeutic cancer vaccines as well as conventional cytotoxic cancer drugs. In addition, non-inferiority trial designs are described; however, because of their complexity, we should consider carefully the use of this method. Furthermore, delayed clinical effects should be anticipated [8], as it is well known that immunotherapy induces a delayed clinical effect that might also delay any survival effects. If the survival curve does not fit the proportional hazard model, it can cause a loss of statistical power even if clinically effective. Chen et al. [16] described this point and recommended the use of the O'Brien and Fleming method.

### 23.3.5 Guidance for Peptide Vaccines for the Treatment of Cancer

Recently, The Japanese Society for Biological Therapy established "Guidance for peptide vaccines for the treatment of cancer" [6], which follows the FDA guidance for industry, but which is more specific for peptide vaccines. In addition, further guidance regarding clinical trials, characteristics of peptide vaccines, nonclinical safety testing of peptide vaccines, and quality assurance in developing peptide vaccine is also described. In this guidance, statistical issues were also described, and unique statistic procedures such as the Harrington-Fleming method were recommended for survival analysis.

## 23.4 Conclusion

In this chapter, novel and unique concepts for developing cancer immunotherapy were described. irRC and guidance for clinical trials have undoubtedly contributed to opening the door to future cancer immunotherapies.

## References


1. Rosenberg SA, Yang JC, Restifo NP (2004) Cancer immunotherapy: moving beyond current vaccines. Nat Med 10(9):909–915. doi:10.1038/nm1100
2. Miller AB, Hoogstraten B, Staquet M, Winkler A (1981) Reporting results of cancer treatment. Cancer 47(1):207–214
3. Therasse P, Arbuck SG, Eisenhauer EA, Wanders J, Kaplan RS, Rubinstein L et al (2000) New guidelines to evaluate the response to treatment in solid tumors. European Organization for Research and Treatment of Cancer, National Cancer Institute of the United States, National Cancer Institute of Canada. J Natl Cancer Inst 92(3):205–216
4. Wolchok JD, Hoos A, O'Day S, Weber JS, Hamid O, Lebbe C et al (2009) Guidelines for the evaluation of immune therapy activity in solid tumors: immune-related response criteria. Clin Cancer Res 15(23):7412–7420. doi:10.1158/1078-0432.CCR-09-1624
5. FGIndustryCancerVaccineFinal110311_508.pdf. http://www.fda.gov/BiologicsBloodVaccines/GuidanceComplianceRegulatoryInformation/Guidances/default.htm
6. Yamaguchi Y, Yamaue H, Okusaka T, Okuno K, Suzuki H, Fujioka T et al (2014) Guidance for peptide vaccines for the treatment of cancer. Cancer Sci 105(7):924–931. doi:10.1111/cas.12443
7. Attia P, Phan GQ, Maker AV, Robinson MR, Quezado MM, Yang JC et al (2005) Autoimmunity correlates with tumor regression in patients with metastatic melanoma treated with anti-cytotoxic T-lymphocyte antigen-4. J Clin Oncol 23(25):6043–6053. doi:10.1200/jco.2005.06.205
8. Suzuki H (2009) Lung cancer. In: Nakamura Y (ed) Peptide vaccine therapy for cancer, 1st edn. Nakayama Shoten, Tokyo
9. Hoos A, Eggermont AM, Janetzki S, Hodi FS, Ibrahim R, Anderson A et al (2010) Improved endpoints for cancer immunotherapy trials. J Natl Cancer Inst 102(18):1388–1397. doi:10.1093/jnci/djq310
10. Hoos A (2012) Evolution of end points for cancer immunotherapy trials. Ann Oncol 23(Suppl 8):viii47–viii52. doi:10.1093/annonc/mds263
11. Lynch TJ, Bondarenko I, Luft A, Serwatowski P, Barlesi F, Chacko R et al (2012) Ipilimumab in combination with paclitaxel and carboplatin as first-line treatment in stage IIIB/IV non-small-cell lung cancer: results from a randomized, double-blind, multicenter phase II study. J Clin Oncol 30(17):2046–2054. doi:10.1200/jco.2011.38.4032
12. Nishino M, Jagannathan JP, Krajewski KM, O'Regan K, Hatabu H, Shapiro G et al (2012) Personalized tumor response assessment in the era of molecular medicine: cancer-specific and therapy-specific response criteria to complement pitfalls of RECIST. AJR Am J Roentgenol 198(4):737–745. doi:10.2214/ajr.11.7483

13. Suzuki H, Owada Y, Watanabe Y, Inoue T, Fukuharav M, Yamaura T et al (2014) Recent advances in immunotherapy for non-small-cell lung cancer. Hum Vaccin Immunother 10 (2):352–357. doi:10.4161/hv.26919
14. Kudrin A (2014) Cancer vaccines: what do we need to measure in clinical trials? Hum Vaccin Immunother 10(11):3236–3240
15. Hoos A, Parmiani G, Hege K, Sznol M, Loibner H, Eggermont A et al (2007) A clinical development paradigm for cancer vaccines and related biologics. J Immunother (Hagerstown, Md:1997) 30(1):1–15. doi:10.1097/01.cji.0000211341.88835.ae
16. Chen TT (2013) Statistical issues and challenges in immuno-oncology. J Immunother Cancer 1:18. doi:10.1186/2051-1426-1-18

# Part IX
# Personalized Immunotherapy

# Chapter 24
# Personalized Cancer Immunotherapy: Immune Biomarkers and Combination Immunotherapy

**Yutaka Kawakami, Boryana Popivanova, Sunthamala Nuchsupha, Taeko Hayakawa, Kenta Nakamura, Haruna Nagumo, Ikumi Katano, Tomonari Kinoshita, Kinya Tsubota, Hajime Kamijuku, Naoshi Kawamura, Junichiro Miyazaki, Ryosuke Satomi, Juri Sugiyama, Hiroshi Nishio, Shinobu Noji, Chie Kudo-Saito, Nobuo Tsukamoto, Toshiharu Sakurai, Tomonobu Fujita, and Tomonori Yaguchi**

**Abstract** Cancer immunotherapies utilizing tumor-specific T-cell responses, immune-checkpoint blockade, and T-cell-based adoptive cell therapy, have recently shown durable responses in advanced patients with various cancers. However, there are still cancer types and patients who do not respond to these immunotherapies. Pretreatment immune status varies in cancer patients, and it correlates with prognosis after various cancer therapies including immunotherapy. The differential T-cell response is defined by positive (e.g., number of immunogenic mutated peptides derived from mainly passenger DNA mutations in cancer cells, polymorphisms of immune-related genes of patients) and negative (e.g., oncogene activation including driver DNA mutations) immune pathways along with environmental factors (e.g., intestinal microbiota, diet, smoking, infection history). These factors could be biomarkers for selection of the patients who are likely to respond to immunotherapy and furthermore could be therapeutic targets to improve efficacy of immunotherapy possibly by combination immunotherapy with interventions on multiple key regulation points in the antitumor T-cell responses. Personalized combination immunotherapy based on the evaluation of T-cell immune status is a promising strategy for cancer treatment.

**Keywords** Cancer immunotherapy • Cancer immunopathology • Biomarkers • Combination therapy • Personalized therapy

---

Y. Kawakami, M.D., Ph.D. (✉) • B. Popivanova • S. Nuchsupha • T. Hayakawa • K. Nakamura • H. Nagumo • I. Katano • T. Kinoshita • K. Tsubota • H. Kamijuku • N. Kawamura • J. Miyazaki • R. Satomi • J. Sugiyama • H. Nishio • S. Noji • C. Kudo-Saito • N. Tsukamoto • T. Sakurai • T. Fujita • T. Yaguchi
Division of Cellular Signaling, Institute for Advanced Medical Research, Keio University School of Medicine, 35 Shinanomachi, Shinjuku-ku, Tokyo 160-8582, Japan
e-mail: yutakawa@keio.jp



Y. Yamaguchi (ed.), *Immunotherapy of Cancer*,
DOI 10.1007/978-4-431-55031-0_24

## 24.1 Introduction

Cancer immunotherapies, utilizing tumor-specific T-cell responses, immune-checkpoint blockade (e.g., anti-PD-1/PD-L1 Ab, anti-CTLA-4 Ab), and T-cell-based adoptive cell therapy (ACT) (e.g., tumor-infiltrating T cells (TIL), TCR (T-cell receptor), or CAR (chimeric antigen receptor)-transduced T cells), have recently shown durable responses even in advanced cancer patients with various cancer types (e.g., metastatic melanoma, renal cell carcinoma (RCC), non-small cell lung cancer (NSCLC), bladder cancer, head and neck (HN) cancer, gastric cancer, ovarian cancer, synovial sarcoma, and B-cell malignancies including lymphoma, ALL, and CLL) [1–6]. The durable response obtained by these immunotherapies is impressive compared with chemotherapies and molecular-targeted drugs which may not result in long survival due to drug resistance [7]. However, not all of the patients responded to the immunotherapy. Therefore, personalized cancer immunotherapy is needed through the identification of biomarkers to predict the patients who are likely to respond immunotherapy. Furthermore, improvement of efficacy of immunotherapies, including changing immune status of the unresponsive patients to responsive status to immunotherapy, is needed possibly by combination interventions targeting multiple key regulating points in the antitumor T-cell responses. The appropriated interventions to use and their combination may be decided based on the individual evaluation of immune status of patients.

## 24.2 Evasion of Cancer Cells During Long Development Process in Patients

Immune surveillance system particularly by T cells and NK cells appears to eliminate cancer cells and their precursors during long cancer developmental process in human [8]. However, eventually cancer cells having genetic instability evade immune defense through various mechanisms (loss of highly immunogenic tumor antigens, dysfunction of antigen processing/presenting machineries such as HLA, and active suppression by various immune-braking mechanisms such as immunosuppressive molecules (e.g., TGF-β, IL10, VEGF, PG-E2, PD-1/PD-L1, CTLA4) and immunosuppressive cells (e.g., Treg, MDSC, tolerogenic DC)) [9–12]. Therefore, cancer cells seen in clinic have already acquired immune-resistant features. The question is whether some of the immune-resistant mechanisms can be overcome by immune interventions. Thus, investigations of these immune-resistant machineries are essential to develop effective cancer immunotherapy.

## 24.3 Individual differences of Immune Status in Cancer Patients

It was recently found that pretreatment immune status varies among cancer patients and appears to correlate with patients' prognosis after various cancer treatments including surgery, chemotherapy, radiation, and immunotherapy [13]. We found that high tumor infiltrations of $CD3^+$ T cells and $CD8^+$ T cells are correlated with favorable prognosis after various treatments of patients with various cancers (e.g., colon cancer, lung cancer, ovarian cancer, head and neck cancer, and melanoma). High $FOXP3^+$ Treg and FOXP3/CD8 ratio in tumors generally correlate with poor prognosis (except colon cancer). We confirmed it in Japanese patients with various cancers including colon cancer, lung cancer, and cervical cancer. International collaboration (immunoscore validation task force) organized by SITC (Society for Immunotherapy of Cancer) is currently in progress first to confirm the prognostic value of tumor-infiltrating T cells (immunoscore: $CD3^+$ T cells and $CD8^+$ T cells) in colon cancer after curative surgery [14]. It may allow us better personalized management of cancer patients. In the PD-1/PD-L1 blockade therapies, $CD8^+$ T-cell infiltration in tumors appears to be essential for clinical responses along with PD-L1 expression in cancer cells and tumor-infiltrating immune cells [15, 16]. Immune status of blood such as cytokine levels also varies among cancer patients. We found that high plasma IL6 and IL8 correlate with poor prognosis after various immunotherapy including cancer vaccines with peptide antigens and DCs. Therefore, these immune factors can be diagnostic markers for personalized cancer therapies including immunotherapy.

## 24.4 Mechanisms for the Differential T-Cell Responses in Cancer Patients

The understanding of the mechanisms for the differential T-cell tumor infiltrations is important for development of personalized cancer immunotherapy. Our previous studies suggested that the T-cell responses and its tumor infiltration may be defined by balance of positive and negative immune pathways in the antitumor T-cell network (Fig. 24.1). We have vigorously studied what kinds of antigens tumor-infiltrating T lymphocytes (TILs) recognize on cancer cells (identification of tumor antigens recognized by tumor-infiltrating T cells) [17]. Various types of antigens including DNA mutation-derived mutated antigens (e.g., β-catenin, hedgehog acyltransferase), cancer-testis antigens (e.g., MAGEs, NY-ESO-1), and tissue-specific shared antigens (e.g., MART-1, gp100, tyrosinase) were identified in melanoma [18–20]. We noticed that TILs which administration resulted in good clinical responses (CR and PR) recognized tumor specific peptides derived from missense DNA mutations [21, 22]. It has recently been shown that melanoma TILs frequently recognize such mutated peptides derived from passenger mutations by

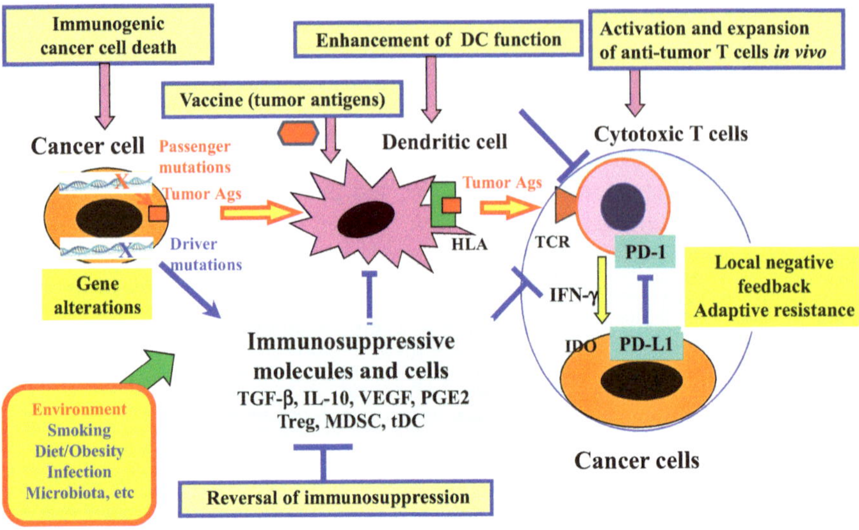


**Fig. 24.1** Personalized combination immunotherapy targeting key regulation points in the antitumor T-cell responses. Balance of the antitumor T-cell induction pathway and immunosuppressive pathway along with environmental factors defines the differential T-cell immune status in cancer patients. Passenger DNA mutations may induce antitumor T cells, while driver DNA mutations rather promote immunosuppressive cascades. Development of immune interventions targeting important regulation points in the antitumor immune responses and their appropriate combination based on the patients' immune status is a key to develop more effective cancer immunotherapy

whole exomic DNA sequencing and that these immunogenic mutated peptides are quite unique antigens among patients [23]. Recently numbers of DNA mutations, particularly mutations which may generate T-cells epitopes (ability to bind the patient's HLAs) were reported to correlate with the clinical responses to immune-checkpoint blockers including anti-PD-1 Ab and anti-CTLA4 Ab in patients with melanoma and lung cancer [24, 25]. In fact, cancers with relatively high DNA mutation numbers, such as UV-induced melanoma, smoking-related lung cancer, and bladder cancer, are cancer types relatively high responsive to PD-1/PD-L1 blockade therapy [26]. It was also reported that the mutations which are possible T-cell targets may be less than expected in colon cancer, suggesting that evasion of cancer cells from mutation-specific T cells might occur [27]. These results indicate that T cells specific for the DNA mutation derived mutated peptide antigens (called neo-antigens) are important for some of the cancer immunotherapies including the immune-checkpoint blockade. In tumor tissues, neo-antigen-specific T cells produce IFN-γ which induces PD-L1 and IDO in cancer cells and infiltrated stromal cells, which in turn counterattack the infiltrated antitumor T cells (local negative feedback, adaptive resistance). For the patients in this immune condition (antitumor T cells were spontaneously induced in infiltrated in tumors), PD-1/PD-L1 blockade appears to work well.

The next question is how quantity and quality of DNA mutations are defined. In lung cancer patients, one of the major factors causing immunogenic DNA mutations appears to be smoking because molecular smoking signature (transversion mutation) correlated with numbers of DNA mutation and clinical responses to PD-1 Ab therapy [25]. It was also shown that dysfunction of DNA repair system caused hypermutations resulting in good response to the PD-1 Ab [25]. We have previously shown that dysfunction of DNA mismatch repair enzymes such as MLH1 causes hypermutations, particularly frameshift mutations by DNA slippage, leading to autologous immune responses to the frameshift-derived c-terminal tumor-specific peptide in MSI (microsatellite instability)$^+$ colon cancers [28]. The patients with MSI$^+$ colon cancer have usually high CD8$^+$ T-cell infiltrations in tumors and relatively good prognosis after surgery even though they show histologically malignant appearance, and it has recently been recognized as a good candidate for the immune-checkpoint blockade. We have recently been working on additional molecular mechanisms causing immunogenic hyper DNA mutations in various cancer types and correlations with antitumor T-cell responses as well as responsiveness to the immunotherapies.

In addition to T-cell epitope-generating DNA mutation status, there may be mechanisms for the differential T-cell infiltrations. It was reported in colon cancer that loss of gene-encoding cytokine (IL15), which promotes proliferation of TILs, and chemokine (CXCL13), which recruits IL21-producing CXCR5$^+$ T cells into tumors, causes less tumor infiltration of CD8$^+$ T cells and B cells [29, 30]. In mouse tumor models, increase of immunosuppressive molecules such as TGF-β in tumor affects immune status of tumor microenvironments (e.g., DC impairment, increase of immunosuppressive Tregs and MDSCs in tumors, and draining lymph nodes) and subsequent decrease of antitumor T-cell induction and accumulation in tumors [31]. In melanoma, we have shown that increased β-catenin activity, which is caused by mutations or Wnt overproduction, may inhibit both induction and effector phases of anti-melanoma T-cell responses, which may result in decreased T-cell infiltration in tumors [32]. Contrary to T-cell epitope generation from passenger DNA mutations, driver DNA mutations such as β-catenin and BRAF in melanoma appear to rather promote immunosuppressive pathways through signal activation such as β-catenin/TCF and MAPK signaling pathways, the common BRAF mutation frequently observed in SSM-type melanoma. We found that mutant BRAF not only promotes proliferation and invasion of melanoma cells but also induces immunosuppression partly through production of immunosuppressive cytokines such as IL6, IL10, and VEGF. STAT3 oncogenic pathway may also contribute to the negative immune pathway on antitumor T-cell responses [33]. Administration of mutant BRAF selective inhibitors increased infiltration of CD8$^+$ T cells in regressing tumors with necrosis, but not in progressing melanoma [34]. The mutant BRAF inhibitor may enhance anti-melanoma T cells through multiple mechanisms, including reduced above immunosuppressive cytokines, induction of melanosomal antigens, and augmentation of T-cell induction via paradoxical activation of MAPK signaling in cells expressing wild-type BRAF. STAT3 activation in melanoma cells also causes production of immune-suppressive cytokines such as IL6, IL10, and VEGF, which activate STAT3 in various immune cells and subsequently made them immunosuppressive immune cells such as tolerogenic DCs, MDSCs, and Tregs [35]. NF-kB activation in ovarian cancer cells strongly promotes production of IL6 and IL8 which suppress dendritic cell functions, and administration of NF-kB inhibitor restored immune status in cancer-bearing hosts [36]. These results illustrate the presence of two major immune-resistant mechanisms: one oncogene-triggered immunosuppression (e.g., IL6, VEGF) and the other antitumor T-cell-triggered immunosuppression (e.g., PD-L1, IDO) (Fig. 24.1).

In addition to these cancer cell factors (e.g., DNA alterations), host patients' immune reactivity defined by polymorphisms of immune-related molecules, including HLA type and cytokine production levels as well as environmental factors including intestinal microbiota which regulate not only intestinal mucosal immunity but also systemic immune responses including antitumor immunity, diet/obesity which promotes chronic inflammation for support of cancer progression, smoking which introduces various chemicals affecting immune system, and infection history which modulates T-cell repertoire, influences antitumor T-cell response and tumor infiltration status before cancer therapy.

## 24.5 Personalized Immunotherapies Based on Evaluation of Patients' Immune Status

Because pretreatment antitumor T-cell status is different in cancer patients, and it correlates with cancer therapy responses, personalized immunotherapy should be exploited based on the evaluation of individual patients' immune status. One simple personalization is selection of patients which are likely to respond to cancer immunotherapy before or early after treatment. As discussed above, T-cell infiltration in tumors and cytokine levels in blood could be biomarkers for cancer immunotherapies. In PD-1/PD-L1 blockade therapy, pretreatment PD-L1 expression on cancer cells or tumor-infiltrating immune cells as well as $CD8^+$ T-cell infiltration can be biomarkers. For the cancer patients with these immune features, usually having hyper DNA mutations, PD-1/PD-L1 blockade may be sufficient for treatment of patients. Since neo-antigen-specific T cells appear to be major effectors in the immune-checkpoint blockade therapy, personalized immunotherapy using vaccines containing immunogenic individual mutations which can be identified by whole exomic DNA sequencing or adoptive cell therapy using T cells specific for such mutated antigens may be possible and has recently been attempted. In contrasts, for cancer cells with almost no immunogenic mutation (very rapidly developed cancer via strong drivers (e.g., translocation/recombination oncogenes) may have much less immunogenic DNA mutations), it may be difficult to induce autologous antitumor T cells. In such cases, adoptive cell therapy using artificially generated antitumor T cells (TCR-/CAR-transduced T cells) may still work. In patients with intermediate immune conditions, various immune interventions may enhance induction of anti-T-cell response and infiltration in tumors, resulting in the responsive status to the immune-checkpoint blockers such as anti-PD-1/PD-L1 Ab. Combination immunotherapy targeting different key regulating points in the antitumor T-cell response and appropriate use of the interventions based on the evaluation of immune condition of each patient are important.

## 24.6 Combination Immunotherapy

Based on the analysis of mouse tumor models and clinical trials using the identified tumor antigens, we have previously proposed combination cancer immunotherapy targeting multiple key regulation points in antitumor T-cell responses [37]. The following issues are particularly important to develop immune interventions for effective combination immunotherapy (Fig. 24.1). (1) Identification of appropriate tumor antigens: The ideal antigens are tumor specific and expressed in cancer initiating cells [38]. Mutation antigens which emerged in early cancer development are attractive antigens [21–23, 39, 40]. It is also important to use appropriate forms of antigens such as long peptides, nanoparticles, and recombinant viruses [41]. (2) In situ tumor destruction to cause immunogenic cancer cell death: Various anticancer drugs (e.g., chemotherapy, molecular-targeted drugs, antitumor Abs, oncolytic viruses, radiation, radiofrequency/cryoablation) may be used [42–45]. (3) Enhancement of dendritic cell (DC) functions: Various adjuvants such as TLR3 agonists, STING agonists, agonistic Abs against co-stimulatory molecules such as CD40, and cytokines such as IL12 and TNF-α may be used [43–47]. (4) Activation and expansion of antitumor T cells in vivo: Cytokine such as IL2, IL7, IL15, IL21, agonistic Abs against co-stimulatory molecules such as CD134 (OX-40) and CD137 (4-1BB), and cultured T-cell transfer (TIL, TCR/CAR-T-cells) may be used [4–6, 48, 49]. (5) Reversal of immunosuppression: Interventions to two types of immunosuppression (oncogene triggered and antitumor T-cell triggered) may be utilized, which include signal inhibitors (e.g., BRAF inhibitors, STAT3 inhibitors) [33–36], blocking and depleting Abs for various immunosuppressive cells and molecules (e.g., anti-CTLA4 Ab, anti-CCR4 Ab), and immune-checkpoint blockers (e.g., anti-PD-1/PD-L1 Abs, anti-CTLA4 Ab) [1–3]. Again, appropriate use of the interventions based on the immunological evaluation of each patient are important (e.g., use of appropriate signal inhibitors according to the immunosuppression-inducing oncogenes in the particular patient). Combination cancer immunotherapy was previously considered around cancer vaccines [50]; however, recent success of PD-1/PD-L1 blockade allows us new concept of combination immunotherapy around PD-1/PD-L1 blockade.

## 24.7 Concluding Remarks

The recent success of cancer immunotherapy along with better understanding of human cancer immunobiology particularly related to antitumor T cells led to the proposal of personalized combination cancer immunotherapy based on the immune evaluation of individual patients for further improvement of cancer immunotherapy. Clinical trials of various combination immunotherapies, particularly with immune-checkpoint blockade, have already been in progress, and some of the combinations have already shown promising clinical results, such as combination of anti-PD-1 Ab and anti-CTLA-4 Ab for patients with melanoma and renal cell cancer. Further investigation of human cancer immunopathology particularly in tumor microenvironments using a variety of new technologies, including systems biological omics approach, new systematic flow cytometric analysis of human immune cell subsets, immunologically humanized mice for in vivo evaluation of human immune responses, and iPS cell technology, may lead to development of effective personalized cancer immunotherapy.

**Acknowledgments** These studies were supported by Grants-in-Aid for Scientific Research (25670506, 23240128, 26221005) from the Japan Society for Promotion of Science (JSPS), a research program of the Project for Development of Innovative Research on Cancer Therapeutics (P-Direct) from Japan Agency for Medical Research and Development (AMED) and the Ministry of Education, Culture, Sports, Science and Technology (MEXT) of Japan. We also thank the technical support and editorial assistance of Ms. Misako Sakamoto and Ms. Ryoko Suzuki.

## References

1. Topalian SL, Hodi FS, Brahmer JR et al (2013) Safety, activity, and immune correlates of anti-PD-1 antibody in cancer. N Engl J Med 366:2443–2454
2. Brahmer JR, Tykodi SS, Chow LQ et al (2012) Safety and activity of anti-PD-L1 antibody in patients with advanced cancer. N Engl J Med 366:2455–2465
3. Hodi FS, O'Day SJ, McDermott DF et al (2010) Improved survival with ipilimumab in patients with metastatic melanoma. N Engl J Med 363:711–723
4. Rosenberg SA, Yang JC, Sherry RM et al (2011) Durable complete responses in heavily pretreated patients with metastatic melanoma using T-cell transfer immunotherapy. Clin Cancer Res 17:4550–4557
5. Robbins PF, Morgan RA, Feldman SA et al (2011) Tumor regression in patients with metastatic synovial cell sarcoma and melanoma using genetically engineered lymphocytes reactive with NY-ESO-1. J Clin Oncol 29:917–924
6. Kalos M, Levine BL, Porter DL et al (2011) T cells with chimeric antigen receptors have potent antitumor effects and can establish memory in patients with advanced leukemia. Sci Transl Med 3:95
7. Wagle N, Emery C, Berger MF et al (2011) Dissecting therapeutic resistance to RAF inhibition in melanoma by tumor genomic profiling. J Clin Oncol 29:3085–3096
8. Schreiber RD et al (2011) Cancer immunoediting: integrating immunity's roles in cancer suppression and promotion. Science 331:1565–1570

9. Yaguchi T, Sumimoto H, Kudo-Saito C, Tsukamoto N, Ueda R, Iwata-Kajihara T, Nishio H, Kawamura N, Kawakami Y et al (2011) Int J Hematol 93:294–300
10. Kawakami Y, Yaguchi T, Sumimoto H et al (2013) Roles of signaling pathways in cancer cells and immune cells in generation of immunosuppressive tumor-associated microenvironments. In: Shurin M, Malyguine A, Umansky V (eds) Tumor immunoenvironment. Springer, Dordrecht Heidelberg New York London
11. Kudo-Saito C, Shirako H, Takeuchi T et al (2009) Cancer metastasis is accelerated through immunosuppression during EMT of cancer cell. Cancer Cell 16:195–206
12. Spranger S, Spaapen RM, Zha Y et al (2013) Up-regulation of PD-L1, IDO, and Tregs in the melanoma tumor microenvironment is driven by CD8(+) T cells. Sci Transl Med 5:200
13. Fridman WH, Pagès F, Sautès-Fridman C et al (2012) The immune contexture in human tumours: impact on clinical outcome. Nat Rev Cancer 12:298–306
14. Galon J, Mlecnik B, Bindea G et al (2014) Towards the introduction of the 'immunoscore' in the classification of malignant tumours. J Pathol 2:199–209
15. Taube JM, Anders RA, Young GD et al (2014) Colocalization of inflammatory response with B7-h1 expression in human melanocytic lesions supports an adaptive resistance mechanism of immune escape. Sci Transl Med 4:127
16. Herbst RS, Soria JC, Kowanetz M et al (2014) Predictive correlates of response to the anti-PD-L1 antibody MPDL3280A in cancer patients. Nature 515:563–567
17. Kawakami Y, Rosenberg SA (1997) Human tumor antigens recognized by T-cells. Immunol Res 16:313–339
18. Kawakami Y, Eliyahu S, Delgado CH et al (1994) Cloning of the gene coding for a shared human melanoma antigen recognized by autologous T cells infiltrating into tumor. Proc Natl Acad Sci U S A 91:3515–3519
19. Kawakami Y, Eliyahu S, Delgado CH et al (1994) Identification of human melanoma antigen recognized by tumor infiltrating lymphocytes associated with in vivo tumor rejection. Proc Natl Acad Sci U S A 91:6458–6462
20. Kawakami Y, Eliyahu S, Sakaguchi K et al (1994) Identification of the immunodominant peptides of the MART-1 human melanoma antigen recognized by the majority of HLA-A2 restricted tumor infiltrating lymphocytes. J Exp Med 180:347–352
21. Robbins PF, El-Gamil M, Li YF et al (1996) A mutated b2-catenin gene encodes a melanoma specific antigen recognized by tumor infiltrating lymphocytes. J Exp Med 183:1185–1192
22. Kawakami Y, Wang X, Shofuda T et al (2001) Isolation of a new melanoma antigen, MART-2, containing a mutated epitope recognized by autologous tumor infiltrating T lymphocytes. J Immunol 166:2871–2877
23. Robbins PF, Lu YC, El-Gamil M et al (2013) Mining exomic sequencing data to identify mutated antigens recognized by adoptively transferred tumor-reactive T cells. Nat Med 19:747–752
24. Snyder A, Makarov V, Merghoub T et al (2014) Genetic basis for clinical response to CTLA-4 blockade in melanoma. N Engl J Med 371:2189–2199
25. Rizvi NA, Hellmann MD, Snyder A et al (2015) Cancer immunology. Mutational landscape determines sensitivity to PD-1 blockade in non-small cell lung cancer. Science 348:124–128
26. Alexandrov LB, Nik-Zainal S, Wedge DC et al (2013) Signatures of mutational processes in human cancer. Nature 500:415–421
27. Rooney MS, Shukla SA, Wu CJ et al (2015) Molecular and genetic properties of tumors associated with local immune cytolytic activity. Cell 160:48–61
28. Ishikawa T, Fujita T, Suzuki Y et al (2003) Tumor-specific immunological recognition of frameshift-mutated peptides in colon cancer with microsatellite instability. Cancer Res 63:5564–5572
29. Bindea G, Mlecnik B, Tosolini M et al (2013) Spatiotemporal dynamics of intratumoral immune cells reveal the immune landscape in human cancer. Immunity 39:782–795
30. Mlecnik B, Bindea G, Angell HK et al (2014) Functional network pipeline reveals genetic determinants associated with in situ lymphocyte proliferation and survival of cancer patients. Sci Transl Med 6:228

31. Nakamura S, Yaguchi T, Kawamura N et al (2014) TGF-β1 in tumor microenvironments induces immunosuppression in the tumors and sentinel lymph nodes and promotes tumor progression. J Immunother 37:63–72
32. Yaguchi T, Goto Y, Kido K, Mochimaru H et al (2012) Immune suppression and resistance mediated by constitutive activation of Wnt/β-catenin signaling in human melanoma cells. J Immunol 189:2110–2117
33. Sumimoto H, Imabayashi F, Iwata T et al (2006) The BRAF-MAPK signaling pathway is essential for cancer immune evasion in human melanoma cells. J Exp Med 203:1651–1656
34. Wilmott JS, Long GV, Howle JR et al (2012) Selective BRAF inhibitors induce marked T-cell infiltration into human metastatic melanoma. Clin Cancer Res 18:1386–1394
35. Iwata-Kajihara T, Sumimoto H et al (2011) Enhanced cancer immunotherapy using STAT3-depleted dendritic cells with high Th1-inducing ability and resistance to cancer cell-derived inhibitory factors. J Immunol 187:27–36
36. Nishio H, Yaguchi T, Sugiyama J et al (2014) Immunosuppression through constitutively activated NF-κB signaling in human ovarian cancer and its reversal by a NF-κB inhibitor. Br J Cancer 110:2965–2974
37. Kawakami Y, Yaguchi T, Sumimoto H et al (2013) Improvement of cancer immunotherapy by combining molecular targeted therapy. Front Oncol 3:136
38. Ueda R, Ohkusu-Tsukada K, Fusaki N et al (2010) Identification of HLA-A2- and A24-restricted T-cell epitopes derived from SOX6 expressed in glioma stem cells for immunotherapy. Int J Cancer 126:919–929
39. Gubin MM, Zhang X, Schuster H et al (2014) Checkpoint blockade cancer immunotherapy targets tumour-specific mutant antigens. Nature 515:577–581
40. Tran E, Turcotte S, Gros A et al (2014) Cancer immunotherapy based on mutation-specific CD4+ T cells in a patient with epithelial cancer. Science 344:641–645
41. Kenter GG, Welters MJ, Valentijn AR et al (2009) Vaccination against HPV-16 oncoproteins for vulvar intraepithelial neoplasia. N Engl J Med 361:1838–1847
42. Zitvogel L, Kepp O, Kroemer G (2011) Immune parameters affecting the efficacy of chemotherapeutic regimens. Nat Rev Clin Oncol 8:151–160
43. Woo SR, Fuertes MB, Corrales L et al (2014) STING-dependent cytosolic DNA sensing mediates innate immune recognition of immunogenic tumors. Immunity 41:830–842
44. Beatty GL, Chiorean EG, Fishman MP et al (2011) CD40 agonists alter tumor stroma and show efficacy against pancreatic carcinoma in mice and humans. Science 331:1612–1616
45. Toda M, Iizuka Y, Kawase T et al (2002) Immuno-viral therapy of brain tumors by combination of viral therapy with cancer vaccination using a replication-conditional HSV. Cancer Gene Ther 9:356–364
46. Ohkusu-Tsukada K, Ohta S, Kawakami Y et al (2011) Adjuvant effects of formalin-inactivated HSV through activation of dendritic cells and inactivation of myeloid-derived suppressor cells in cancer immunotherapy. Int J Cancer 128:119–131
47. Udagawa M, Kudo-Saito C, Hasegawa G et al (2006) Enhancement of immunologic tumor regression by intratumoral administration of dendritic cells in combination with cryoablative tumor pretreatment and Bacillus Calmette-Guerin Cell Wall Skeleton Stimulation. Clin Cancer Res 12:7465–7475
48. Chapuis AG, Ragnarsson GB, Nguyen HN et al (2013) Transferred WT1-reactive $CD8^+$ T cells can mediate antileukemic activity and persist in post-transplant patients. Sci Transl Med 5:174
49. Aranda F, Vacchelli E, Eggermont A et al (2014) Trial watch: immunostimulatory monoclonal antibodies in cancer therapy. Oncoimmunology 3:e27297
50. Rosenberg SA, Yang J, Schwartzentruber D et al (1998) Immunologic and therapeutic evaluation of a synthetic peptide vaccine for the treatment of patients with metastatic melanoma. Nat Med 4:321–327

FSC
www.fsc.org
MIX
Papier | Fördert gute Waldnutzung
FSC® C083411

Kolibri 360 GmbH
Ferdinand-Jühlke-Straße 7
99095 Erfurt, Deutschland
produktsicherheit@kolibri360.de